Dentin and Dentinogenesis

Volume I

Editor

Anders Linde, D.D.S., Odont.Dr.
Associate Professor of Histology and Oral Diagnosis
Assistant Dean of Research Training
University of Göteborg
Gothenburg, Sweden

CRC Press, Inc.
Boca Raton, Florida

Library of Congress Cataloging in Publication Data

Main entry under title:

Dentin and dentinogenesis.

Includes bibliographical references and index.
1. Dentin. 2. Dentinogenesis. I. Linde, Anders.
[DNLM: 1. Dentin—Anatomy and histology.
2. Dentinogenesis. WU 220 D413]
QM569.D38 1984 599′.013 83-7714
ISBN 0-8493-5200-2
ISBN 0-8493-5201-0 (pbk.)

Direct all inquiries to CRC Press, Inc., 2000 Corporate Blvd., N.W., Boca Raton, Florida, 33431.

International Standard Book Number 0-8493-5200-2(v. 1)
International Standard Book Number 0-8493-5201-0(v. 2)

Library of Congress Card Number 83-7714
Printed in the United States

PREFACE

Dentin and Dentinogenesis represents an attempt to concisely present the current state of knowledge on the structure of dentin, the chemistry and morphology of dentin formation, and the recent advances in dentin pathology. It is hoped that this volume will prove to be of value to anyone carrying out research both in this field and in other related areas, and that it will provide instructive reading and relevant information to advanced students and other interested persons.

For obvious reasons, the subject of this volume should be of central interest to the dental profession. In addition, tooth formation has attracted increased interest as an experimental system for investigation of the detailed biochemical and cytological mechanisms underlying two important developmental processes: the ectodermal-mesenchymal interaction during organ differentiation and morphogenesis and the calcification process. Advances in our understanding of these processes in other tissues has been due to major progress made in the study of tooth formation.

Developing dental organs are relatively easy to dissect out in large numbers and they can be cultivated in vitro. Accurate timing of the developmental stages can be made, and it is possible to study separately the substructures of ectodermal and mesenchymal origin.[1]

Due to the metabolic simplicity of dentin compared to bone, dentinogenesis is the preferred experimental model for many investigators studying the detailed mechanisms of the calcification process. As far as is known to date, there is no turnover of dentin after it has been formed, and no resorptive processes occur normally. Furthermore, there is a distinct morphology, dentinogenically active cells are easily dissected out for analysis,[2] and a well-defined final product, dentin, is readily obtained with virtually no contamination problems.

The main emphasis in this publication is thus twofold. Primarily, the chapters describe the morphology and chemical characteristics of both the cells and the structural elements of the tissue. Tissue structure is the product of a prior developmental process. Secondarily, an important and integral part of this volume is the discussion about how the different constituents are presumed to take part in the formation of dentin. Pathological alterations and chemical changes may give valuable hints about physiologically occurring processes, and a proper understanding of these is a prerequisite for understanding cause-relationships in pathogenesis.

One aim with this volume has hence been to integrate biochemical and morphological knowledge. It cannot be overemphasized how important this is for a realistic, in-depth understanding of the processes taking place during dentin formation.

Some areas of *Dentin and Dentinogenesis* have been investigated quite thoroughly, while little is known about others. This fact will be obvious to the intent reader when going through this volume and, hopefully, it may stimulate increased research in such sparse areas.

A certain amount of overlapping between different chapters is inevitable in any publication. However, to have the same thing discussed by authors with different points of view has not been regarded as a disadvantage. Moreover, it was found to be essential to let the different contributors freely present their theories and their interpretations of the data, even though some of these may be controversial and may not necessarily be shared in every detail by the editor. On the other hand, the choice of authors for the chapters guarantees that the overall picture of *Dentin and Dentinogenesis* follows the editor's intentions. In this regard, the editor would be very pleased to hear from readers with their comments and criticisms.

Every editor has to acknowledge regretfully the fact that reviews of specific scientific areas have a tendency to become outdated. The importance with this is not only that, in some cases, certain facts and findings are found to be incorrect, but rather that the research emphasis may change rather abruptly. Views either become broadened or totally renewed, and unexpected factors reallocate the research emphasis. This risk is even more pronounced with a rapidly accelerating field such as dentinogenesis and represents one of the thrilling challenges within this research area. As a result, the selection of subjects for the present volume reflects the research areas where interest has been concentrated during the last decade. It must be understood, furthermore, that some of these areas, viewed retrospectively, may seem to have a less relevant role in future research.

The area of dentin and dentinogenesis has not been comprehensively and extensively reviewed since the publication by A. E. W. Miles, the editor of the two-volume *Structural and Chemical Organization of Teeth* (1967)[3] and the conference proceedings *Dentine and Pulp: Their Structure and Reactions* (1968), as edited by N. B. B. Symons.[4] Exactly how rapidly the field has progressed since these two publications can be seen by comparison with the present work. Several of the chapters in these books are excellent and deserve thorough reading; some areas, such as the biochemistry, are less well covered. Embryonic tooth formation was eloquently reviewed by H. C. Slavkin,[1] and another more recent monograph further discusses several aspects of the pulp-dentin complex.[5] Shorter articles also have been published recently reviewing dentinogenesis[6] and dentin and pulp,[7] the latter from a more clinical approach. In the present publication, the literature has been reviewed up to summer, 1982. For the latest and most specialized information available with a review character, the reader is referred to proceedings from meetings and congresses. At the time of preparation of this book, see appropriate References 8-9.

It is a privilege for me, as editor, to be able to present, in two volumes, the contributions of such outstanding authors, each being a prominent scientist in a research sub-area of dentin and dentinogenesis. I want to thank these authors for their most important contributions and their willingness to cooperate. Valuable support has been given by the Swedish Medical Research Council and the Faculty of Odontology, University of Göteborg.

Anders Linde

REFERENCES

1. **Slavkin, H. C.,** *Embryonic Tooth Formation. A Tool for Developmental Biology,* Munksgaard, Copenhagen, 1974.
2. **Linde, A.,** A method for the biochemical study of enzymes in the odontoblastic layer during dentinogenesis, *Arch. Oral Biol.,* 17, 1209, 1972.
3. **Miles, A. E. W., Ed.,** *Structural and Chemical Organization of Teeth,* Vol. 1 and 2, Academic Press, New York, 1967.
4. **Symons, N. B. B., Ed.,** *Dentine and Pulp: Their Structure and Reactions,* Livingstone, Edinburgh, 1968.
5. **Baume, L. J.,** *The Biology of Pulp and Dentine. A Historic, Terminologic-Taxonomic, Histologic-Biochemical, Embryonic and Clinical Survey,* S. Karger, Basel, 1980.
6. **Linde, A.,** Calcium metabolism in dentinogenesis, in *The Role of Calcium in Biological Systems,* Vol. 3, Anghileri, L. J. and Anghileri, A. M., Eds., CRC Press, Boca Raton, Fla., 1982, 55.
7. **Mjör, I. A.,** Dentin and pulp, in *Reaction Patterns in Human Teeth,* Mjör, I. A., Ed., CRC Press, Boca Raton, Fla., 1983, 63.
8. **Veis, A., Ed.,** *The Chemistry and Biology of Mineralized Connective Tissues,* Elsevier/North-Holland, New York, 1981.
9. **Ascenzi, A., Bonucci, E., and de Bernard, B., Eds.,** *Matrix Vesicles,* Wichtig Editore, Milano, 1981.

THE EDITOR

Anders Linde, D.D.S., Odont.Dr., is Associate Professor of Histology and Senior Scientist at the Laboratory of Oral Biology at the Faculty of Odontology, University of Göteborg (Gothenburg), Sweden. Since 1979 he has served as Assistant Dean with responsibility for the Faculty's research training program.

Dr. Linde is the odontological representative on the Swedish Medical Research Council and the chairman of its Priority Committee for Dental Research.

He received his D.D.S. degree from the University of Göteborg and his Odont.Dr. degree in Histology there in 1973. During the years 1971—1978 Dr. Linde held different research career positions at the Swedish Medical Research Council, during 1975—1978 combined with clinical duties and teaching at the Department of Oral Diagnosis. In 1978—1979 he was a visiting scientist at the Institute of Dental Research, University of Alabama in Birmingham. Dr. Linde is a member of several national and international scientific societies.

Dr. Linde has authored or coauthored more than 100 scientific articles, primarily in the field of calcification biology and connective tissue biochemistry. In addition, he has maintained an interest in clinical dentistry, and he has published several articles within the field of oral diagnosis.

CONTRIBUTORS

James K. Avery, D.D.S., Ph.D.
Professor
School of Dentistry and Medical School
The University of Michigan
Ann Arbor, Michigan

Ermanno Bonucci, Ph.D.
Professor of Pathology
First Institute of Pathological Anatomy
University of Rome
Rome, Italy

Alan Boyde, Ph.D.
Professor of Dental Anatomy
Department of Anatomy and Embryology
University College London
London, England

William T. Butler, Ph.D.
Professor
Department of Biochemistry
Senior Scientist
Institute of Dental Research
University of Alabama in Birmingham
Birmingham, Alabama

Daniel J. Chiego, Ph.D.
Assistant Research Scientist
Department of Oral Biology
School of Dentistry
The University of Michigan
Ann Arbor, Michigan

Charles F. Cox, M.S.
Associate Research Scientist
Department of Oral Biology
School of Dentistry and Medical School
The University of Michigan
Ann Arbor, Michigan

H. G. Fromme, Dr. phil. nat.
Professor for Medical Physics
Institute of Medical Physics
Westfälische Wilhelms-Universität
Münster, West Germany

Harold M. Fullmer, D.D.S.
Director, Institute of Dental Research
Associate Dean and Professor of Pathology
School of Dentistry
University of Alabama in Birmingham
Birmingham, Alabama

H. J. Höhling, Dr. rer. nat.
Professor for Medical Physics
Institute of Medical Physics
Westfälische Wilhelms-Universität
Münster, West Germany

Sára Karjalainen, D. Odont.
Department of Cariology
Institute of Dentistry
University of Turku
Turku, Finland

Sheila J. Jones, Ph.D.
Senior Lecturer
Department of Anatomy and Embryology
University College London
London, England

Ivar A. Mjör, Ph.D.
Director
Scandinavian Institute of Dental Materials
Oslo, Norway

Aaron S. Posner, Ph.D.
Associate Director of Research
The Hospital for Special Surgery
Professor of Biochemistry
Cornell University Medical College
New York, New York

J. V. Ruch, Dr. med., Dr. ès Sc.
Professor and Head
Institut de Biologie Médicale
Faculté de Médecine
Strasbourg, France

Paul J. Tannenbaum, Ph.D.
Consultant
The Hospital for Special Surgery
Research Associate
Cornell University Medical College
New York, New York

Roy E. Wuthier, Ph.D.
Professor
Coordinator of Medical Biochemistry
Department of Chemistry
School of Medicine
University of South Carolina
Columbia, South Carolina

TABLE OF CONTENTS

Volume I

Volume II

Chapter 1

THE MORPHOLOGY OF DENTIN AND DENTINOGENESIS

Ivar A. Mjör

TABLE OF CONTENTS

I. INTRODUCTION

Dentin is a mineralized connective tissue (Figures 1 and 2). Similar to all other mineralized tissues, it is laid down as an organic matrix which subsequently mineralizes. The organic matrix is formed by the odontoblasts. The initial and main mineralization occurs during dentinogenesis. A gradual mineralization also continues with age. Species differences are found. The present text will focus on human dentin.

The average inorganic content of dentin is considered to be approximately 70% by weight, while the organic components constitute approximately 18%, and water 12% (Figure 1). The inorganic component comprises mainly hydroxyapatite while the organic matrix is chiefly collagen, noncollagenous proteins including proteoglycans, glycosaminoglycans, lipids, and citrate. Due to the difference in specific gravity of the inorganic material (3.0), the organic components (1.6), and water (1.0), the volume distribution of the various fractions differs from that of the weight distribution (Figure 1).

II. BASIC STRUCTURE

The *odontoblasts* are the cells of the dentin. The cell body is located in the pulp (Figure 2), and it has a long, cellular extension into the dentin, called the odontoblast process. The *dentinal tubules* contain either the odontoblast processes or their remnants and tissue fluid (also called "dentin liquor"). The odontoblast layer is an integral part of the dental pulp. This intimate relationship between the cells of the dentin and the pulp (Figures 2 and 3) represents one of several reasons why the dentin and the pulp should be considered as one functional entity, sometimes referred to as the pulp-dentin organ.[1] The pulpal aspect of the dentin is bordered by an unmineralized matrix, the *predentin*. It is present during dentinogenesis and throughout the life of the tooth. Coronal dentin is bordered peripherally by enamel, and root dentin by cementum.

The mineralized entities comprise the *intertubular* and *peritubular dentin*. The term *mantle dentin* is used to denote the initially formed dentin, located adjacent to the enamel, while the main part of dentin is referred to as *circumpulpal dentin*.

A. Odontoblasts

The odontoblasts line the entire pulpal aspect of the predentin. It comprises one layer of cells, but in fully formed teeth it often appears pseudostratified (Figure 3). This is due to a crowding of the cells as they move in a pulpal direction during dentinogenesis.

The odontoblasts are tall columnar cells or sometimes somewhat cuboidal in shape, especially in the root. The nucleus is oval, has one or two nucleoli, and is located in the proximal end of the cell (Figure 3). The cytoplasm of the cell body contains numerous organelles (Figure 4), rough surfaced endoplasmic reticulum arranged in longitudinally running cisternae, a well-developed Golgi apparatus, mitochondria, vesicles, vacuoles, electron dense bodies, microtubules, and fibrils. Their frequency is dependent on the matrix-producing activity of the odontoblasts. A number of different types of contact areas exist between odontoblast cell membranes, e.g., gap, tight, or intermediate junctional complexes (Figure 5).

The *odontoblast process* extends from the cell body into the dentin and is located in the dentinal tubules. Much controversy exists regarding how far peripherally it extends as a cytoplasmic process. Ultrastructural studies indicate that it may be found in the inner half[3] or the inner third[4] of the dentin. The structure of its peripheral end or its continuation as remnants of a process is poorly understood. Its ultrastructure is characterized by cytoplasm which contains microtubules and filaments without major organelles.[5,6] Branching of the odontoblasts is sometimes seen, and is particularly frequent at the amelodentinal and ce-

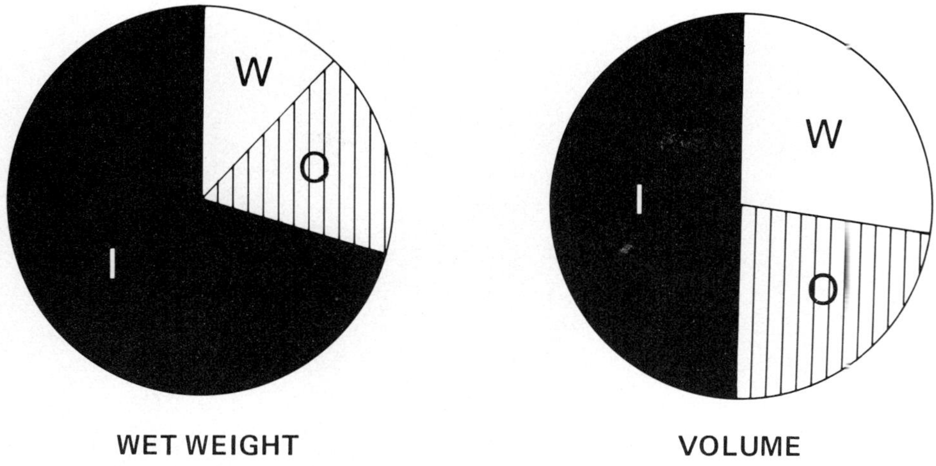

FIGURE 1. Diagram showing wet weight and volume composition of dentin. I, inorganic component; O, organic component; W, water.

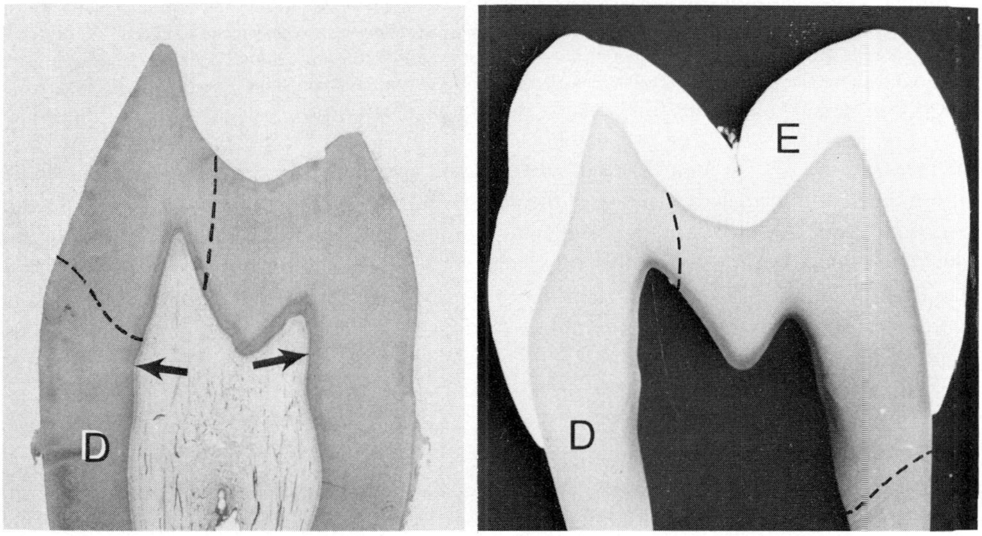

FIGURE 2. Dentin (D) in demineralized, hematoxylin-eosin stained section (left) and in a microradiograph of a ground section of a premolar (right). Arrows point to odontoblast layer. The direction of the tubules is indicated by dotted lines. E, enamel.

mentodentinal junction. A special type of fine branching is regularly seen in root dentin (Figures 5 and 6). One portion of the odontoblast process in newly erupted teeth, about 150 to 200 μm from the predentin, stains intensely (Figure 7).

B. Dentinal Tubules

The most striking feature of dentin is probably the dentinal tubules. They lodge the odontoblast processes. The size of their lumen is dependent on their location within the dentin and the age of the tooth. Measurements of the diameter of the tubules indicate similar dimensions in different species,[7] i.e., up to 3 μm near the pulp and less than 1 μm in the peripheral dentin. In old teeth tubules may be completely obturated by highly mineralized

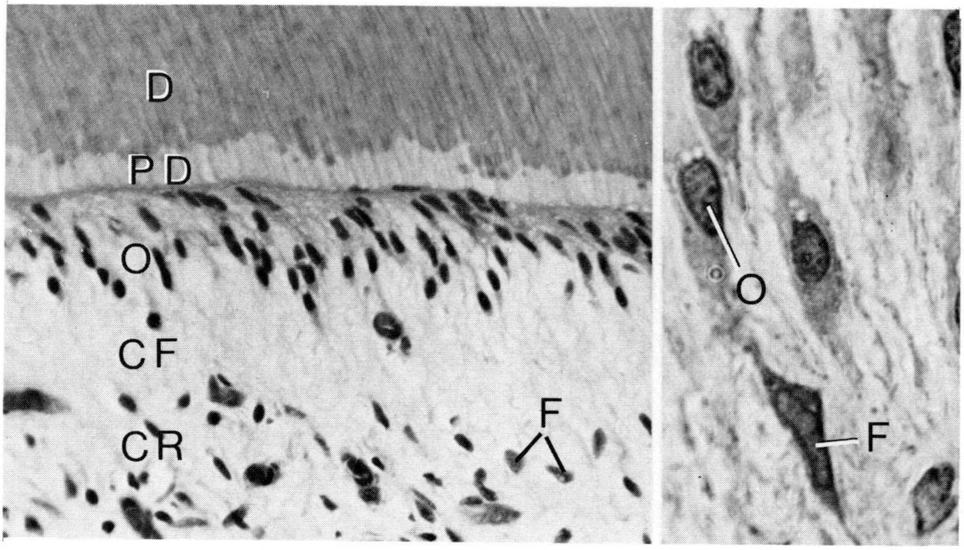

FIGURE 3. Odontoblasts (O) form a layer of cells which lines the predentin (PD). They are tall columnar cells which appear pseudostratified. The odontoblast nuclei are located in the proximal or basal end of the cell. CF, cell-free zone; CR, cell-rich zone; F, fibroblast. The left section is 6-μm thick from a demineralized tooth and it is stained with hematoxylin-eosin. The section on the right is 1-μm thick and shows the pulp/dentin interface of a tooth split immediately after extraction, and it is stained with toluidine blue.

material (Figure 8). The number of tubules per unit area will vary depending on the location within the dentin, primarily because of the decreasing size of the dentin surface in a pulpward direction, especially in the crown. Depending on the species, 50,000 to 90,000 tubules per mm^2 have been recorded near the pulp, and 10,000 to 25,000 peripherally.[7] The corresponding figures for human teeth are about 65,000 and 15,000 tubules per mm^2 with an average of 30,000 to 35,000 in the middle of the dentin. The dentinal tubules run from the amelodentinal and cementodentinal junction in a slightly curved fashion (Figure 2), and they may sometimes take on a S-shaped curvature.

C. Peritubular Dentin

The highly mineralized structure which lines the dentinal tubules in almost their entire length is called the peritubular dentin (Figure 9). The only part of the dentin devoid of this structure is in the pulpal 150 to 200 μm of the coronal part of newly erupted teeth (Figure 10). This transition between the presence and absence of peritubular dentin corresponds to the intense staining of the tubular content (Figure 7). The peritubular dentin has a scanty organic matrix, and its few collagen fibers are continuous with those of the intertubular matrix (Figure 9).

A membranous, hypomineralized structure considered to line the inner aspect of the peritubular dentin, has been described.[8] It appears as a tube in demineralized sections and may correspond to Neumann's sheath.[9]

D. Periodontoblastic Space

The potential space between the wall of the dentinal tubule and the odontoblast process is called the periodontoblastic space (Figure 11).[10] It contains tissue fluid and a few collagen fibers. This interface is important for secondary intratubular changes, e.g., growth of the peritubular dentin. The transition between the hypomineralized structure lining the tubules[8] and the periodontoblastic space has not been clarified.

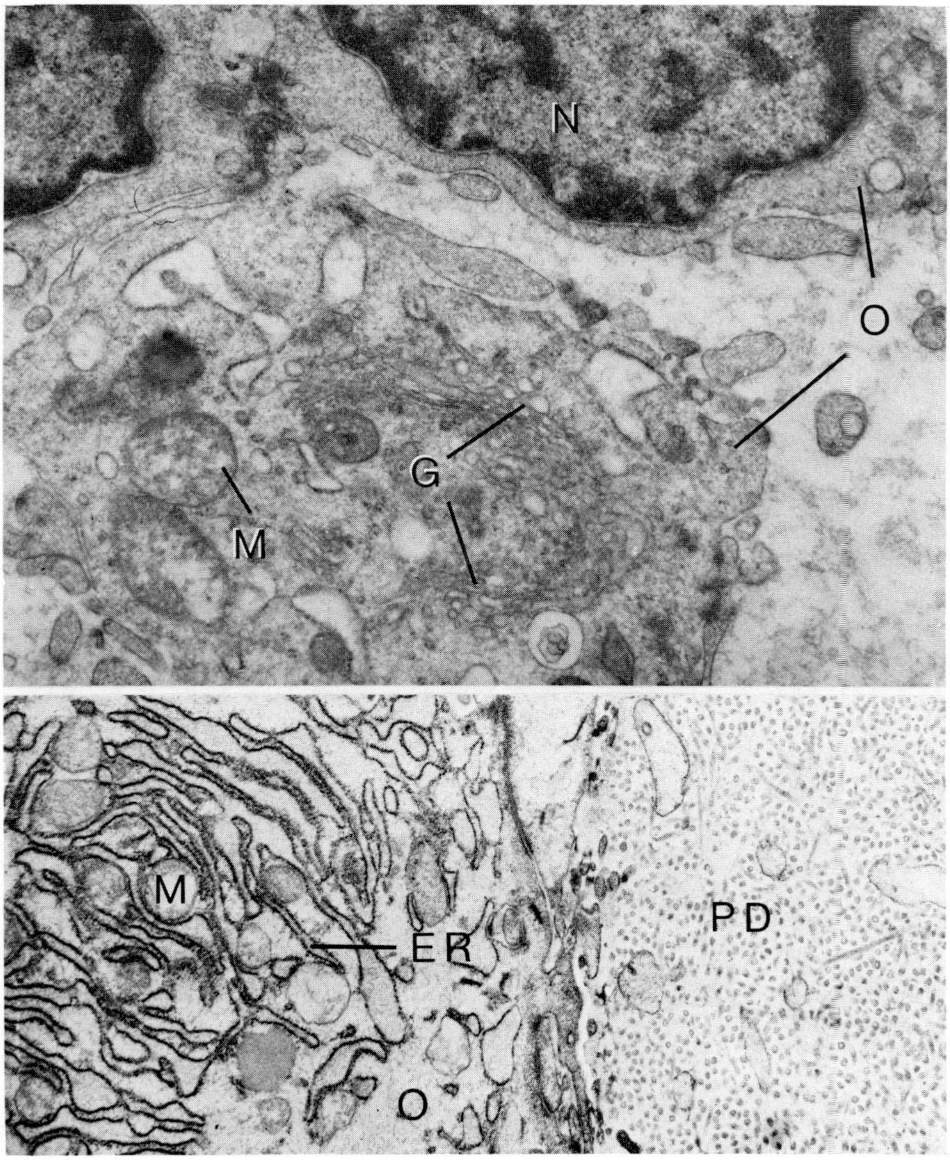

FIGURE 4. Electron micrographs of human odontoblasts (O) showing Golgi apparatus (G), mitochondria (M), and endoplasmic reticulum (ER). PD, predentin; N, nucleus. (Top, × 24,000; bottom, × 16,000.) Top micrograph from Dahl, E. and Mjör, I. A., *Acta Odontol. Scand.*, 31, 349, 1973. With permission; bottom micrograph courtesy of Furseth.[6])

E. Intertubular Dentin

The mineralized intertubular areas constitute the main part of the dentin. The collagen which is the major organic component, is considered to be oriented roughly parallel to the incremental pattern, but it is irregular in the other two dimensions. The intertubular dentin stains intensely close to the predentin (Figure 7) and remains practically unstained in the rest of the dentin.

The amount of intertubular dentin decreases in a pulpward direction. It is evenly mineralized, except in one area of coronal dentin located a slight distance from the predentin, where it is somewhat less mineralized than in the rest of the dentin (Figure 10). This area

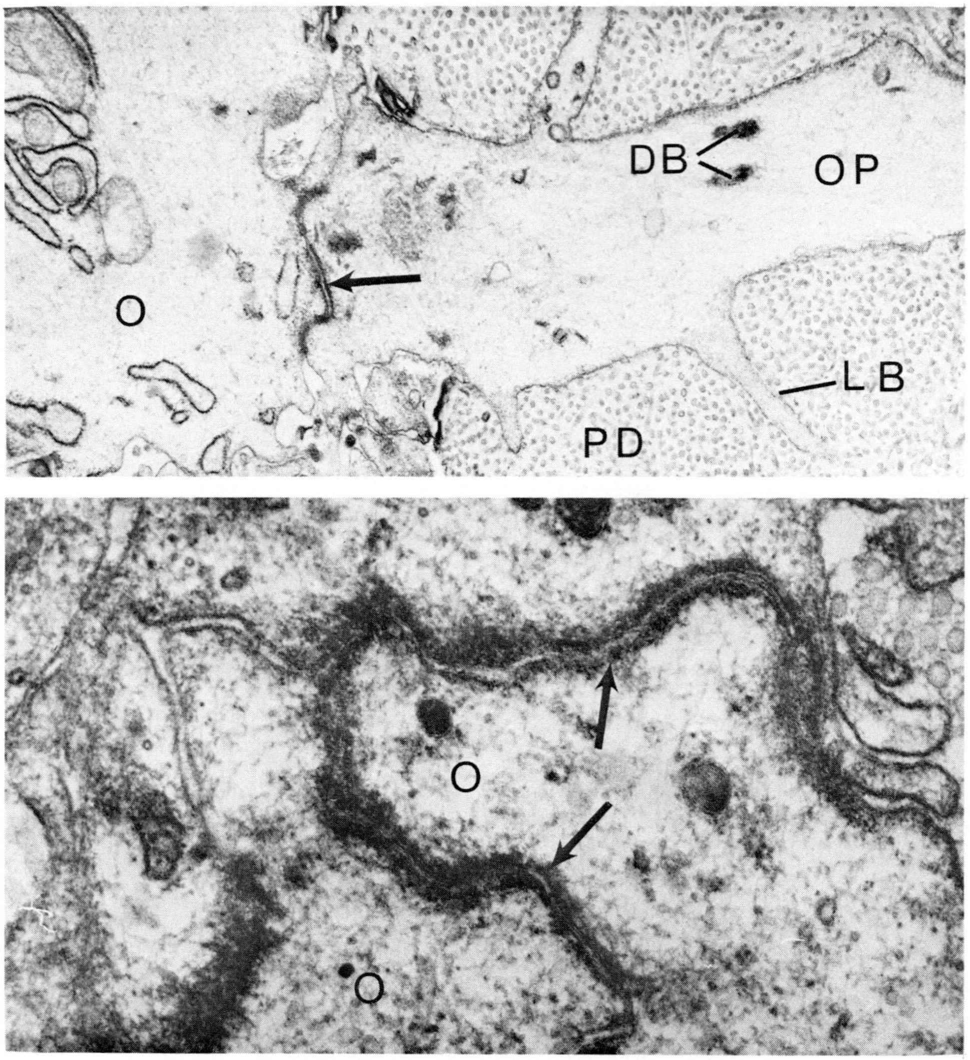

FIGURE 5. Electron micrographs of odontoblast/predentin interface from human root dentin. Electron dense junctional complexes (arrows) are found between odontoblasts (O). The cytoplasm of the odontoblast process (OP) contains microtubules and dense bodies (DB). LB, lateral branches of the odontoblast process; PD, predentin, (Top, × 20,000; bottom, × 65,000.) (Courtesy of Furseth.[6])

is just pulpal to the extension of the peritubular dentin in newly erupted teeth. The relative hypomineralization occurs during dentinogenesis and it is also recognized in teeth from older individuals[11]

F. Interglobular Dentin

Unmineralized islands within the dentin (Figure 12) are called interglobular areas. They reflect any type of disturbance in mineralization during dentinogenesis and are particularly frequent at the border between mantle and circumpulpal dentin. The disturbance noted as a result of the breaking down of Hertwig's epithelial root sheath results in the appearance of *Tomes' granular layer* which is therefore only located in the root (Figure 10). This type of minor disturbance is often globular rather than interglobular in appearance.

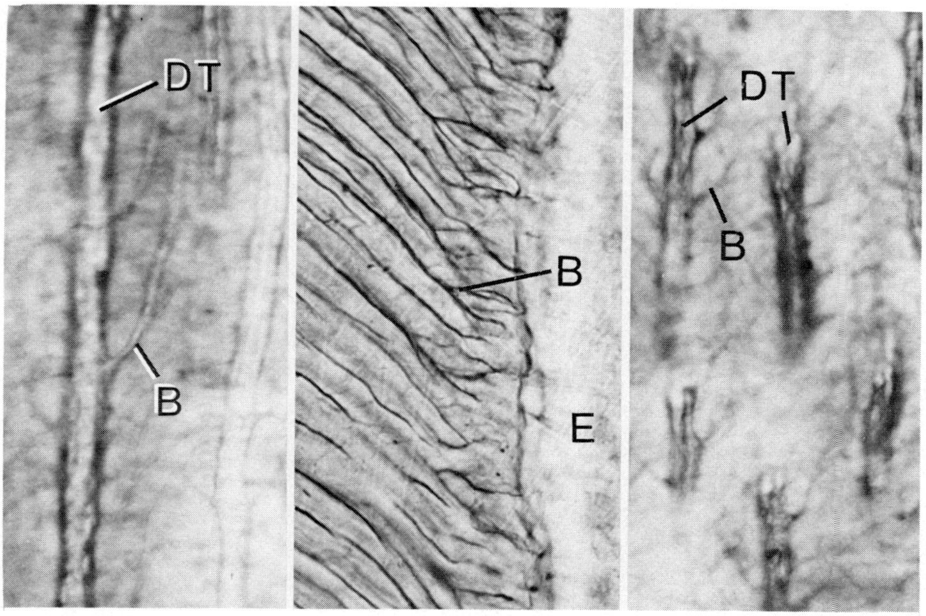

FIGURE 6. Branching (B) of dentinal tubules (DT) in hematoxylin-stained, demineralized sections (left: coronal dentin, right: root dentin) and undemineralized dentin at the amelodentinal junction (middle). (From Mjör, I. A., *Histology of the Human Tooth,* Mjör, I. A. and Fejerskov, O., Eds., Munksgaard, Copenhagen, 1979, 43. With permission.)

G. Predentin

The unmineralized dentin matrix, approximately 15 μm wide and lining the entire pulpal aspect of the dentin, is called predentin. Morphologically, it may be differentiated into two layers (Figure 13), old and new predentin.[12] The oldest is adjacent to the dentin. The dentin/predentin interface is characterized by calcospherites (Figure 13). These globular structures represent mineralization foci which fuse during mineralization.

A localized or generalized lack of predentin is occasionally found, and it reflects a pathological condition. This presence of predentin may be important for the prevention of internal resorption of dentin, because odontoblasts apparently only attack mineralized tissues.[13]

H. Innervation

Controversy, undoubtedly based on inadequate techniques, has existed regarding the presence of nerves in the dentin. Up until about 1960, most of the work on the innervation of dentin was based on silver impregnation techniques applied to histologic sections of demineralized teeth.[14] The conclusions reached indicated that nerves may be found anywhere in dentin.

Electron microscopic studies have demonstrated that nerves are found in the periodontoblastic space (Figure 11) of predentin and dentin.[15,16] However, uncertainty still exists regarding how far peripherally the nerves extend. It is generally agreed that they do not extend beyond the pulpal third of the dentin. Their frequency is also low and they can only be demonstrated in one out of several hundred dentinal tubules.

III. DENTINOGENESIS

Dentin and pulp develop from the dental papilla (Figures 14 and 15) which is mesodermal in origin. It has been claimed that ectomesenchymal cells may be present in the dental

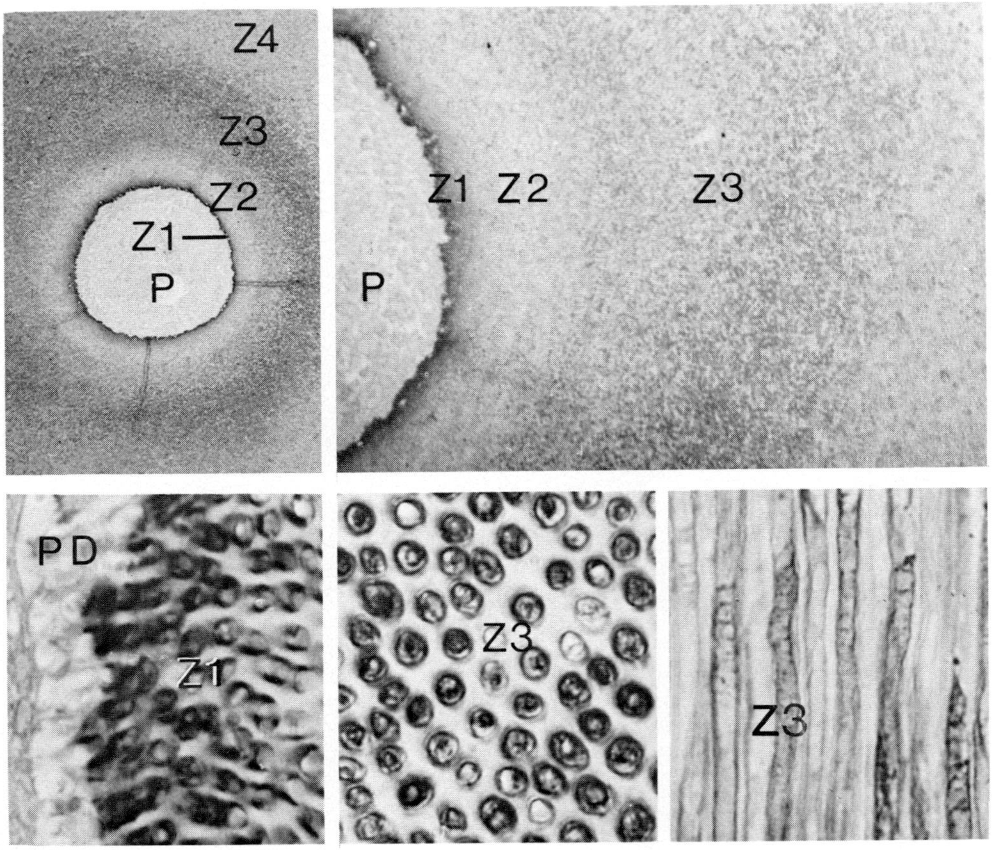

FIGURE 7. All illustrations are from demineralized sections of dentin stained with alcian blue. Note zonated staining pattern (top left and right). The dentin adjacent to the predentin (Z1) stains intensely (lower left) due to staining of the periphery of the tubules and the intertubular matrix. The next area is lightly stained (Z2). Further peripherally (bottom center) a fairly intensely stained area (Z3) is found due to staining of the periphery and the contents of the tubules, but without stainable components in the intertubular matrix. A granular structure of the contents of the tubules is noted in Z3 in longitudinally sectioned tubules (bottom right). The main bulk of the dentin (Z4) stains lightly.

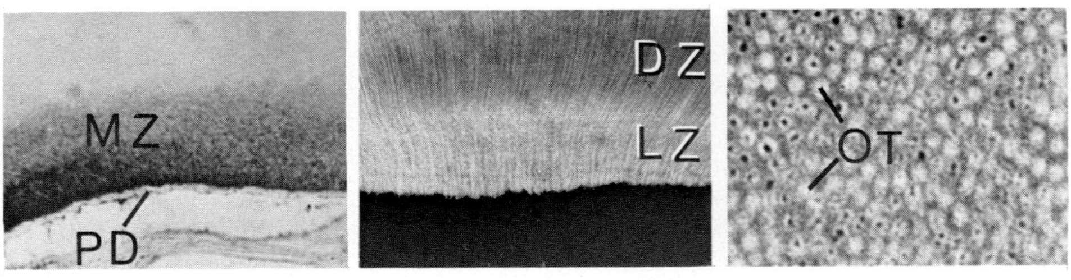

FIGURE 8. Toluidine blue-stained demineralized section (left) and microradiograph of ground section (middle) of the same tooth and at the same magnification from a 71-year-old individual. Compare with Figures 7 and 10. DZ, dark zone; LZ, light zone; MZ, metachromatic zone; PD, predentin. Microradiograph on the right shows several obturated tubules (OT) from a ground section of a tooth from the same patient.

papilla, i.e., cells which originate from the neural crest.[18,19] They can only be differentiated from mesodermal cells by special histochemical methods. These ectomesenchymal cells, rather than those of mesodermal origin, may be the precursors of the odontoblasts.

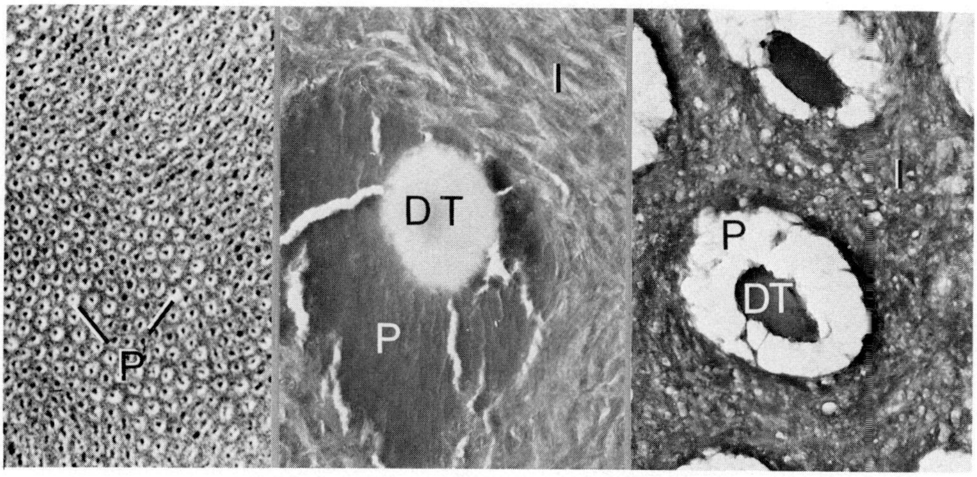

FIGURE 9. Peritubular dentin (P) from the main bulk of dentin in a microradiograph of an undemineralized section (left) and in electron micrographs (courtesy of Furseth) of undemineralized (middle, × 12,000) and phosphotungstic acid demineralized (right, × 6500) dentin. It is highly mineralized and contains a scanty organic matrix. DT, dentinal tubule; I, intertubular matrix.

A. Cytodifferentiation

During early tooth development the cells of the dental papilla are similar in size, shape, and structure (Figure 14). They have large nuclei and little cytoplasm which contains few organelles, i.e., typical undifferentiated cells. At the bell stage of tooth development (Figure 15) a differentiation of odontoblasts takes place, starting at the cuspal or incisal region. This cytodifferentiation is under the control of the cells in the inner dental epithelium The cells become cylindrical in shape and are sometimes referred to as *predontoblasts*. The number of organelles markedly increases, and the cells become tall and columnar with the nucleus located at the end farthest from the basement membrane of the inner dental epithelium (Figure 16). These cells are the odontoblasts and they are responsible for predentin formation. Concomitant with the formation of predentin at the cuspal/incisal region, continued differentiation of new odontoblasts takes place further apically in the dental papilla. After the crown is fully formed, the rate of dentin deposition slows down markedly (up to 2 to 3 years for permanent teeth) until root formation starts. The root shape is mapped out by proliferation of Hertwig's root epithelium which consists of the inner and outer dental epithelium. Similar to the cytodifferentiation in the crown, odontoblasts develop from the dental papilla under the influence of the inner dental epithelium.

B. Matrix Formation

The odontoblasts exhibit all the characteristics of matrix-producing cells, i.e., an abundance of rough surfaced endoplasmic reticulum, a well-developed Golgi apparatus, mitochondria, and secretory granules. Procollagen is synthesized in the rough-surfaced endoplasmic reticulum, transferred to the Golgi apparatus, and finally appears in secretory granules.[20] It is released by exocytosis and transformed to tropocollagen, which is the collagen molecule made up of several polypeptide chains. The tropocollagen molecules make up the collagen fibrils. A basically similar process is involved in proteoglycan and glycoprotein formation. In the synthesis of carbohydrate-protein complexes, sugar may be added to the protein both in the cisternae of the rough-surfaced endoplasmatic reticulum and in those of the Golgi apparatus.

The collagen, glycoprotein, and proteoglycan complexes constitute the organic matrix of

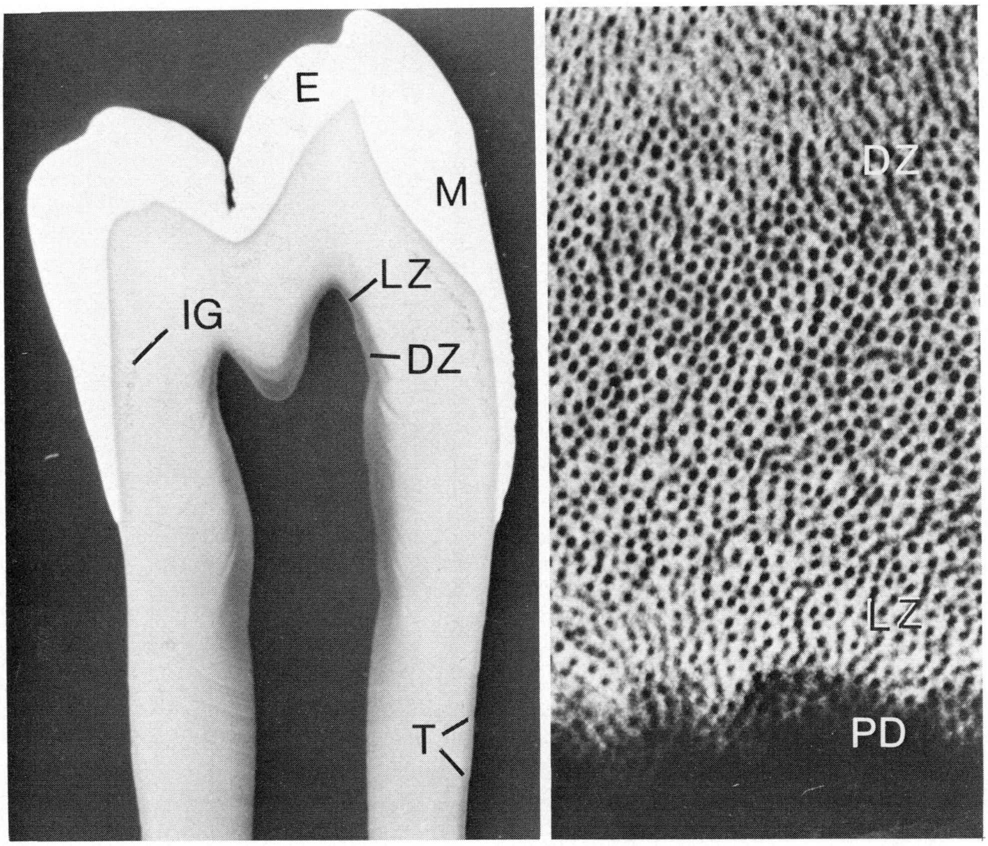

FIGURE 10. Microradiograph of undemineralized sections of newly erupted premolars. At low magnification (left) the following areas with relatively low mineral content are noted: M, mantle dentin; DZ, dark (less mineralized) zone near the pulp; IG, interglobular dentin; T, Tomes' granular layer. Higher magnification (right) of dentin adjacent to predentin (PD) shows that only the intertubular matrix is mineralized, both in the light (LZ) and in the dark (DZ) zones, and to a lesser degree in the dark than in the light zone. E, enamel. (From Mjör, I. A., *Arch. Oral Biol.*, 11, 225, 1966. With permission.)

the dentin. Prior to mineralization two layers in the predentin may be differentiated (Figure 13). The fibers involved in the formation of the initial (mantle) predentin are argyrophilic (Figure 13) and are called von Korff's fibers.

During initial dentinogenesis, i.e., the formation of the mantle dentin, the odontoblasts have several cytoplasmic projections at the formative end. At a later stage in the development, one cytoplasmic process, sometimes with branches (Figure 5), extends from the odontoblast cell body. This condition prevails throughout the formation of the rest of the dentin, the circumpulpal dentin. After the predentin reaches a certain width its oldest part will mineralize, but a predentin zone normally remains throughout the life of the tooth. The odontoblast will form more predentin and move in a pulpal direction at a speed of about 4 μm/day in humans.[21]

The odontoblasts which form the root dentin are structurally slightly different from those in the crown in that they have several fine branches giving the dentinal tubules a rather brush-like appearance (Figure 6). At the time of the normal breaking up of Hertwig's root epithelium, a disturbance in dentinogenesis occurs, i.e., small interglobular areas form in larger numbers than usual for a short time. This part of the root dentin is referred to as *Tomes' granular layer*.

The important role of the odontoblast in dentin matrix production is virtually undisputed.

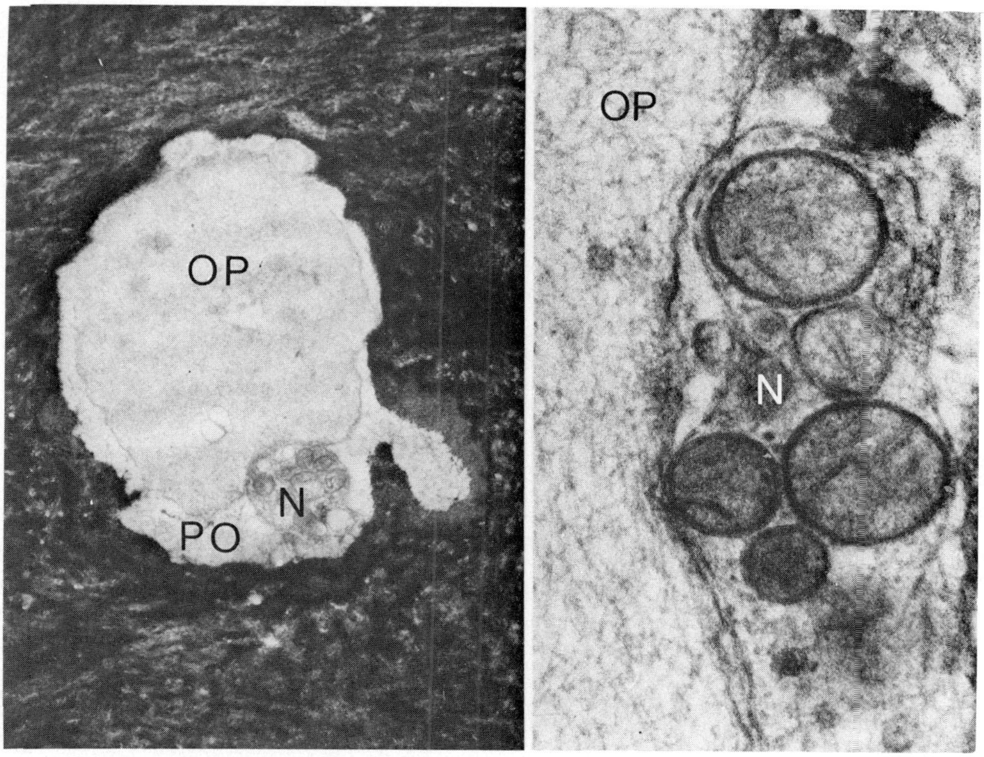

FIGURE 11. Cross-sectioned dentinal tubule in mineralized dentin (left) and in predentin (right) showing odontoblast process (OP) and nerve (N) in periodontoblastic space (PO). (Left, × 17,000; right, × 52,000.) (From Dahl, E. and Mjör, I. A., *Acta Odontol. Scand.*, 3, 349, 1973. With permission.)

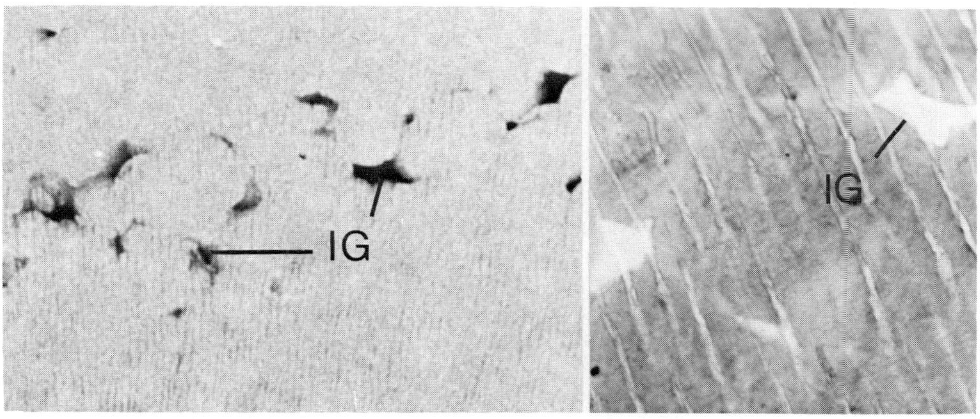

FIGURE 12. Microradiograph of undemineralized section (left) and hematoxylin-eosin-stained demineralized section (right) showing interglobular areas (IG).

However, the first formation of dentin occurs at a time prior to complete cytodifferentiation of odontoblasts. The initial von Korff's fibers may, therefore, originate from the *subodontoblastic cells*. The subodontoblastic cells may also play a role in the circumpulpal dentinogenesis. The presence of a *cell-free zone* subjacent to the odontoblasts is dependent on the dentinogenic activity.[22] The lack of a cell-free zone during irregular secondary dentin for-

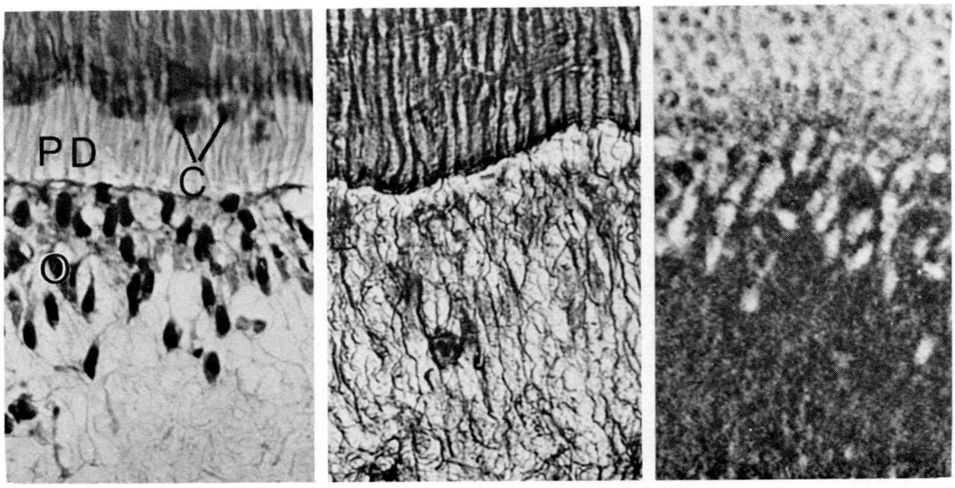

FIGURE 13. Predentin (PD)/odontoblast (O) area in sections from demineralized dentin stained with hematoxylin-eosin (left), silver stain (middle), and in a microradiograph (right) at the same magnification. Note argyrophillic (von Korff's) fibers in the odontoblast region. The predentin close to the odontoblasts contains less mass than the old predentin as seen on the microradiograph (right). C, calcopherites.

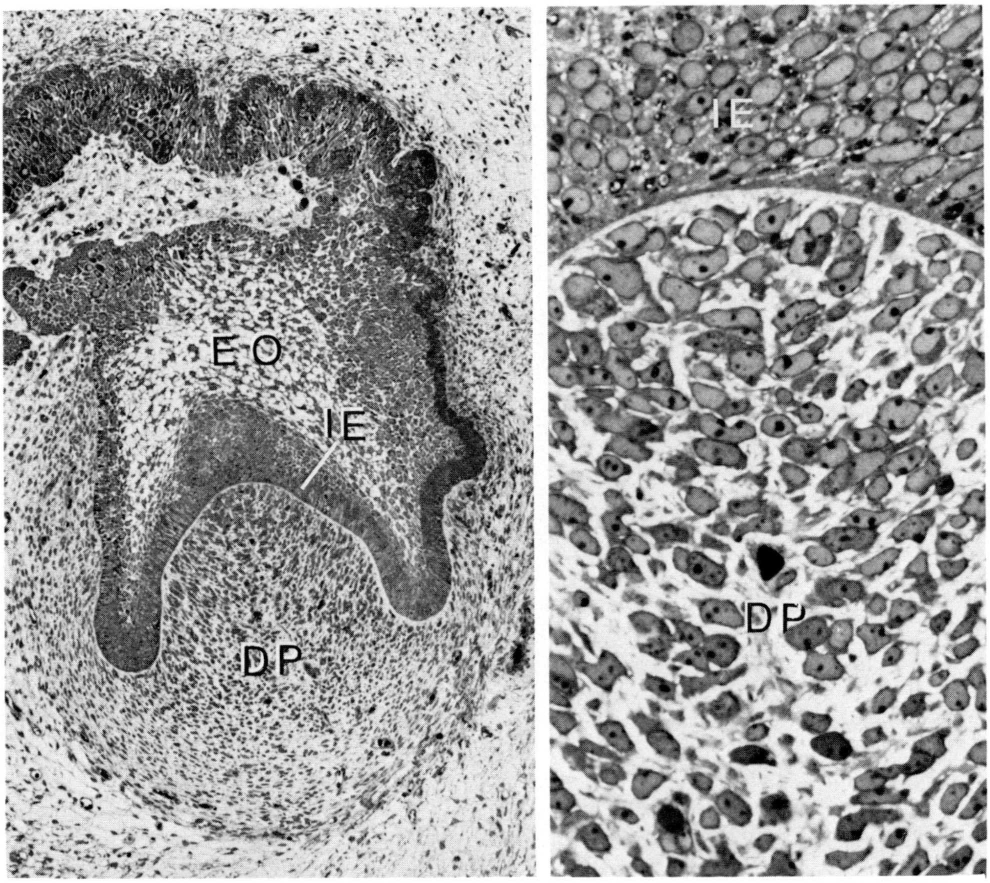

FIGURE 14. Cap stage of tooth development. Dentin and pulp are formed from the dental papilla (DP) which comprises large, similar mesenchymal cells. EO, enamel organ; IE, inner dental epithelium. (Courtesy of Fejerskov.[17])

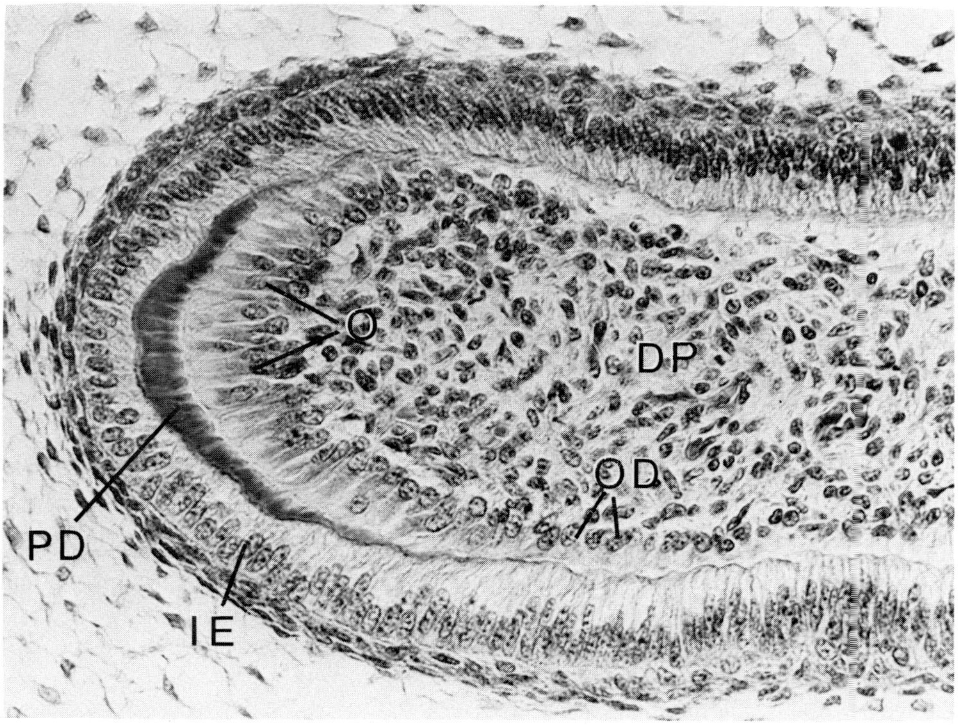

FIGURE 15. Bell stage of tooth development. DP, dental papilla; O, odontoblasts; OD, differen iating odontoblasts; PD, predentin; IE, inner dental epithelium.

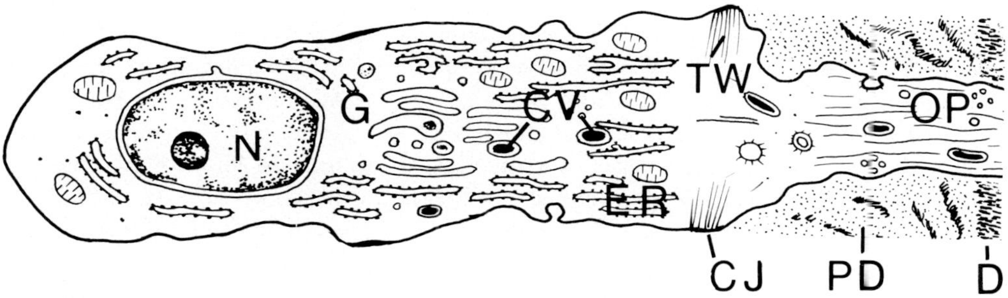

FIGURE 16. Diagram of odontoblast (O) showing the arrangement of organelles. G, Golgi apparatus; CV, condensing vacuoles; RER, rough endoplasmic reticulum; M, mitochondria; TW, terminal web; C., cell junctions; PD, predentin; OP, odontoblast process; D, dentin. (Courtesy of Fejerskov.[17])

mation is also a characteristic feature.[13] The fact that cells under these conditions are present in the subodontoblastic area, which normally is relatively cell-free, suggests that this particular structural arrangement may be functionally important.

C. Mineralization

Mineralization of dentin is closely associated with its collagen. The mechanism involved in the initial crystal formation, often termed *nucleation*, is difficult to explain. It is probably initiated through cellular activity and by specific interactions between regularly spaced groups in the matrix which attract calcium and phosphate ions. After the initial mineral nuclei are formed, a growth of crystals occurs. Although the nature or the mechanisms of the nucleation

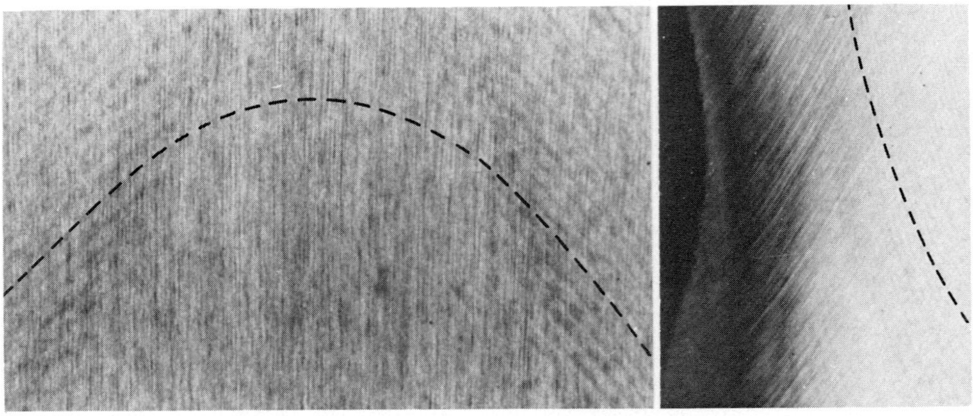

FIGURE 17. Incremental lines, direction indicated by dotted lines, in hematoxylin-eosin-stained, demineralized section (left) and in microradiograph of undemineralized section (right).

and crystal growth are not known in detail, it is apparent that collagen, proteoglycans, phosphoproteins, as well as cellular activities, may play important roles in initiating and regulating mineralization of dentin and other mesodermal mineralized tissues.

Hydroxyapatite — $Ca_{10}(PO_4)_6(OH)_2$ — is the main inorganic component of dentin as in other mineralized tissues. The crystals are needle shaped with a thickness of about 5 nm and a length of about 20 nm, but varying from 10 to 50 nm. A small portion of the calcium phosphates of dentin may also be in an amorphous form.

The foci of mineralization grow into spherical structures, often called *calcospherites* (Figure 13) which fuse with neighboring spheres. If this fusion does not take place, small unmineralized islands, *interglobular areas*, will remain in the dentin. They show the typical structure of the calcospherites at their boundary (Figure 12). Their number will increase if dentinogenesis occurs during severe systemic diseases. Apart from this spherical type of mineralization, dentin is also under the influence of a linear type of mineralization. This is reflected in the presence of incremental lines (Figure 17). Accentuated incremental lines, *Owen's contour lines*, may be noted and are considered to reflect disturbances in mineralization. In teeth where dentinogenesis takes place at the time of birth, an accentuated incremental line, the *neonatal line*, signifies the dramatic changes which occur at birth.

Mineralization of the intertubular and peritubular dentin takes place simultaneously during dentinogenesis of the main part of coronal dentin.[23] The highly mineralized peritubular dentin is, therefore, in these locations a primary structure. In the most pulpally located coronal dentin, only mineralization of the intertubular dentin occurs.[12] A similar pattern of mineralization may also be found in the incisal/cuspal areas.[24] The appearance of highly mineralized peritubular dentin in these locations is, therefore, a result of secondary formation, i.e., after the dentin per se has formed. The situation in human root dentin has not been fully clarified, but it appears as if a thin layer of highly mineralized peritubular dentin forms as a primary structure during dentinogenesis.

D. Incisal/Cuspal Dentin

The structure of the incisal and cuspal dentin is different from that of the circumpulpal dentin (Figure 18).[24,25] It would seem likely, therefore, that its development is different. However, the central area of the incisal/cuspal dentin may represent an extension of the pulp chamber.[24,25] If its structure is considered on this basis, the distribution of inorganic components is similar to that seen in the pulpal aspect of the coronal dentin.[12]

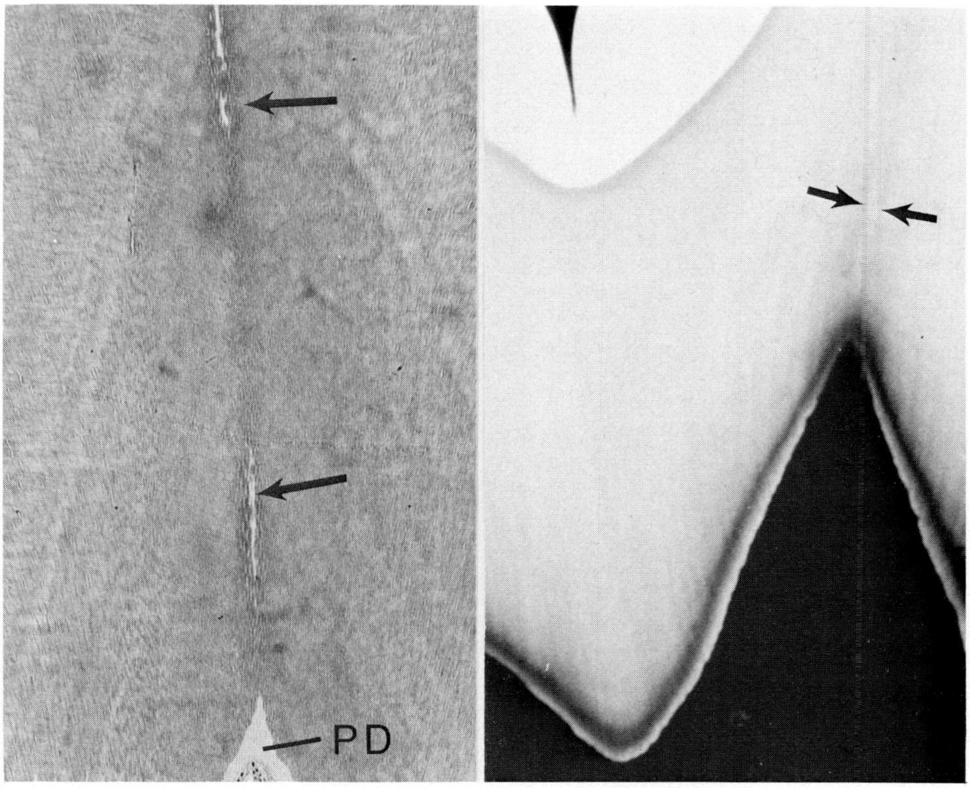

FIGURE 18. The dentin structure in the incisal/cuspal region. Note predentin (PD)-like tissue in the incisal area (arrows) of demineralized, hematoxylin-eosin-stained section of unerupted monkey canine (left). Microradiograph (right) of ground section of a newly erupted premolar shows a zonated appearance (arrows) in the cuspal region.

E. Secondary Dentin

Dentin formed after the teeth are fully developed is called *secondary dentin*. It has been claimed that an irregularity in the smooth S-shaped curvature of the tubules may mark the transition between primary and secondary dentin, but such a transition is very rarely noted. Secondary dentin which is formed without any special reason apart from normal use of the teeth, is called physiological or regular secondary dentin. It forms on the entire pulpal aspect of the dentin, but somewhat more on the ceiling and the floor of the pulp chamber than on the side walls. The reduction in the size of the pulp is, therefore, somewhat asymmetrical compared to its original shape. Secondary dentin which is formed in a localized area subjacent to caries, attrited areas, or restorations is called *irregular secondary dentin* (or *reparative dentin*, irritation dentin, and tertiary dentin). The interface between primary and irregular secondary dentin often exhibits a very irregular structure, including cellular inclusions (Figure 19).[13]

IV. AGE CHANGES

The formation of regular secondary dentin is a typical age change. Its rate of formation in monkey teeth has been found to be 0.8 μm/day as compared to almost 3 μm/day for irregular secondary dentin[26] and 4 μm/day during tooth development.[21] The result is a gradual reduction in the size of the pulp.

The stainability of sections of demineralized dentin from young and old teeth differs. The

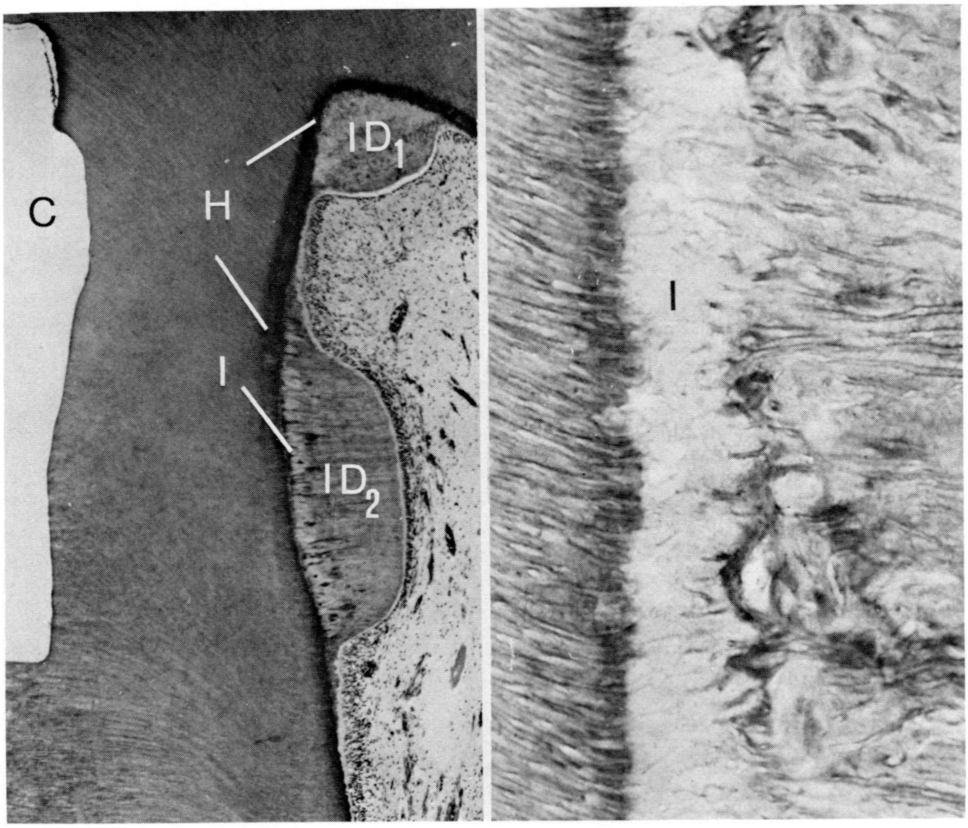

FIGURE 19. Irregular secondary dentin subjacent to an attrited area (ID_1) and subjacent to a restoration (ID_2) which had been placed in the cavity (C). Note the irregular structure at the interface (I) between primary and secondary dentin at ID_2, shown in higher magnification on the right side. No such irregularities are found at ID_1. Hematoxyphilic line (H) is not limited to the primary/irregular secondary dentin interface.

typical zonated staining pattern, which is characteristic in young teeth is not found in teeth from older individuals. The only stainable portion in older teeth is the dentin adjacent to the predentin (Figure 7). The dentin immediately adjacent to the predentin is markedly stained, and the staining is probably located in the intertubular areas. The adjacent, somewhat lighter stained area, is due to staining of the periphery of the tubules. In other words, the slow forming, regular secondary dentin is probably formed in the same way as the most pulpal coronal dentin, but the two zones in young teeth which stain markedly (Figure 7) are immediately adjacent to each other without an intervening, light-stained zone (Figure 8). The peripheral dentin is practically unstained.

A continued growth of the peritubular dentin resulting in partial or complete obturation of the tubules (Figure 8) is the most common age change in dentin. It changes its physical properties, e.g., the dentin becomes harder, more brittle, and translucent. The terms sclerosis (hardening) or *sclerotic dentin* are commonly used to describe these changes. *Secondary intratubular mineralization* would probably be a more meaningful term. The periodontoblastic space plays an important role in the growth of the highly mineralized peritubular dentin.

V. SPECIES DIFFERENCES

The dentin described in this introductory chapter is of the typical *orthodentin* type, i.e.,

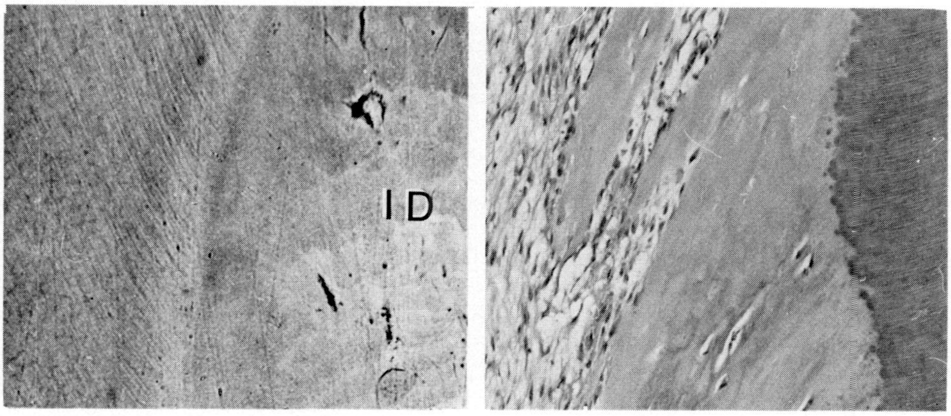

FIGURE 20. Microradiograph of a ground section of a tooth from a 68-year-old individual with irregular secondary dentin (ID), including unmineralized areas in the coronal pulp (left). The demineralized section on the right shows irregular secondary dentin with cellular inclusions from a replanted tooth. (Courtesy of Breivik.[28])

it contains tubules which run parallel. A number of other types of dentins have also been identified,[27] e.g., vasodentin, plicidentin, fibrodentin, and osteodentin.

Vasodentin contains blood vessels and *plicidentin* (or plicadentin) is characterized by infoldings of tubular dentin which sometimes fill most of the pulp chamber. Both types have phylogenic interest and are common in certain fishes and lower reptiles.

Fibrodentin and *osteodentin* are intrapulpal dentins and may be basically similar; fibrodentin being acellular while osteodentin has cellular inclusions.[27] They are normally found in lower vertebrates, but may also be found in the pulps of human teeth during repair (Figure 20). The dentin at the interface between primary and irregular secondary dentin is often of the fibrodentin (Figure 19) or osteodentin types. Thus, a potential to form these primitive types of dentins apparently exists in pulp cells. This is important to keep in mind in evaluating the biologic reactivity of the dental pulp. Furthermore, the specialized structure of the dentin in certain commonly used experimental animals should be recognized, e.g., the osteodentin in the central area of the anterior portion of rat incisors.[29] Marked variations in the extent of the peritubular dentin have also been reported, including the absence of this structure.[30] The significance of such structural variations has not been established, but it is at least theoretically possible that the reaction patterns of dentins with and without highly mineralized peritubular areas may be quite different.

REFERENCES

1. **Mjör, I. A.,** Dentin and pulp, in *Histology of the Human Tooth,* Mjör, I. A. and Fejerskov, O., Eds., Munksgaard, Copenhagen, 1979, 43.
2. **Dahl, E., and Mjör, I. A.,** The structure and distribution of nerves in the pulp dentin organ *Acta Odontol. Scand.,* 31, 349, 1973.
3. **Holland, G. R.,** The extent of the odontoblast process in the cat, *J. Anat.,* 121, 133, 1975.
4. **Thomas, H. F. and Payne, R. C.,** The ultrastructure of dentinal tubules from erupted human premolar teeth, *J. Dent. Res.,* 60, (Abst. 161), 351, 1981.
5. **Frank, R. M. and Nalbandian, J.,** Comparative aspects of development of dental hard structures, *J. Dent. Res.,* 42, 422, 1963.

6. **Furseth, R.,** The fine structure of the odontoblast predentin area in the root, *Scand. J. Dent. Res.*, 79, 141, 1971.
7. **Forssell-Ahlberg, K., Brännström, M., and Edwall, L.,** The diameter and number of dentinal tubules in rat, cat, dog, and monkey. A comparative scanning electron microscopic study, *Acta Odontol. Scand.*, 33, 243, 1975.
8. **Thomas, H. F. and Carella, P.,** Correlation of SEM and TEM appearance of peritubular dentin, *J. Dent. Res.*, 61 (Abstr. 1033), 293, 1982.
9. **Bradford, E. W.,** The interpretation of decalcified sections of human dentin, *Br. Dent. J.*, 98, 153, 1955.
10. **Frank, R. M.,** Ultrastructure of human dentine, in *Calcified Tissues 1965*, Hirsh, H., Blackwood, H. J. J., and Owen, M., Eds., Springer-Verlag, Berlin, 1965, 259.
11. **Mjör, I. A.,** Microradiography of human coronal dentin, *Arch. Oral Biol.*, 11, 225, 1966.
12. **Mjör, I. A. and Shackleford, J. M.,** Microradiography of human pulp tissue and decalcified coronal dentine, *Arch. Oral Biol.*, 11, 1307, 1966.
13. **Mjör, I. A.,** Dentin and pulp, in *Reaction Patterns in Human Teeth*, Mjör, I. A., Ed., CRC Press, Boca Raton, Fla., 1983.
14. **Arwill, T.,** Some morphologic aspects of dentinal innervation, in *Sensory Mechanisms in Dentine*, Anderson, D. J., Ed., Pergamon Press, Oxford, 1963, 3.
15. **Arwill, T.,** The ultrastructure of the pulpodentinal border zone, in *Dentine and Pulp: Their Structure and Reactions*, Symons, N. B. B., Ed., Churchill Livingstone, Edinburgh, 1968, 147.
16. **Frank, R. M.,** Ultrastructural relationship between the odontoblast, its process and the nerve fibers, in *Dentine and Pulp: Their Structure and Reactions*, Symons, N. B. B., Ed., Churchill Livingstone, Edinburgh, 1968, 115.
17. **Fejerskov, O.,** Odontogenesis, in *Histology of the Human Tooth*, Mjör, I. A., Ed., Munksgaard, Copenhagen, 1979, 21.
18. **Avery, J. K. and Rapp, R.,** An investigation of the mechanism of neural impulse transmission in the teeth, *Oral Surg.*, 12, 190, 1959.
19. **Gaunt, W. A. and Miles, A. E. W.,** Fundamental aspects of tooth morphogenesis, in *Structure and Chemical Organization of Teeth*, Vol. 1, Miles, A. E. W., Ed., Academic Press, New York, 1967, 151.
20. **Frank, R. M.,** Etude autoradiographique de la dentinogenese en microscopie electronique a l'aide de la proline tritiee chez le chat, *Arch. Oral Biol.*, 15, 583, 1970.
21. **Avery, J. K. et al., Eds.,** Development of the teeth-crown formation, in *Oral Histology*, The University of Michigan Dental Publications, Ann Arbor, 1981, 1.
22. **Gotjamanos, T.,** Cellular organization in the subodontoblastic zone of the dental pulp. I. A study of cell-free and cell-rich layers in pulps of adult rat and deciduous monkey teeth, *Arch. Oral Biol.*, 14, 1007, 1967.
23. **Takuma, S.,** Ultrastructure of dentinogenesis, in *Structure and Chemical Organization of Teeth*, Vol. 1, Miles, A. E. W., Ed., Academic Press, New York, 1967, 325.
24. **Tronstad, L.,** Optical and microradiographic appearance of intact and worn human coronal dentine, *Arch. Oral Biol.*, 17, 847, 1972.
25. **Orban, B.,** Biologic considerations in restorative dentistry, *J. Am. Dent. Assoc.*, 28, 1009, 1941.
26. **Wennberg, A., Mjör, I. A., and Heide, S.,** Rate of formation of regular and irregular secondary dentin in monkey teeth, *Oral Surg.*, 54, 232, 1982.
27. **Baume, L. J.,** Definitions and classifications of the pulpdentinal tissues, in *The Biology of Pulp and Dentine. A Historic, Terminologic-Taxonomic, Histologic-Biochemical, Embryonic and Clinical Survey*, S. Karger, Basel, 1980, 41.
28. **Breivik, M.,** Human odontoblast response to tooth replantation, *Eur. J. Orthod.*, 3, 95, 1981.
29. **Takuma, S., Kurahashi, Y., and Tsuboi, Y.,** Electron microscopy of the osteodentine in rat incisors, in *Dentin and Pulp: Their Structure and Reactions*, Symons, N. B. B., Ed., Churchill Livingstone, Edinburgh, 1968, 169.
30. **Takuma, S. and Eda, S.,** Peritubular matrix in mammalian dentin, *Bull. Tokyo Dent. Coll.*, 1, 20, 1960.

Chapter 2

STRUCTURAL AND PHYSIOLOGIC ASPECTS OF DENTIN INNERVATION

James K. Avery, Charles F. Cox, and Daniel J. Chiego, Jr.

TABLE OF CONTENTS

I. INTRODUCTION

The morphology of the peripheral tooth pulp, the odontoblasts, their processes, and the dentinal tubule complex imparts a unique relationship whereby both tissues act in concert as a vital, perceptive tissue which is sensitive to external stimuli. Pain transmission in dentin has concerned scientific investigators and clinicians alike since the mid-1800s. Dentin is one of the few tissues in the body from which only pain is perceived; whether the stimulus is due to temperature changes, mechanical cutting or grinding, pressure, a direct stream of air, electrical or chemical stimuli, all produce a nociceptive response.

Dentin is a highly mineralized tissue, with approximately 68% inorganic content, second only to enamel. The sensitivity of teeth is believed to arise in part from intradental receptors, some of which exist in the dentinal tubules. In young individuals, there are approximately 70,000 to 80,000 dentinal tubules per μm^2 at the pulp-dentin interface. Older teeth, subjected to occlusal wear and trauma demonstrate less tubules per μm^2, 30,000 to 40,000 at the pulp-dentin interface. In human teeth the tubule diameter is approximately 0.3 to 1.0 μm at the dentino-enamel junction (DEJ) and 4.0 to 5.0 μm at the pulpal interface. Although some investigators have demonstrated nerve fibers and endings in the predentin and juxtaposed to odontoblast processes within the pulpal third of the dentinal tubules, none have demonstrated neural structures at or near the DEJ where pain is most clinically intense. In this respect, the precise mechanism of pain perception in dentin has not yet been determined. It is the objective of this chapter to discuss the development, structure, and mechanism of action of pain transmission in dentin.

II. CENTRAL PATHWAYS

All somatosensory afferent nociceptive information is carried from the peripheral oral-facial complex via the maxillary and mandibular branches of the *trigeminal V cranial nerve* to the *trigeminal nuclei* of the brain stem.[1] This trigeminal nuclear complex is divided into the *principal sensory pontine nucleus* and the *descending spinal nucleus* which runs through the medulla to the second cervical spinal cord segment (Figure 1). Nerve fibers exiting the tooth apex are characterized as A-delta myelinated 1- to 6-μm diameter fibers and small unmyelinated C-type of 0.25- to 1.5-μm diameter fibers, which also run with the proprioceptive fibers of the adjacent periodontal ligament. The somatosensory afferent fibers pass through the *Gasserian ganglion* where the primary ganglion cells are located.[2]

The caudal extent of the ganglion cells enter the brain stem at the level of the pons where these first order sensory fibers run to the descending trigeminal tract (Figure 2). This long descending nucleus is subdivided into the *oralis, interpolaris,* and *caudalis nuclei.* Recent evidence by Gobel and Binck[3] has demonstrated different strata within the subnucleus caudalis, which is homologous to the various laminae (layers) of the dorsal horn of the spinal cord I, III, and V, laminae. The outer marginal I lamina receives small A-type myelinated nociceptive afferents. The middle II and III laminae receive small C-type unmyelinated afferents and the inner IV magnocellular lamina receives tactile information from large A-type myelinated primary afferent nociceptors.[4] Some of these laminae project (ascend) directly to the thalamus via second order neurons while other laminae send collaterals to other nuclei in the same ipsilateral descending trigeminal complex.[5,6] Recent data have shown that the subnucleus caudalis has two general types of neurons; one neuron responds to a narrow spectrum of noxious stimuli while the other neuron responds to a wide range of nociceptive stimuli. Sessle[7] has suggested that the subnucleus caudalis participates in the localization and discrimination of pain. However, the main sensory nucleus and the nucleus oralis appear to be the major site for presynaptic facilitation and inhibition.[8]

Fibers from the long descending tract send collaterals at varying levels which synapse on

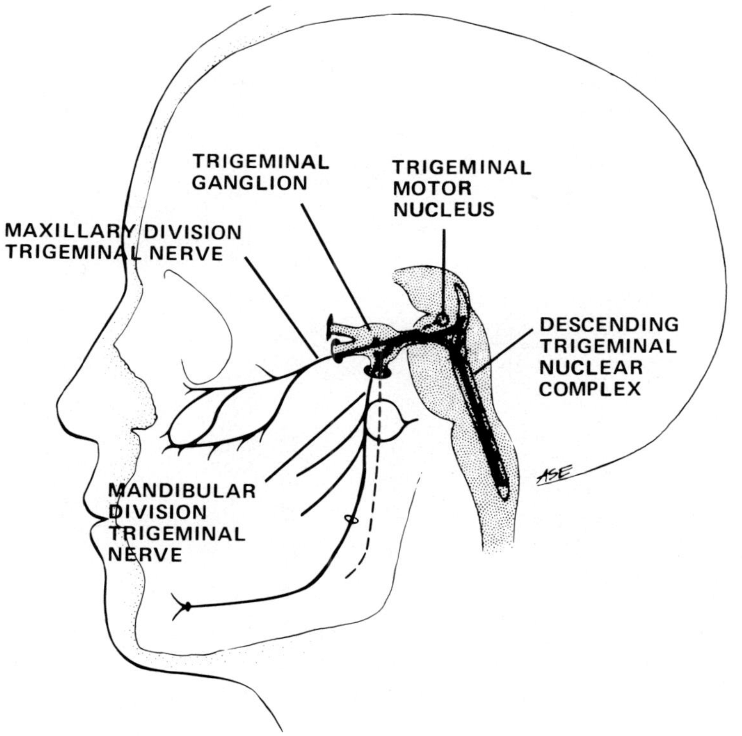

FIGURE 1. This diagram illustrates the central and peripheral components of the trigeminal nerve involved in the sensory innervation of the teeth.

the neurons of an adjacent associated descending trigeminal nucleus, containing fibers from the ophthalmic, maxillary, and mandibular divisions of the trigeminal nerve. The trigeminal ganglion, the descending tract, and trigeminal nucleus are each organized somatotopically, with the ophthalmic lying most caudal, the mandibular most rostral, and the maxillary intermediate. After reaching the descending trigeminal nucleus, second order fibers cross the midline to the opposite side of the brain stem and ascend rostrally as the *ventral trigeminothalamic tract*. There are, however, collateral fibers to the dorsolateral reticular formation which are given off before a small number of fibers reach the ventroposterior medial nucleus of the thalamus and thalamic nuclei. Neurons of the dorsal trigeminal tract do not decussate, as they remain ipsilateral projecting to the ventroposterior nucleus of the thalamus.

From clinical and research data, investigators consider that the tooth perceives only pain whereby the periodontal ligament perceives touch and pressure. As a consequence, many physiologic studies have employed this model to study the location of cells in the trigeminal nuclei as they respond to nociceptive stimuli. Sessle and Greenwood[9] have recently demonstrated that noxious stimuli elicit the most responses to the main sensory and oralis nuclei of the trigeminal nuclear complex. In addition, the same investigators suggested that the rostral portions of the descending complex are involved in the localization of the dental pulp stimulus.[10] Whenever a nuclear portion of the trigeminal complex is stimulated the medial reticular formation is simultaneously stimulated. Consequently, there is convergence of both maxillary and mandibular tooth input, with some neurons receiving input from both tooth pulp and periodontal ligament.[11] Adding even more confusion is the fact that stimuli from other areas of the oral-facial complex will elicit responses from the same pulpal afferents that respond to noxious stimuli to the tooth.

In addition to pain, investigators have reported that teeth respond to modalities such as

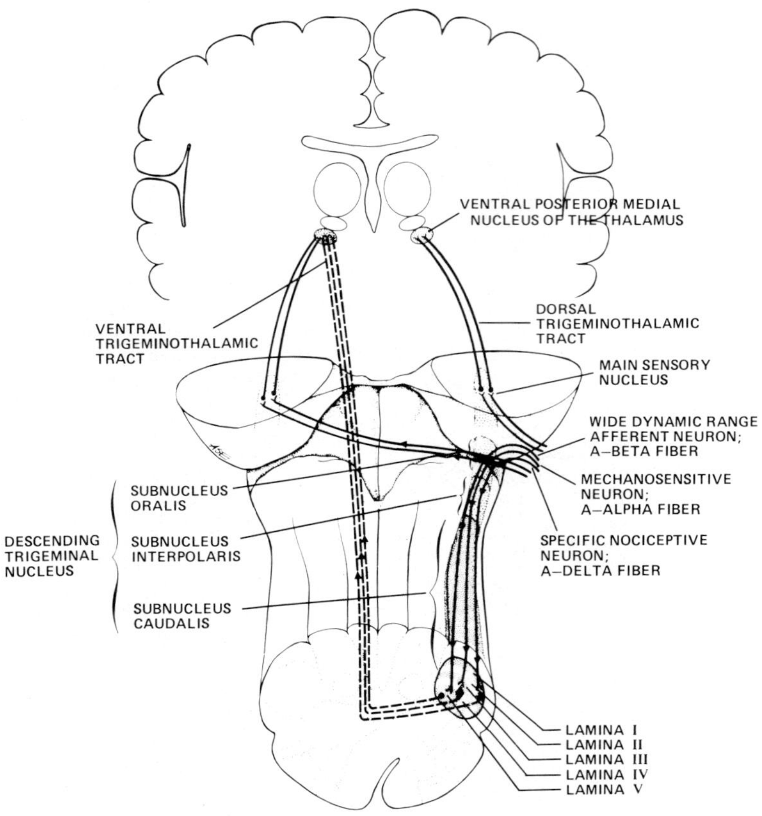

FIGURE 2. This is a diagram of the first and second order neurons which are involved in the relaying of sensory information from the teeth to the thalamus.

pressure, proprioception, and various thermal sensations.[12-14] These studies, employing injection of radioisotopes into trigeminal ganglia, have demonstrated the presence of large terminals in the dental pulp and inner third of the tubules, similar to the morphology of cutaneous mechanoreceptors. However, some question regarding specificity of proline labeling relates to the possible spillover of proline into the blood pool, becoming bound into the developing predentin, thereby masking labeling of neural elements.

The autonomic nervous system was demonstrated by histochemical fluorescence along the vessels of monkey pulps by Pohto.[15] The sympathetic modulation of pain intensity, originating in the dental pulp, has been reported by Edwall and Scott[16] and Matthews.[17] Avery et al.[18] have recently demonstrated adrenergic endings in the pulp and predentin by the use of a false neurotransmitter (5-OH-dopamine). Whether the modification of the neural response is modulated through the release of a neurotransmitter or through a vascular tone is not known. Dellows and Morgan[19] reported that stimulation of pulpal nerves results in a decrease in blood pressure, indicative of a reflexive sympathetic neural activity. Centrally these effects can be seen upon the stimulation of the trigeminal nucleus and tract,[20] suggesting an efferent pathway, possibly through the tenth cranial nerve (Vagus). Whether these sympathetic nerve activities effects are direct or secondary to vascular changes at the adrenergic terminals, superior cervical ganglion, brain stem, or hypothalamus are not known at this time.

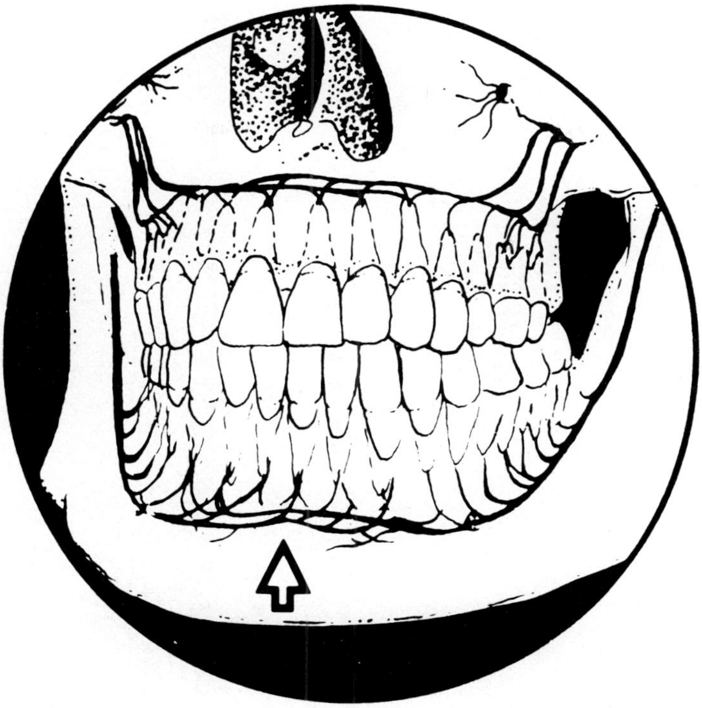

FIGURE 3. A diagram of transmedian innervation of the incisor and cuspid teeth. Crossover of both of the maxillary anterior superior and mandibular inferior alveolar nerves is seen.

III. PERIPHERAL PATHWAYS

The *mandibular* and *maxillary nerves* arise from the trigeminal ganglion, exiting through the base of the skull at the foramen ovale and rotundum. The maxillary branch V-2 supplies the maxillary teeth as the *superior alveolar nerves* with some small auxillary branches. The mandibular V-3 branch divides into the *lingual, buccal,* and *inferior alveolar branches*. The latter courses on the medial aspect of the mandible and enters into the mandibular foramen with accompanying vessels proceeding through the bony canal, giving rise to smaller dental branches to the apical root canal of each tooth.

The teeth are innervated by the superior and inferior alveolar branches of the trigeminal nerves. Recent studies have reported accessory innervation to the molar teeth from the *mylohyoid nerve branch* that enters the inferior retromolar foramen. This mylohyoid branch terminates directly in the incisor teeth and gingiva or joins the ipsilateral or contralateral incisive nerve to provide a limited transmedian innervation.[21] Other investigators have reported small accessory or supplemental branches from the lingual, cervical plexus, long buccal, auriculotemporal nerves.[22-28] Clinical data have demonstrated that incisor teeth have the largest proportions of anesthesia failures when an inferior dental block is performed.[29] In any case, complete anesthesia to anterior teeth may be affected by a buccal injection including the lingual nerve. Anderson and Pearl[30] have described transmedian innervation of the anterior teeth (Figure 3).

IV. GENERAL PULP CONSIDERATIONS

As the superior and inferior alveolar nerves leave the main trunks from their bony canals,

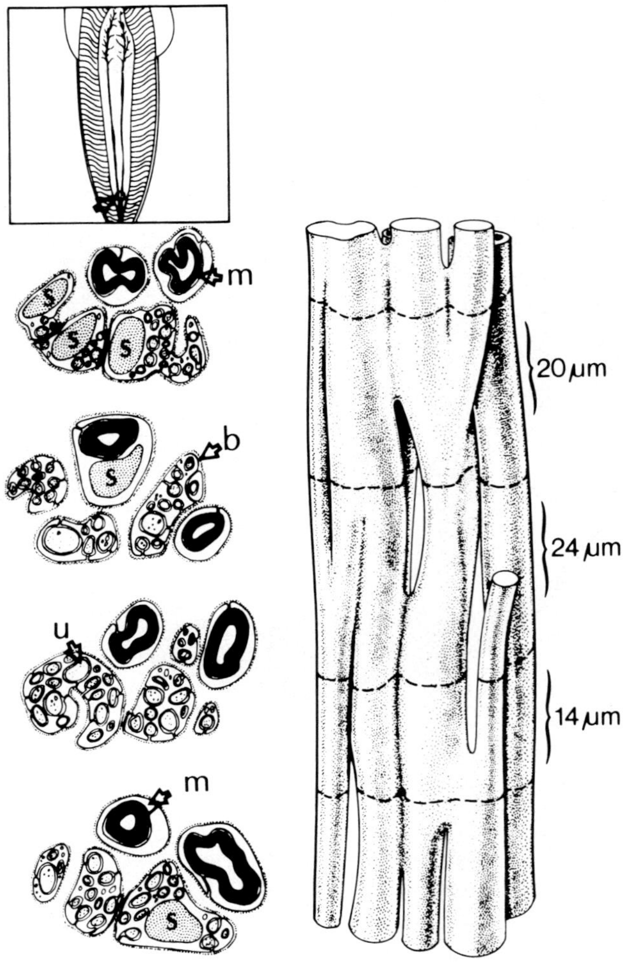

FIGURE 4. A diagram of a nerve plexus from the apical (central core) region of a human pulp as it appears from an ultrastructural reconstruction. On the left are schematic cross sections, representing various relationships which myelinated and unmyelinated nerves have to each other. Associated Schwann cells are seen surrounding the axons. (b) Basal lamina, (m) myelinated axon, (u) unmyelinated axon, (S) Schwann cell nucleus.

smaller branches of nerve fiber groups enter the root pulp through the apical canals. For the most part, these nerves are composed of trigeminal and autonomic sources. Two or three branches enter the molar and premolar root apices whereas single fiber bundles generally enter the incisor and canine pulps (Figure 4). Johnsen and Johns[31] have shown that human premolar teeth may have from 1000 to 2500 unmyelinated and 350 to 700 myelinated axons which enter into their respective root pulp apex. These nerve trunks are composed of myelinated and unmyelinated nerves which run as bundles coursing adjacent to the vascular components of the pulp. Recent studies by Johnsen and Harschbarger[32] in human teeth have demonstrated that the myelinated and unmyelinated nerves do not lie within a distinct neural-vascular connective tissue bundle, but are seen lying throughout the stroma of the root pulp. A high magnification picture (Figure 5) demonstrates A-delta and C-type axons appearing in groups enveloped by a single Schwann cell or as part of a much larger bundle of myelinated axons completely enveloped by one Schwann cell and its investing layers; or the axon(s) may be immediately adjacent to another axon with no intervening Schwann cell. When

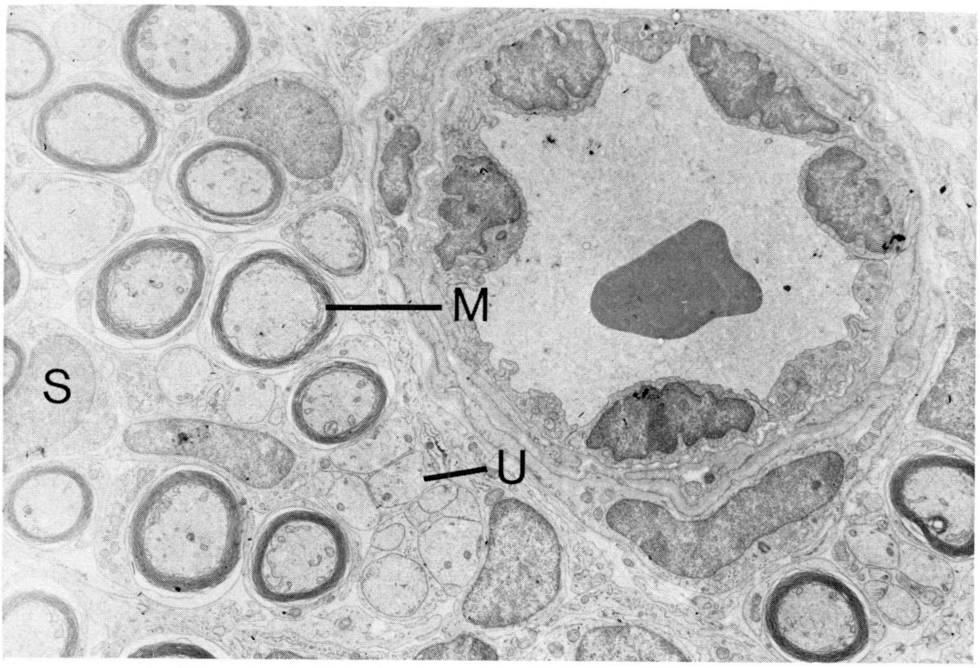

FIGURE 5. An area of the pulp near the subodontoblastic plexus showing both myelinated (M) and unmyelinated (U) axons adjacent to a precapillary. Note the Schwann cell nuclei (S) adjacent to the axons.

human tooth pulps are viewed longitudinally, the myelinated axons are similar to other peripheral nerves found elsewhere in the body. Lack of branching, nodes of Ranvier, and Schmidt-Lantermann clefts are also present. Each myelin sheath lies in close approximation to that of adjacent axons. However, in a few instances, myelin loops may be seen which do not encircle the axoplasm and as a consequence may pass through such a Schwann cell plexus without having direct contact with the cells of the plexus.[32] The larger A-delta conducting myelinated fibers of the root pulp range from 2.0 to 6.0 μm in diameter.

Unmyelinated axons seldom branch, but the Schwann cell wrappings may form elaborate anastomoses. A single network of Schwann cell(s) can envelop several hundred unmyelinated axons within the human pulp. These unmyelinated axon groups may appear to be separate in a single section, but they are joined at some point while traversing the root pulp canal.

The Schwann cell junction for myelinated axons differs from the configuration seen for unmyelinated axons. A butt-joint arrangement of two Schwann cells characterizes a node of Ranvier for myelinated axons, whereas an overlapping arrangement is common with many Schwann cells contributing to the envelopment of groups of unmyelinated axons. The result is that a series of overlapping adjacent Schwann cells may meet at any angle from parallel to 90°, relative to the axon. Enclosing the entire plexus is a basal lamina. As each tooth matures and ages the nerve plexuses may break up and some fibers will degenerate. It is thought that these Schwann cell plexuses serve to maintain large groups of axons in a relatively stable spatial relationship as each root canal decreases in diameter during secondary dentin formation.

Both myelinated and unmyelinated nerves arborize throughout the pulp and branch as a *parietal plexus* of nerves at the periphery of the cell rich zone of the coronal pulp. The large myelinated nerves of the pulp lose their outer myelin sheaths as they branch and enter the cell free zone and project to the subjacent juxta-odontoblastic cell layer (Figure 6). Lilja[33] reported that the majority of nerves within the circumpulpal area are located in the roof of

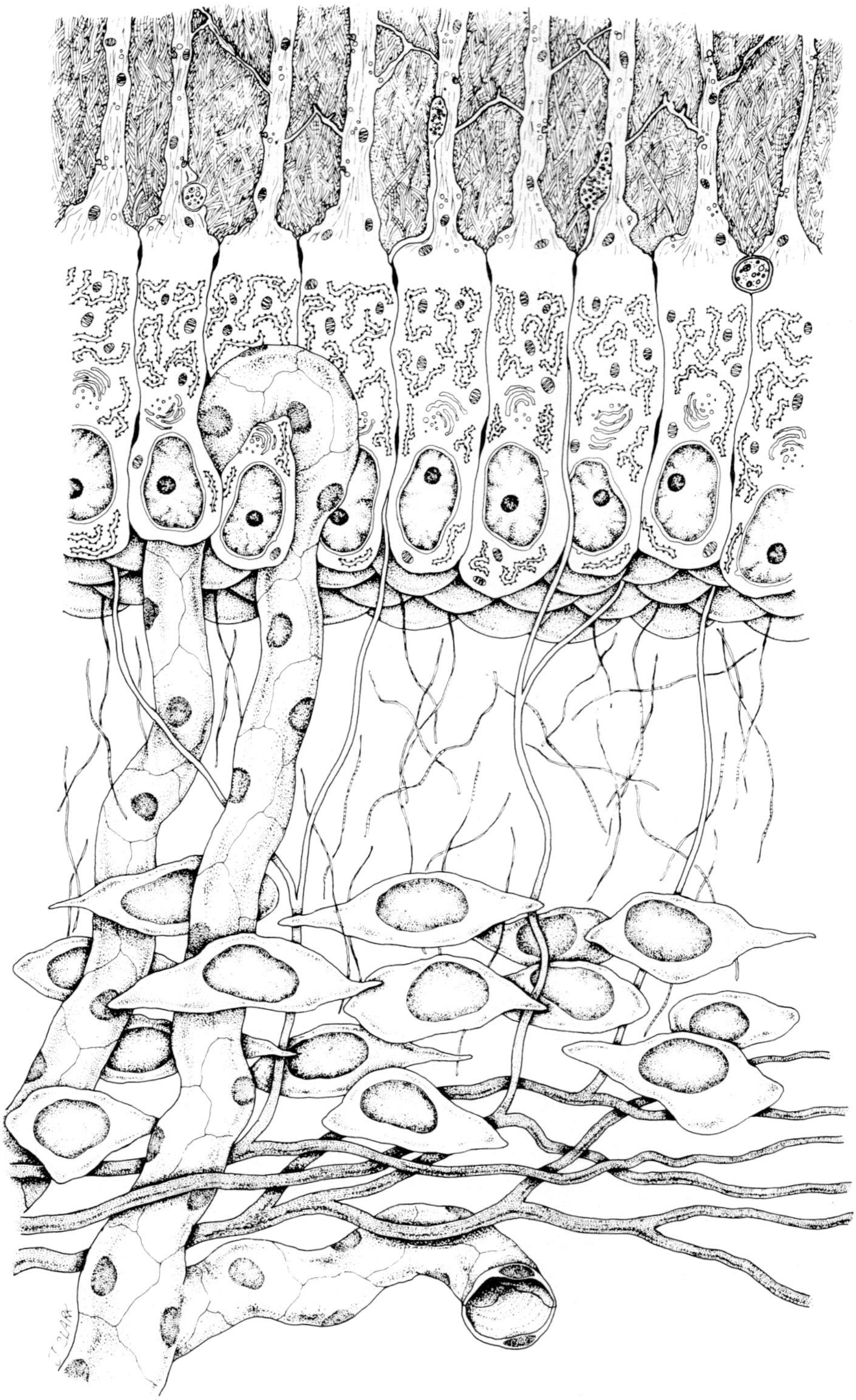

FIGURE 6. A diagram of the odontoblastic zone and predentin illustrating nerves and nerve endings in the region of the odontoblasts and their processes in the dentinal tubules.

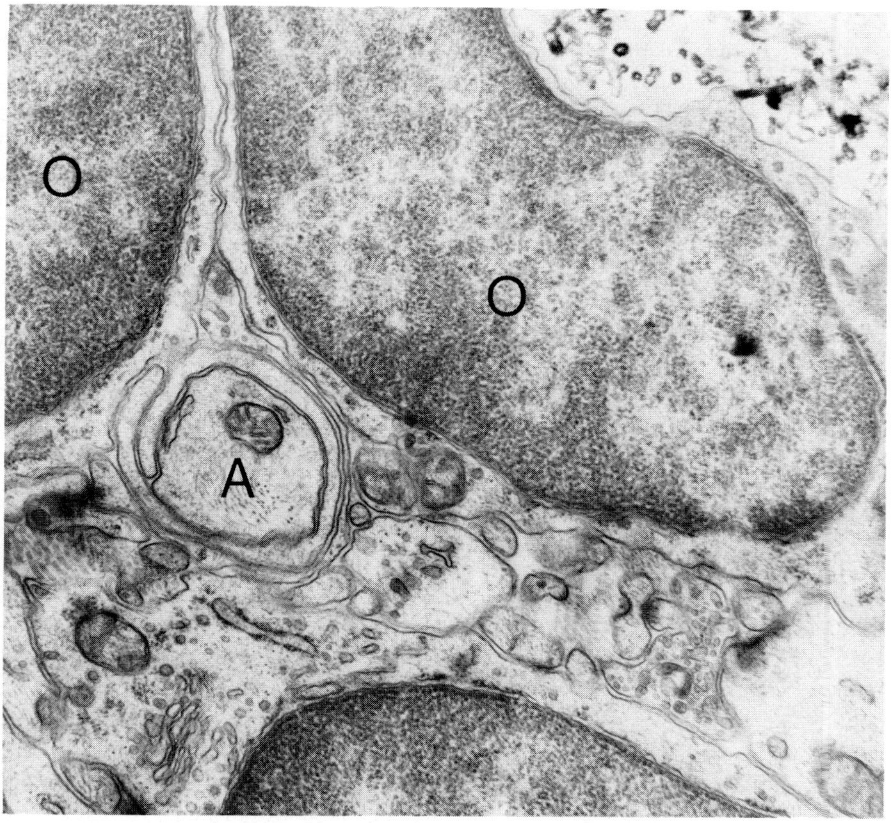

FIGURE 7. A Schwann cell-enveloped axon (A) located adjacent to the plasma membrane of two odontoblasts (O) in the upper part of the field and one in the lower part of the field.

the coronal pulp chamber horns of human teeth. Fewer endings are found along the lateral walls and floor of the coronal aspects of primary teeth. Fearnhead,[34] employing light microscopy, reported that the most concentrated density of nerves is approximately one ending per every eight or ten odontoblasts/tubules in the coronal pulp horn, whereas the distribution of endings is one per 200 odontoblasts/tubules in the root area. Unmyelinated nerves pursue a course that is closely adjacent to the odontoblast cell body (Figure 7).

V. IDENTIFICATION OF NERVE ENDINGS

One technique of demonstrating nerve endings in the dental pulp was that of Pohto,[35] who used a fluorescence histochemical technique to demontrate the presence of adrenergic endings along the blood vessels of monkey and human dental pulp tissues. Larsson and Linde[36] administered a monamine oxidase inhibitor followed by noradrenalin which resulted in an increase in the fluorescence of the pulp by the technique of Falk et al.[37] Avery et al.,[38] Nakano et al.,[39] and Pohto et al.[40] quantitated the level of noradrenalin in the dental pulp by various procedures.

Several of the earliest ultrastructural studies by Frank,[41] Arwill,[42] and Corpron et al.[43] demonstrated electron micrographs of nerves and endings in the area of the odontogenic layer as well as in the inner third of the dentinal tubules. The majority of nerve endings in the pulp have been classified by their type of vesiculated terminals.[44] Small endings contain many small homogeneous light- to moderate-staining vesicles. The larger terminals or endings contain large dense core staining vesicles with occasional mitochondria. Based on the appearance of these vesicles, the terminals with small, light-staining vesicles (Figure 8) are believed to be cholinergic and the terminals with dense core staining vesicles (Figure 9) are believed to be adrenergic in nature. Richardson[45] found that potassium permanganate fixation improved the preservation of the dense core granules over that of the glutaraldehyde or osmium, which was the typically used fixative. According to Hökfelt and Johnsson[46] an electron-dense precipitate of manganese dioxide is formed when noradrenalin is reduced by permanganate. More recent studies by Hand[47] employed a potassium permanganate fixative which was able to differentiate the cholinergic from the adrenergic nerve terminals in the parotid gland of the rat. Examination of the odontogenic region with this technique led to the conclusion that some of the nerve ending terminals contained large, dense core staining vesicles of from 300 to 700 Å in diameter.[48] Some of these terminals were observed as large endings which interdigitated with several odontoblasts at their basal ends.

Numerous investigators have described the tortuous path the fine unmyelinated fibers take as they pass through the cell-free and cell-rich zones juxtaposed to the odontoblasts.[49-53] Ultrastructural studies have described both naked and Schwann cell-covered fibers, approximately 0.3 to 0.5 μm in diameter, in close approximation to the odontoblast cell layer terminating adjacent to an odontoblast or to its process in a dentinal tubule. The presence of nerves in the tubules has been reported extending some 100 to 150 μm into the dentinal tubules from the pulp in a number of animals.[44,54-56] These unmyelinated axons appear to have alternating dilations and constrictions which interdigitate with the odontoblast and its processes. Frank[57] reported nerves as coiling around the odontoblasts and their processes in the tubules, while others noted them traversing adjacent to the process (Figure 10). The nerves may be described as containing mitochondria, filaments, and microtubules. The vesicular granules of nerve endings and beadings appear as concentrations in the dilated portions of the nerve, whereas the constricted portions are devoid of them. The morphological relationship of the nerve terminal and the odontoblast demonstrates that as much as 50% of the structure may be enfolded by the cell or its process[50] (Figures 11 and 12). Lilja[56] reported that degenerating neural structures were a common feature in the root predentin.

In summary, both myelinated nerves as well as Schwann cell-covered and/or naked axons lie in close association to the cell bodies of odontoblasts as well as their processes. The small axons lie adjacent to the plasma membrane of the odontoblast. Although the majority of these small axons lie close to the basal nucleated region of the odontoblasts, others pass between the cells to terminate at the apical level of the cell along the pulpal-predentin junction. Some extend into the dentin as far as 200 μm, although the axons appear to have no relationship. The terminals may be enfolded by the cell body. This relationship of the nerve ending is especially true in the tubule producing an interdigitating relationship. Holland[58] reported gap junctions between the nerve and odontoblast; however, Cox et al.[59] and Byers[60] have not been able to confirm this observation. Recent studies by Gunji[61] have reported that all nerve fibers terminate as free endings, being confined adjacent to the odontoblastic process in the predentin region.

VI. ODONTOBLAST RELATIONSHIPS

Odontoblasts maintain a somewhat different relationship to each other throughout the various regions of the root pulp, such as the bifurcation zone, the central pulp, and the coronal pulp. Along the root pulp-dentin interface, the odontoblasts are seen as cuboidal- to low columnar-appearing cells with some extracellular spaces between them. In the central and coronal pulps, the odontoblasts appear crowded together, having a pseudostratified columnar appearance. In the pulp horns, the odontoblasts are densely packed together with many junctional complexes evident between the cells (Figure 13).

Early light microscopic observations by Kolliker[62] described the membrane eboris as a

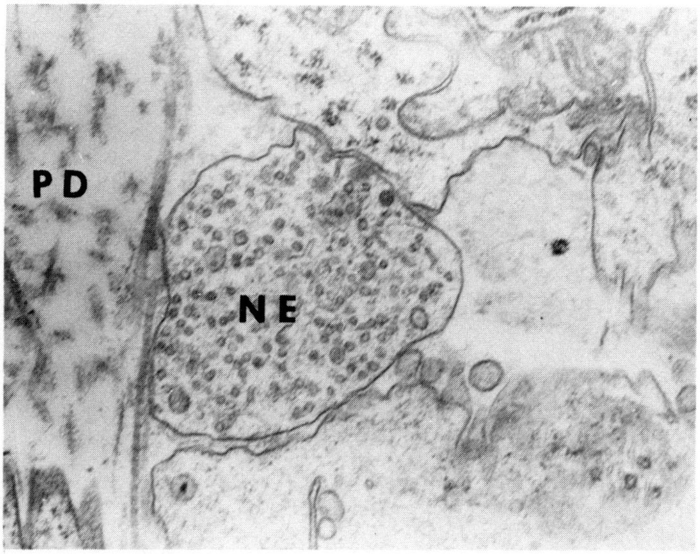

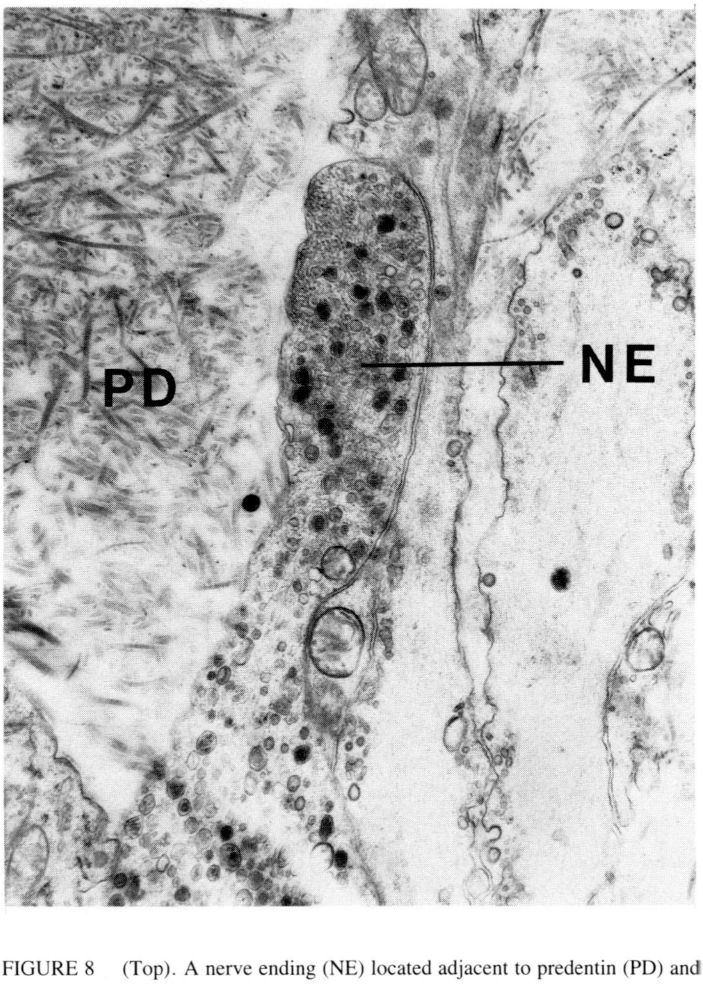

FIGURE 8 (Top). A nerve ending (NE) located adjacent to predentin (PD) and cytoplasm of odontoblasts on the right. This nerve ending has numerous small light-staining vesicles. FIGURE 9 (Bottom). A large nerve ending (NE) located in the predentin (PD) zone. The majority of vesicles have dense core staining.

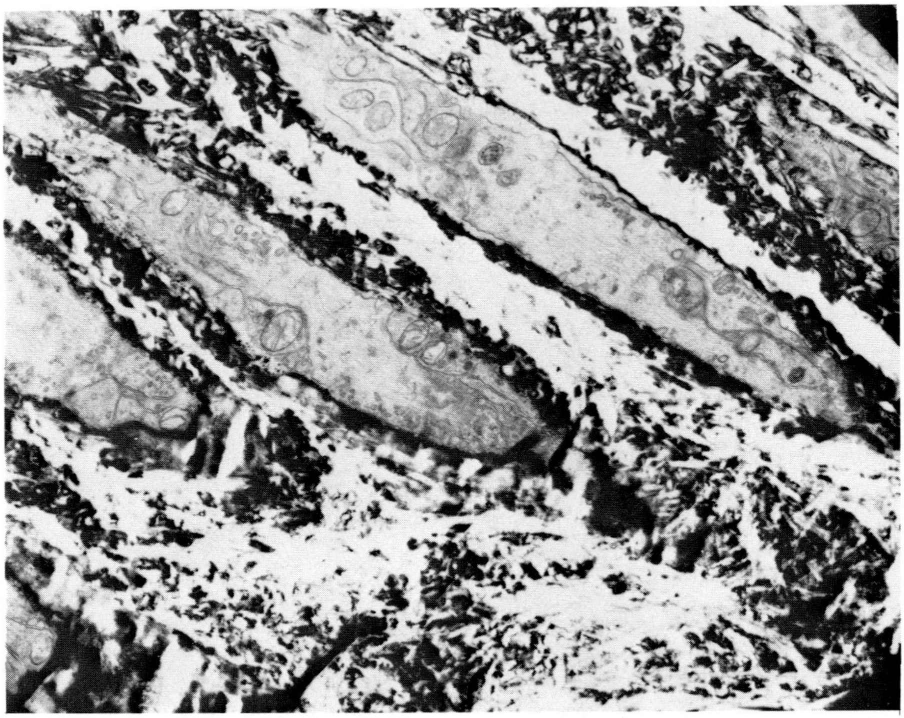

FIGURE 10. Nerves may extend 200 μm into the dentinal tubules from the pulp. The nerve ending in the tubule is seen to interdigitate with the odontoblast process.

layer of cells at the periphery of the tooth pulp arranged like a palisade up to three cells deep. This layer was described as having intercellular relationships only to those cells formative of true dentin. Paul[63] reported that odontoblasts in the early stages of growing exhibited a collar, while mature odontoblasts did not possess it. Mummery[64] interpreted the dense zone as lateral attachments directly along the apical portion of the odontoblasts. It was speculated that these lateral processes gave rise to small tubes that exited into the calcified dentin. A later theory by Bernard[65] described adherence attachments which were seen between odontoblasts only at the time of embryological development and not at later maturation stages. Orban[66] reported that odontoblasts were separated by terminal bars which were interpreted as intercellular condensations appearing as fine dots or lines between the apex of the odontoblasts. Bradford,[67] on the other hand, described the zone separating the odontoblasts from the predentin as a pulpo-dentinal membrane which appeared as a synctium throughout the odontoblasts of the pulp.

Ultrastructural observations by Watson and Avery[68] described an osmophilic interrupted broken line at the predentin border which separated the cell body of the odontoblast from its process. Quigley[69] reported that this incomplete terminal bar boundary separated the odontoblast cells from their processes; however no intercellular bridges were seen between odontoblasts. Frank[70] described "desmosome like" structures in the nuclear regions of odontoblasts connecting their lateral surfaces and defined the terminal bar as a continuous "belt-like" attachment apparatus which joined the odontoblasts at their predentin border.

FIGURE 11. A cross section of terminals (NE) in adjacent dentinal tubules. Observe the increased surface area of the odontoblast process (P) and terminal due to the enfolding of the two structures. FIGURE 12. Odontoblasts can be seen above and on the left of the fie!d. One odontoblast partially surrounds a vesiculated nerve ending (NE).

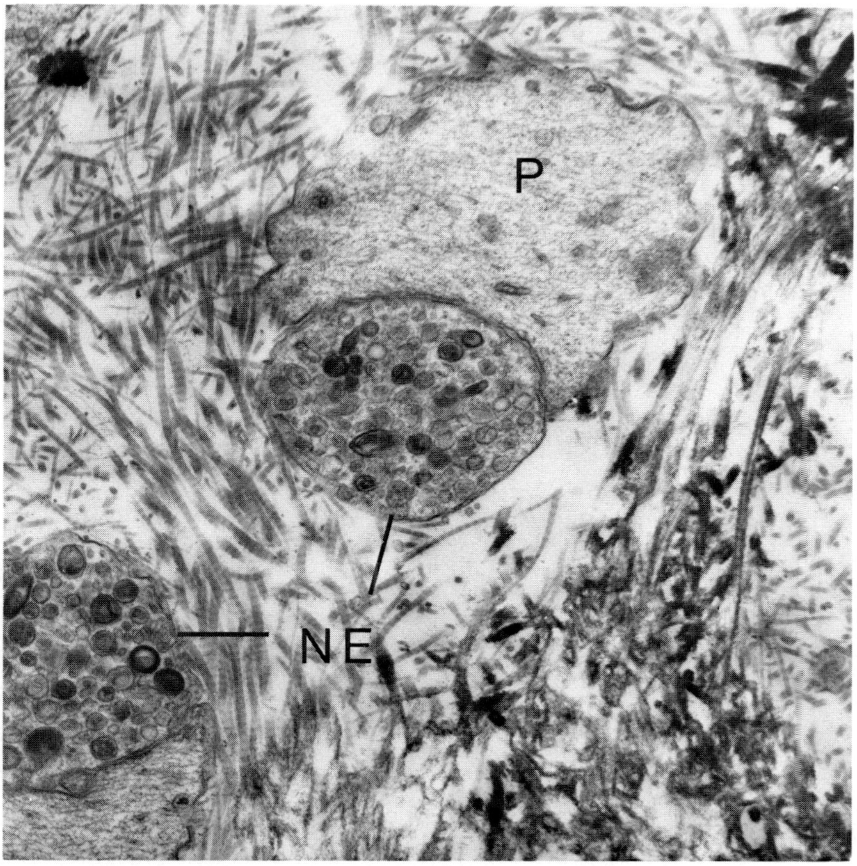

FIGURE 11 .

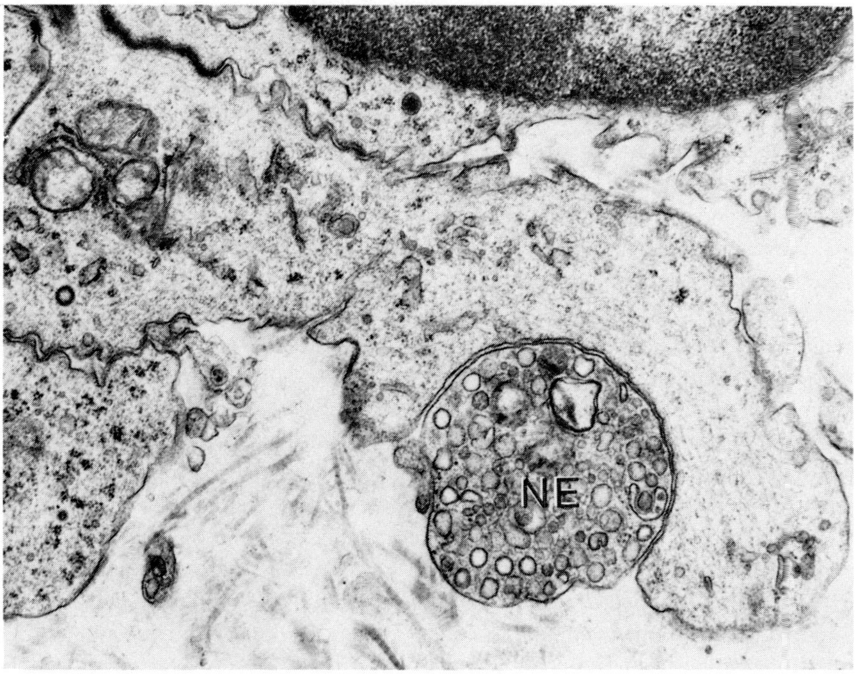

FIGURE 12 .

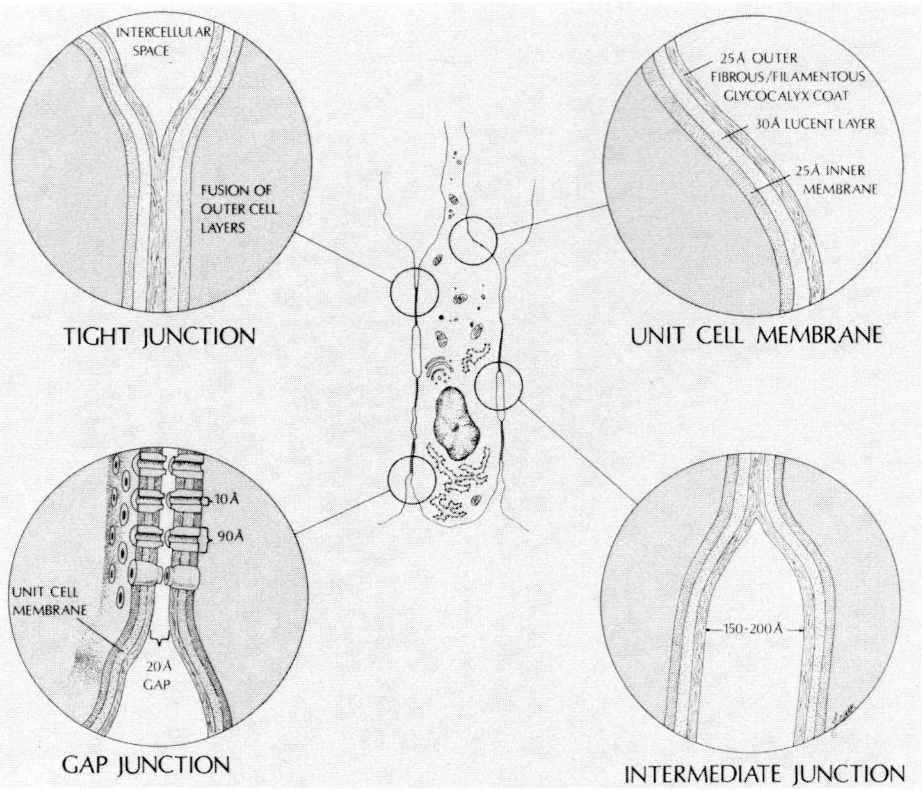

FIGURE 13. A diagram of the various types of junctional complexes that have been identified on odontoblasts. The upper left schematic shows a tight junction with the fusion of two adjacent odontoblast plasma membranes. The upper right schematic delineates the layers of a unit cell membrane of an odontoblast. The lower left schematic shows the 20 Å gap which takes up the lanthanum as a staining precipitate. This gap junction complex has a field of 20 Å pores which allow the direct electrochemical exchange of proteins between two or more cells. The intermediate junction is a 200-Å space that composes a glycocalyx beltway between and around cells.

Arwill[71] described long desmosomal contact attachment plaques between human odontoblasts in a crowded state and further described a triple-layered membrane with a gap between odontoblast processes as well as between associated cells. Other types of junctional complexes were also independently described by Frank,[70] Garant et al.,[72] and Jessen[73] as tight junctions, zona adherens, filament cuffs, as well as desmosomes and terminal bars. Observations by Reith,[74] Tsubo,[75] and Takuma and Nagai[76] defined a well-developed cell web in the clear distal area of functional odontoblasts of rodent incisors. Cell contacts were judged to be a series of microtubules which ran parallel to the filaments of the webs. Stockinger[77] speculated that the long tight junctional cell contacts and shorter desmosomes were membrane fusion zones for low resistance electrical conduction between cells. Corpron and Avery[44] noted areas of constrictions and dilatations between intratubular nerves and odontoblastic processes, while Dahl and Mjör[78] reported tight junctions between cytoplasmic invaginations of nerves and odontoblast cell bodies. Holland[79] described desmosomal junctions between some of the odontoblasts at the predentinal border, and the presence of small subunit junctions of low electrical resistance based on the presence of pale and dark staining processes. Cox et al.,[80] using colloidal tracers, reported the differentiation of both tight and gap junctions between odontoblasts. Cohen and Kramer[81] stated that odontoblasts and ameloblasts exhibited both tight, intermediate, and desmosome junctional complexes; however, gap junctions were not mentioned. Studies by McNutt and Weinstein[82] have characterized gap junctions in

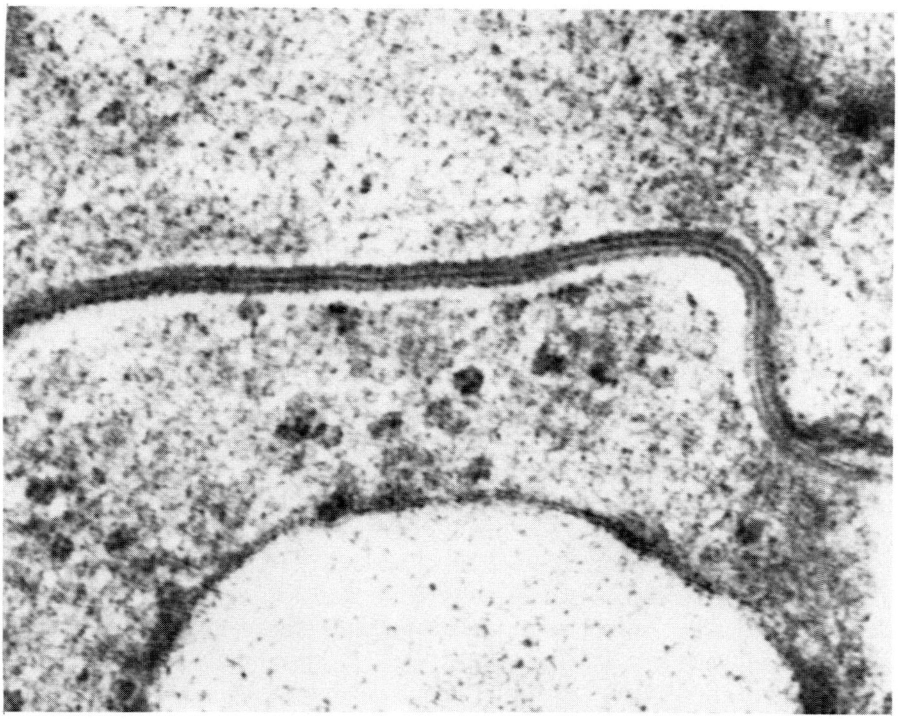

FIGURE 14. A transmission electron micrograph of a gap junction between two odontoblasts after staining the 20-Å space with lanthanum nitrate. Note the appearance of the electron dense precipitate along the adjacent plasma membranes of the odontoblasts.

various mammalian systems as providing both cell-to-cell adhesion and direct intercellular communication of a metabolic nature.

Most important to this discussion is the presence of *junctional complexes* which are located on the surface of the odontoblasts and their processes (Figure 14). Recent studies have characterized these junctional complexes as gap, tight, and intermediate complexes. The most numerous junctional complex is the *gap junction*. These are characterized by the presence of 20- to 30-Å pores located in the center of long pentalaminar 20 Å lamina between cells. These gap junctions are specialized complexes which pass impulses of an electrochemical nature from cell to cell. When teeth are fixed with various metal stains, a small 20 Å gap is seen to separate the cells from each other. It has been speculated that these gap junctions play an important role in the regulation of cell growth and differentiation as well as in the coordination of function between a few or many of the cells. Recent data implicate gap junctions as low-resistance pathways over which nociceptive information passes very rapidly from cell to cell, which may allow the odontoblasts to act as a synctium.[83] The *tight junctions* (zona occludens) provide a physical mechanical attachment plaque between odontoblasts and their processes. Tight junctions have five layers which provide a bonding between cells as well as translating electrical information over their surfaces. *Intermediate junctions* (zona adherens) are 150- to 200-Å thick spaces which contain a glycoprotein-rich material beltway between the cells. These beltways have been postulated to provide for the transport of extracellular materials, e.g., collagen, glycosaminoglycans, and fibronectin. Several researchers have speculated that odontoblasts have desmosome complexes. However, the recent data have not confirmed this as these are seen primarily between epithelial types of cells.

VII. THEORIES OF DENTINAL INNERVATION

There are three basic theories of pain conduction through dentin. The first one is that of *direct neural stimulation*. This theory presumes the presence of nerves and endings in the predentin and dentinal tubules. The nociceptive stimuli are picked up at or below the DEJ and carried to the pulp via nerve ending activation and then directly without synapse to the descending nucleus of the trigeminal system. The second is the fluid or *hydrodynamic theory*. Various stimuli such as heat, cold, air blast, desiccation, mechanical pressure, and other factors affect the fluid movement within the dentinal tubule. It is this fluid flow, inward or outward, which stimulates the nociceptive mechanism within the dentinal tubules, predentin, and/or odontogenic zone, ultimately resulting in a painful response at higher centers. The third *transduction theory* presumes that the odontoblastic process which is located at, or near to the DEJ, is the primary structure excited by a stimulus, causing a mechanoreceptor-like effect at the nerve endings located in the tubules and odontogenic zone. Each of these theories of pain transmission has supportive factors as well as information that is nonsupportive in regard to that mechanism of conduction through dentin (Figure 15).

The *direct neural stimulation theory* implies that nerves and endings are present in the dentinal tubules, at or near the DEJ. Stella and Fuentes[84] claimed to have seen nerves near the DEJ using the optical microscope, however, it has not been confirmed by various ultrastructural studies.[43,85] Nerves are reported to enter the circumpulpal dentin of the crown and penetrate the tubules to a depth of approximately 150 μm from the pulp. It is possible, but not probable, that external nociceptive stimuli could reach these nerves directly when they are located so far from the DEJ without an intermediary system such as the tubule wall. Clinical experience indicates that the DEJ of the crown and cervical region is the most sensitive area of the tooth in regard to pain. The electrophysiologic studies of Ogawa et al.[86] did not indicate nerves in the outer dentinal tubules. Further evidence that nerves penetrate only the inner circumpulpal dentinal tubules is shown by the radiolabeled proline injection studies of Byers and Kish[87] as seen in Figure 16.

The recent findings do not appear to lend support to the direct neural stimulation concept. A strong proponent of this theory in the 1960s was Scott[88] who assumed the electrophysiological responses recorded in dentin were derived from afferent nociceptors in the dentinal tubules. Horiuchi and Matthews[89] failed to obtain the same recording data after removing the pulp and flushing Formalin® through the pulp chamber. Matthews[90] suggested that dentinal recordings represent pulpal neural activity, as neural activity recorded from the pulp has similar characteristics to responses obtained in dentin. Horiuchi and Matthews[91] suggest that some stimuli act on dentinal nerve endings, but the event cannot be recorded. Obviously, further research is necessary. Recent findings by Lilja et al.[92] have demonstrated nerves in the dentinal tubules of human teeth. Lilja completed studies to abolish the nerves and the odontoblasts and yet did not abolish the sensitivity of the dentin.

The *fluid hydrodynamic theory* was first suggested by Gysi[93] who attempted to explain dentinal pain on the basis of fluid movement in the dentinal tubules. More recent work by Brännström[94] carried out studies that clarified and supported the hydrodynamic principle. Further studies by Brännström[95] and Brännström and Åström[96] indicated that the inward and/or outward movement of fluid tubule contents produces a mechanical disturbance in the odontogenic zone affecting the nerves of that region. In essence, these nerves function as mechanoreceptors. Support of this theory is demonstrated when histamine or substance P are placed on cut dentin; no nociception (pain) is recorded. However, when aconitine, a substance that excites cutaneous mechanoreceptors is used, activation of receptors in the dentinal tubules occurs.[97,98]

Brännström et al.[99] pointed out that dentinal fluid movement must occur at a rapid rate to elicit pain. They pointed out that even when the juxta-odontoblastic zone was necrotic,

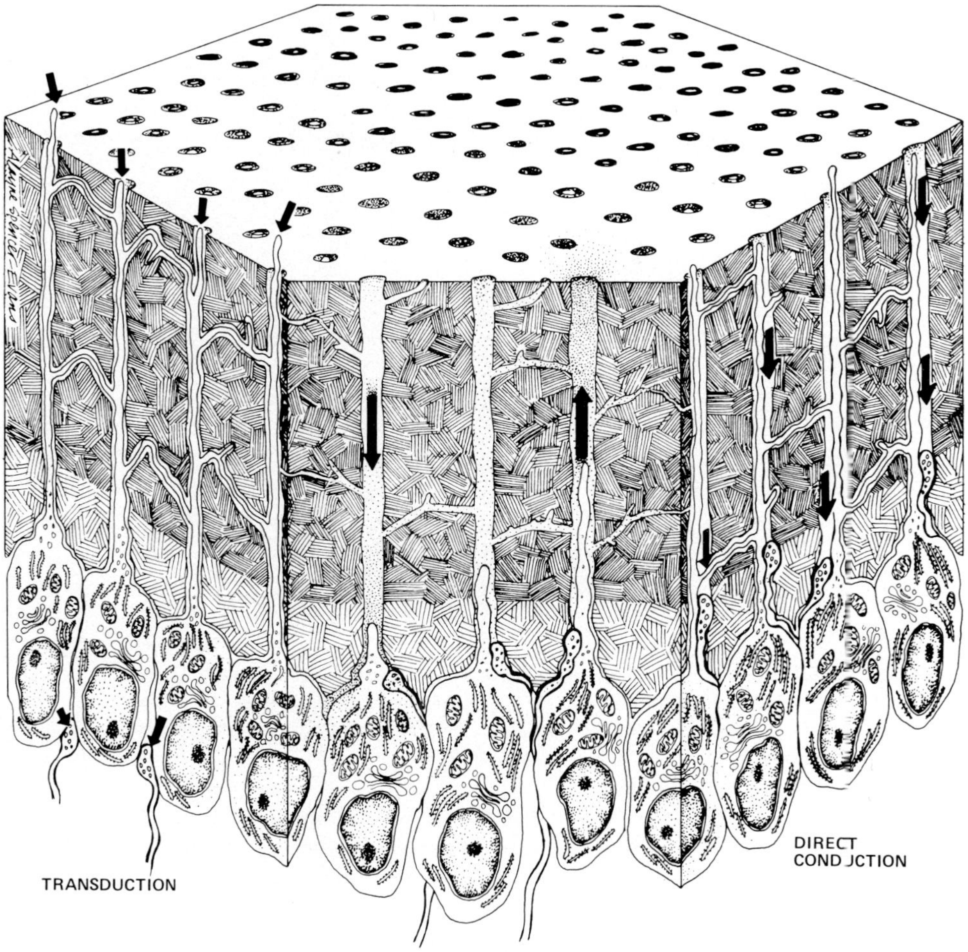

FIGURE 15. A diagram of the three main explanations of pain perception through dentin. On the left is shown the transduction theory in which the membrane of the odontoblast process conducts an impulse to the nerve endings in the predentin, odontoblast zone, and pulp. In the center is the hydrodynamic theory. Stimuli cause an inward or outward movement of fluid in the tubule which in turn produces movement of the odontoblast and its process. This in turn stimulates the nerve endings. On the right is the direct conduction theory in which stimuli directly effect the nerve endings in the tubules.

pain could still be provoked by a dental probe. They theorized that this cell could not function as a primary nociceptor. Drilling, drying with absorbent paper, pressure, or scraping with an explorer, and direct air blasts all produce pain as does inflammation of the subjacent pulp. According to Horiuchi and Matthews[100] calcium chloride and sugar produce an outward flow of tubule fluid resulting in pain. A repeated application of these substances causes a decrease in fluid movement, which in turn results in a decreased dentinal sensitivity. To explain this theory, they suggested that the dentinal tubule changes are a result of a buildup of the solutes that were used in their studies. Anderson and Matthews[101] suggested that a relationship was evident between the osmotic pressure of substances such as sugar, salt, ammonium chloride, and urea and their ability to produce pain when applied to cut dentinal tubules. These phenomena have subsequently not been found to be true for all substances. The general applicability of the hydrodynamic theory is questioned because solutions such as dextrose and ammonium chloride, which both have the same osmotic pressure and produce

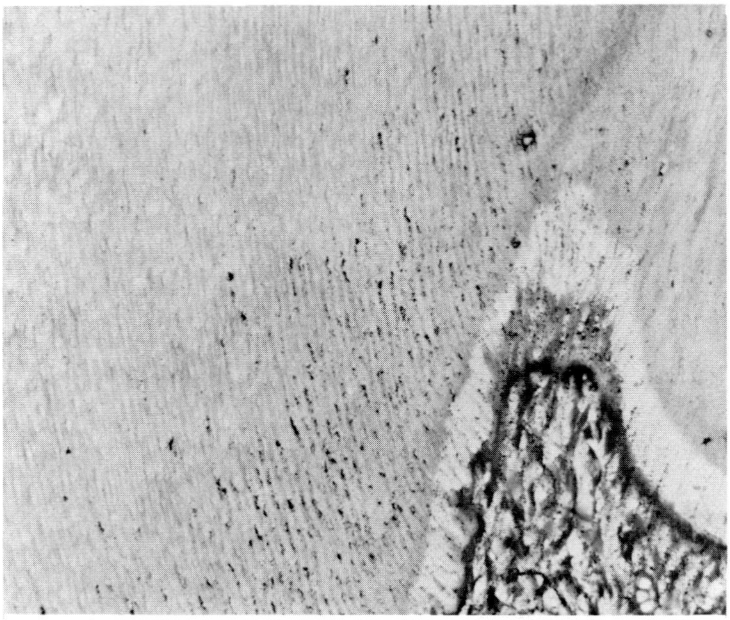

FIGURE 16. Note the linear array of silver grains in the dentinal tubules; [^{3}H]proline had previously been injected into the trigeminal ganglion. Anterograde axoplasmic flow resulted in the migration of the labeled protein within the nerve to its terminals in the dentin.

the same level of pain, cause a vastly different fluid flow movement pattern.[102,103] Since these substances cause excitability when directly applied to nerves, it appears that they are acting directly on the nerves in the dentinal tubules and pulp. Horiuchi and Matthews[104] and Horiuchi[105] have suggested that hot and cold may act directly on pulpal nerves. In addition, Dubner et al.[106] have also suggested the same manner of action by electrical stimuli. Thus peripheral nerve endings may act as mechanoreceptors as they are affected by mechanical displacement of the tubular fluid.

The *transduction theory* is based on the premise that the odontoblast process acts as the primary nociceptor and is further capable of transmitting this impulse to the nerves in the dentinal tubules or odontogenic zone. The evidence that the odontoblast is of neural crest origin[107,108] is supportive of this view. Several studies support the transducer theory by the demonstration of odontoblastic processes in the dentinal tubules of various species.[109-111] Avery[109] demonstrated membrane-bound eosinophilic structures running the length of dentinal tubules in mice and monkey dentin and provided transmission electron microscopy (TEM) data that reconfirmed membrane-bound structures within the tubules as well as some at the DEJ. Kelley[112] presented scanning electron microscopy (SEM) data of odontoblastic processes in the inner and outer third of the dentinal tubules of monkey dentin (Figures 17 and 18) and demonstrated odontoblast processes crossing the DEJ into the enamel as spindles. They theorized that the absence of processes in the middle third was due to the trauma of freeze fracturing resulting in the breaking out of some of the processes along the longitudinal axis of the middle third of dentinal tubules. Gunji et al.[113] demonstrated both nerve fibers and odontoblast processes lying in close contact in the dentinal tubules. The treatment of dentin with a HCl-collagenase method has demonstrated by SEM, that the odontoblast processes extend throughout the whole thickness of inner carious dentin and normal dentin of intact human teeth.[114] Other studies by Brännström and Garberglio,[115] Holland,[116] and

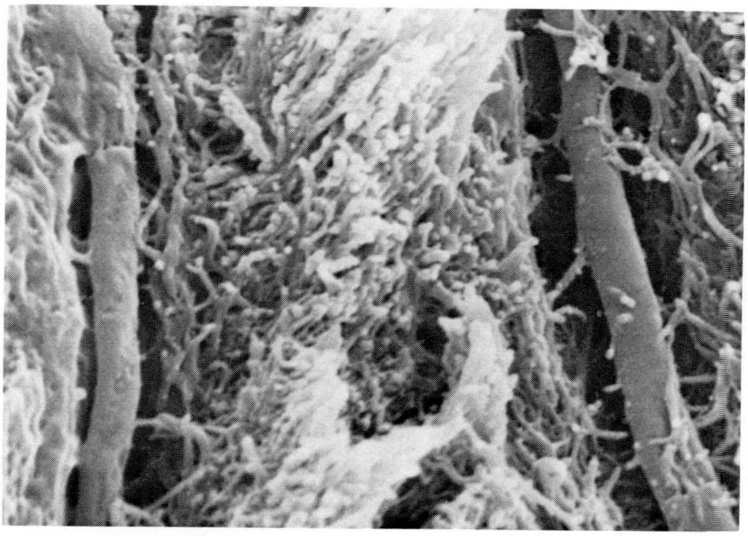

FIGURE 17. A scanning electron micrograph of odontoblast processes lying in dentinal tubules from a primate tooth. Observe the occasional lateral processes. This specimen was acquired after perfusion, demineralization, and freeze-fracturing.

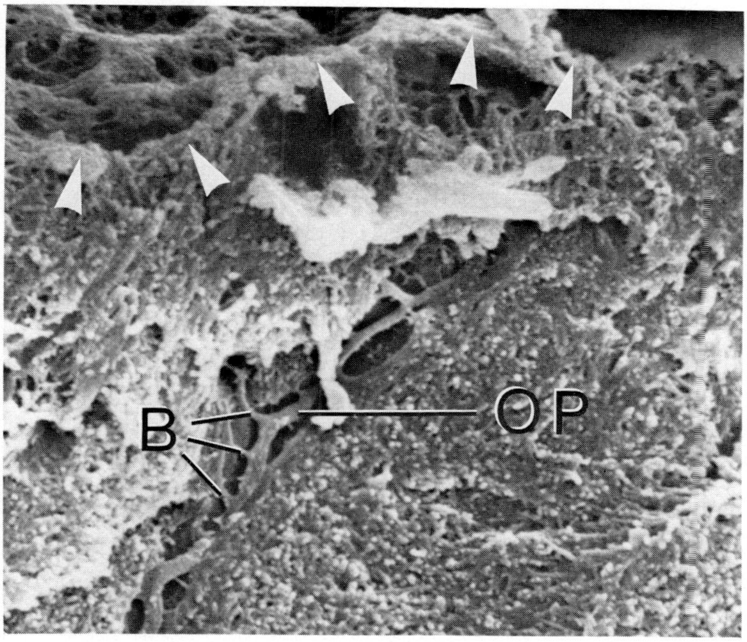

FIGURE 18. This scanning electron micrograph shows an odontoblast process (OP) in a dentinal tubule at the dentinoenamel junction (arrowheads). Note the branching (B) of the process at the terminal portion with small side branches.

Thomas[117] have suggested that the processes do not in fact traverse the length of the dentinal tubule, but are confined to the inner third of the dentinal tubule.

Important to the theory of transduction are the findings of Kroeger et al.[118] who found the intracellular potentials of cells in the odontogenic region of cats and dogs, as well as cultured mouse pulpal cells, to be as high as 45 mV. Winter et al.[119] found similar results as did Yamada et al.[120,121] Although these are low potentials for neural cells, they are similar to other cells which function in transduction.[122] However, there is no certainty they were measuring the odontoblasts and not the adjacent nerves or fibroblast cells. Winter et al.[119] applied a stimulus between the enamel and the DEJ and produced a response in the inferior alveolar nerve, but no change was recorded in the potential of the odontoblasts. Winter felt this confirmed lack of odontoblast involvement in the transduction theory. However, as Dubner et al.[106] stated, the electrical stimulus may have spread to the adjacent periodontal structures, negating the odontogenic response.

The evidence for odontoblastic transduction is therefore inconclusive, although the concept remains quite viable based on recent TEM and SEM data which demonstrate odontoblast processes extending the length of the dentinal tubules as well as extending into enamel.

VIII. NEUROREGULATORY ROLE OF NERVES IN TEETH

A number of investigators have demonstrated the effects of presence or absence of nerves and their effects on growth and regeneration of tissues. Moss[123] has stated that neurotrophism is the main control mechanism which regulates the growth of the oral-facial complex. Bone, cartilage, and dentin can differentiate without nerves, but nerves have been shown to be important in the early inductive mechanism of various organs. An internal axon protein transport occurs at various rates of flow.[124] More specifically, these proteins have been characterized as moving or flowing within the axon from a slow to a fast or rapid rate. Several investigators[125-130] have characterized this fast rapid moving protein as being associated with the smooth surface endoplasmic reticulum. On the other hand, Lasek et al.[131] reported a slow transport occurring at the rate of a few millimeters per day, primarily involving the renewal of axoplasmic microtubules and neurofilaments. It has been reported that rapid transport occurs at a similar rate in peripheral sensory axons.[132,133]

Apart from the conventional neural function of relaying information to and from the central nervous system, the peripheral nerves are also known to aid in the regulation of growth, maintenance, and repair of specific target organs and cells. The exact way this auxiliary function is accomplished is not known at this time, although it is presumed to be mediated by a specific chemical substance, a *neurotrophic factor*. The concept of a trophic function is relatively recent and is derived from evidence involving denervation of muscle,[134,135] taste buds,[136,137] and the amputation and regeneration of amphibian limbs. More recently, investigators have demonstrated autonomic, sympathetic, and sensory neurotrophic activity in alveolar bone.[138-140]

The literature provides some controversy as to the effects of denervation on the development and formation of dental tissues as well as the eruption of teeth. Taylor and Butcher[141] demonstrated that the eruption rate of continuously erupting incisors in rats was increased after resection of the inferior alveolar nerve. This was also demonstrated by Brown et al.[142] and Devoto et al.[143] Resection of the superior cervical ganglion, however, did not seem to have any effect on the eruption rate of incisor teeth.[144] Although the presence of sensory or autonomic nerves does not seem to significantly affect the eruption of the incisor teeth, it does affect the secretion of the dentinal matrix. Weatherred[145] demonstrated irregular calcification patterns, while Rehak[146] reported entrapped odontoblasts in a widened predentin zone after inferior alveolar nerve resection. Avery et al.[147] demonstrated that the rate of reparative dentin was dramatically increased after inferior alveolar nerve and inferior alveolar nerve plus superior cervical ganglion denervation plus cavity preparation. Chiego et al.[148] demonstrated that inferior alveolar nerve denervation produced an altered pattern of cellular proliferation in the progenerative compartment of the mouse incisor, while Klein et al.[149] reported that superior cervical ganglion resection only has a minor effect on cellular proliferation. More recent studies by Chiego et al.[150] have shown that inferior alveolar nerve

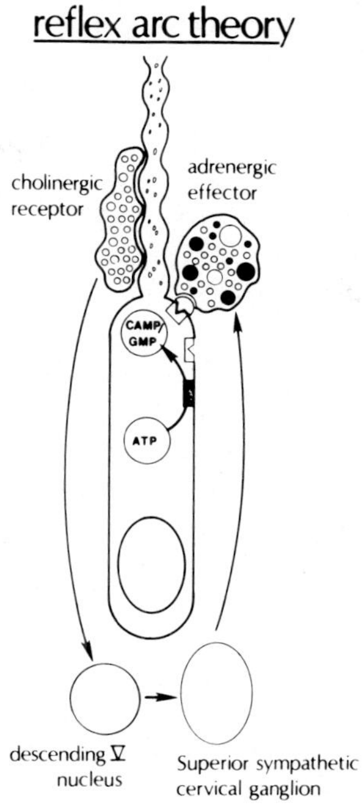

FIGURE 19. A theoretical model suggesting how the sensory nerves may modulate the formation and deposition of dentin through interaction with the sympathetic nerves.

resection produces large fluctuations in the uptake of [^{3}H]proline in the mouse incisor odontoblast. Mouse molar odontoblasts demonstrated large increases of [^{3}H]fucose after inferior alveolar nerve and/or superior cervical ganglion resection.[151]

Several laboratories have reported the labeling of sensory nerve endings in teeth both among the odontoblasts and in the dentinal tubules.[87,128,152] Byers has reported that the biochemistry of proteins in the trigeminal axons are the same as those leading to sensory terminals. The axoplasmic transport of protein is confined to within the axon. In the odontogenic region, the axoplasmic flow is limited to the sensory nerves in the peripheral pulp and in the dentinal tubules. However, the radioautographic techniques are not sensitive enough to detect those small amounts of labeled protein that may have escaped into the adjacent extracellular matrix, becoming incorporated into nonneural tissue A theoretical model is thus presented as a means to express various biochemical changes that may be occurring on the odontoblasts that are underneath a zone of remaining dentin that has been cut and restored by some sort of medicament (Figure 19).

IX. CLINICAL TREATMENT OF DENTINAL PAIN

The control of dentinal pain is a major concern of the clinician as well as the patient. In that we have discussed the several theories of transmission of dental pain it is necessary for us to briefly comment on the various restorative materials and their placement effects upon the sensory elements of the tooth. A number of dental materials have been employed for the treatment and relief of dental pain. However, the most common medicament of clinical choice is a zinc oxide and eugenol (ZOE) compound. Early ZOE formulations reported that an ''obtundant'' effect usually resulted in the remission of the patient's pain. More recent commercially available ZOE medicaments have appeared on the market, each with their claims of success in pain remission. In fact, some of the claims equated remission of pain with an anti-inflammatory effect on the pulpal healing. As a consequence of these various ZOE treatment regimens, it has gained a respectable place in the clinician's armamentarium for treatment of dental pain.

Recent studies by Ozeki[153] have shown that 200 ppm of eugenol will anesthetize a crayfish. He demonstrated that eugenol increased the nerve axons permeability of potassium while depressing the rate of sodium during membrane excitation. A study by Kozam[154] demonstrated that concentrations of eugenol in excess of 100 ppm blocked transmission in the sciatic nerve of the bullfrog. Higher concentrations of eugenol will have a toxic effect upon the neural tissues.

A recent study comparing the effect of ZOE and calcium hydroxide on intradental nerve activity was completed by Trowbridge et al.[155] The placement of a ZOE into a cavity which had been previously irritated with a nerve stimulating compound (48/80) demonstrated that the nerve impulse firing activity was rapidly eliminated. However, a mixture of zinc oxide powder and paraffin oil did not cause a rapid drop in nerve impulse firing. The placement of eugenol on stimulated cavities produced an immediate nerve impulse firing, whereas the application of a calcium hydroxide paste did not effectively decrease impulse firing.

As a consequence of these studies demonstrating the mechanism of ZOEs or more specifically eugenol's effectiveness in relieving dental pain, additional studies should be carried out to identify at what level (ppm) eugenol may be incorporated into the various restorative medicaments without provoking or initiating pulpal inflammation. Perhaps the generation of newer calcium hydroxide materials may provide sedative or obtundant effects as well as benefiting pulpal healing.

X. SUMMARY

The primary afferent somatosensory nerves of the dentin and pulp project to the main sensory nucleus of the midbrain. The greatest representation of pulpal dentinal receptors is in the main sensory, caudalis, and oralis nuclei. The nerve supply to the teeth is carried by the maxillary and mandibular divisions of the fifth nerve. Autonomic efferent innervation to the vascular elements of the pulp is by sympathetic fibers arising from the superior cervical ganglion. As the myelinated and unmyelinated nerves enter the tooth pulps, they course in various sized myelinated and unmyelinated axon bundles, the latter in greater numbers than the former. Nerves arborize throughout the pulp and branch into a parietal plexus of nerves adjacent to the cell-rich zone of the subodontoblastic plexus. Schwann cell-covered axons pass from this plexus and the nerves and endings may terminate either among the odontoblasts, in the predentin, or within the dentinal tubules adjacent to the processes. The greatest number of nerve endings are in the coronal pulp horns.

Odontoblasts have junctional complexes that are seen as gap, tight, and intermediate junctions. Gap junctions demonstrate electrotonic coupling as electrical and/or chemical communication between cells. Vesiculated nerve endings extend into human dentinal tubules no more than 100 to 150 μm and appear between odontoblasts and their processes in the tubules. There is a close association of these terminals with the odontoblast and its intratubular process by means of interdigitating dilatations and constrictions. The highly vesiculated endings appear to be of two types: one group having large electron dense core vesicles, the second group having smaller lucent vesicles. Recent data implicate the small lucent vesiculated endings as afferent sensory endings and the dense core endings as adrenergic.

Three main theories of nociception (pain) conduction through dentin are evident. The most probable one may be a combination of the fluid flow and transducer theories. The close contact of the odontoblast and nerve terminals may be a factor in the movement of the cell with the nerve. The development, maintenance, and renewal of the odontoblasts are interesting to speculate upon. The odontoblasts lay down dentin in a rhythmic fashion and appear to be controlled by their surrounding environment. Neurotrophic factors are present and may act on the odontoblast through the adjacent nerve processes.

ACKNOWLEDGMENTS

The authors wish to thank Drs. Margaret Byers, Keith W. Kelley, and Soo Duk Lee for their contribution of various transmission and scanning electron micrographs; to Ms. Alayne Spencer-Evans for the illustrated diagrams and figures, which are presented within this text; and to Warren Wheeler and John Viery for photographic assistance.

REFERENCES

1. **Iwata, N., Kitai, S. T., and Olson, S.,** Afferent component of the facial nerve: its relation to the spinal trigeminal and facial nucleus, *Brain Res.*, 43, 662, 1972.
2. **Piminidis, M. and Hinds, J.,** An autoradiographic study of the sensory innervation of teeth, *J. Dent. Res.*, 56, 827, 1977.
3. **Gobel, S. and Binck, J. M.,** Degenerative changes in primary trigeminal axons and in neurons in the nucleus caudalis following tooth pulp extirpation in the cat, *Brain Res.*, 132, 347, 1977.
4. **Fukushima, T. and Kerr, F. W. L.,** Organization of the trigeminothalamic tracts and other thalamic afferent systems of the brainstem in the rat: presence of gelatinosa neurons with thalamic connection, *J. Comp. Neurol.*, 183, 169, 1979.
5. **Hu, J. W., Lucier, G. E., and Sessle, B. J.,** Presynaptic modulation of tooth pulp afferents: a compound action potential analysis. Second World Congr. on Pain, *Pain Abstrs.*, 1, 65, 1978.
6. **Price, D. D., Dubner, R., and Hu, J. W.,** Trigeminothalamic neurons in nucleus caudalis responsive to tactile, thermal and nociceptive stimulation of monkeys face, *J. Neurophysiol.*, 39, 936, 1976.
7. **Sessle, B. J.,** Sensory regulation of brain stem motorneurons: physiological and clinical implications, in *Oral Physiology and Occlusion*, Perryman, J. H., Ed., Pergamon Press, New York, 1977, 91.
8. **Young, R. F. and King, R. B.,** Excitability changes in trigeminal primary afferent fibers in response to noxious and non-noxious stimuli, *J. Neurophysiol.*, 35, 87, 1972.
9. **Sessle, B. J. and Greenwood, L. F.,** Inputs to trigeminal brain stem neurons from facial, oral, tooth pulp and pharyngeal tissues. I. Responses to innocuous and noxious stimuli, *Brain Res.*, 117, 211, 1976.
10. **Sessle, B. J. and Greenwood, L. F.,** Role of trigeminal nucleus caudalis in the modulation of trigeminal sensory and motor neuronal activities, in *Advances in Pain Research and Therapy,* Bonica, J. J. and Albe-Fessard, D., Eds., Raven Press, New York, 1976.
11. **Anderson, K. V., Rosling, H. S., and Pearl, G. S.,** Physiological and anatomical studies revealing an extensive transmedian innervation of the feline canine teeth, in *Pain in the Trigeminal Region,* Anderson, D. J. and Matthews, B., Eds., Elsevier, Amsterdam, 1977.
12. **Byers, M. R. and Holland, G. R.,** Trigeminal nerve endings in the gingiva, junctional epithelium and periodontal ligament of rat molars as demonstrated by autoradiography, *Anat. Rec.*, 188, 509, 1977.
13. **Piminidis, M. Z. and Gianelly, A. A.,** Class II malocclusion produced by oral facial sensory deprivation in the rat, *Am. J. Orthod.*, 71, 94, 1977.
14. **Mumford, J. and Bowsher, D.,** Pain and protopathic sensibility. A review with particular reference to the teeth, *Pain,* 2, 223, 1976.
15. **Pohto, P.,** Sympathetic adrenergic innervation of permanent teeth in the monkey (Macaca irus), *Acta Odontol. Scand.*, 30, 117, 1972.
16. **Edwall, L. and Scott, D.,** Influence of changes in microcirculation on the excitability of the sensory unit in the tooth of the cat, *Acta Physiol. Scand.*, 82, 555, 1971.
17. **Matthews, B.,** Effects of sympathetic stimulation on the response of intradental nerves to chemical stimulation of dentin, in *Advances in Pain Research and Therapy,* Vol. 1, Bonica, J. J. and Albe-Fessard, D., Eds., Raven Press, New York, 1976.
18. **Avery, J. K., Cox, C. F., and Chiego, D. J., Jr.,** Presence and location of adrenergic nerve endings in the dental pulps of mouse molars, *Anat. Rec.*, 198, 59, 1980.

19. **Dellows, P. G. and Morgan, M. J.,** Trigeminal nerve inputs and central blood pressure change in the cat, *Arch. Oral Biol.,* 14, 295, 1969.
20. **Kamuda, M., Dampney, R. A. L., and Reis, D. J.,** The trigeminal depressor response: a cardiovascular reflex originating from the trigeminal system, *Brain Res.,* 92, 485, 1975.
21. **Madeira, M., Percinoto, C., and Silva, M.,** Clinical significance of supplemental innervation of the lower incisor teeth: a dissection study of the mylohyoid nerve, *Oral Surg.,* 46, 608, 1978.
22. **Rood, J. P.,** The analgesia and innervation of mandibular teeth, *Br. Dent. J.,* 140, 237, 1976.
23. **Carter, R. B. and Keen, E. N.,** The intramandibular course of the inferior alveolar nerve, *J. Anat.,* 108, 433, 1971.
24. **Sutton, R. N.,** The practical significance of mandibular accessory foramina, *Austr. Dent. J.,* 86, 167, 1974.
25. **Frommer, J., Mele, F. A., and Monroe, C. W.,** The possible role of the mylohyoid nerve in mandibular posterior tooth sensation, *J. Am. Dent. Assoc.,* 85, 113, 1972.
26. **Cook, W. A.,** The cervical plexus and its probable role in the oral operator's field, *Modern Dent.,* 18, 7, 1951.
27. **Yax, G. L., Cox, C. F., and Avery, J. K.,** Supplemental innervation of the mandibular mouse molar teeth, *J. Dent. Res.,* Abstr., 446, 1977.
28. **Chiego, D. J., Jr., Cox, C. F., and Avery, J. K.,** H3-HRP analysis of the nerve supply to primate teeth, *J. Dent. Res.,* 59, 736, 1980.
29. **Howe, G. L. and Whitehead, F. I. H.,** *Local Anesthesia in Dentistry,* J. Wright, Bristol, 1972.
30. **Anderson, K. V. and Pearl, G. S.,** Transmedian innervation of canine tooth pulp in cat, *Exp. Neurol.,* 44, 281, 1974.
31. **Johnsen, D. C. and Johns, S.,** Quantification of nerve fibers in the primary and permanent canine and incisor teeth in man, *Arch. Oral Biol.,* 23, 825, 1978.
32. **Johnsen, D. C. and Harschbarger, J.,** Unmyelinated axon networks in root portions of human primary canines, *Neurosci. Lett.,* 6, 311, 1977.
33. **Lilja, J.,** Innervation of different parts of the predentin and dentin in young human premolars, *Acta Odontol. Scand.,* 37, 339, 1974.
34. **Fearnhead, R. W.,** The neurohistology of human dentine, *Proc. R. Soc. Med. (London),* 54, 877, 1961.
35. **Pohto, P.,** Sympathetic adrenergic innervation of permanent teeth in the monkey (Macaca irus), *Acta Odontol. Scand.,* 30, 117, 1972.
36. **Larsson, P. A. and Linde, A.,** Adrenergic vessel innervation in the rat incisor pulp, *Scand. J. Dent. Res.,* 79, 7, 1971.
37. **Falk, B., Hillarp, N. A., Thieme, G., and Torp, A.,** Fluorescence of catecholamines and related compounds condensed with formaldehyde, *J. Histochem. Cytochem.,* 10, 348, 1962.
38. **Avery, J. K., Strachan, D. S., Corpron, R. E., and Cox, C. F.,** Morphological studies of the altered pulps of the New Zealand white rabbit after resection of the inferior alveolar nerve and/or the superior cervical ganglion, *Anat. Rec.,* 171(4), 495, 1971.
39. **Nakano, G. H., Kuzuya, and Nagatsu, T.,** Catecholamines in the dental pulp, *J. Dent. Res.,* 49(16), 1549, 1970.
40. **Pohto, P. R., Antila, R., and Klinge, E.,** Quantitation of transmitter noradrenalin in the pulps of cat canine teeth, *Proc. Finn. Dent. Soc.,* 68, 20, 1972.
41. **Frank, R. M.,** Attachment sites between the odontoblast process and the intradental nerve fiber, *Arch. Oral Biol.,* 13, 833, 1968.
42. **Arwill, T.,** Studies on the ultrastructure of dental tissue. II. The predentine-pulpal border zone, *Odontol. Rev.,* 18, 191, 1967.
43. **Corpron, R. E., Avery, J. K. and Cox, C. F.,** Ultrastructure of intradentinal nerves after resection of the inferior alveolar nerve in mice, *J. Dent. Res.,* 51(2), 673, 1972.
44. **Corpron, R. E. and Avery, J. K.,** The ultrastructure of intradentinal nerves in developing mouse molars, *Anat. Rec.,* 173(3), 585, 1973.
45. **Richardson, K. C.,** Electron microscopic identification of autonomic nerve endings, *Nature (London),* 210, 756, 1966.
46. **Hökfelt, T. and Johnsson, G.,** Studies on reaction and binding of monoamines after fixation and processing for electron microscopy with special reference to fixation with potassium permanganate, *Histochemie,* 16, 45, 1968.
47. **Hand, A. R.,** Adrenergic and cholinergic neural terminals in the rat parotid gland, *Anat. Rec.,* 173, 131, 1973.
48. **Avery, J. K. and Cox, C. F.,** Role of nerves in teeth relative to pain and dentinogenesis, in *Pain in the Trigeminal Region,* Anderson, D. J. and Matthews, B., Eds., Elsevier, Amsterdam, 1977.
49. **Bernick, S.,** Innervation of the human tooth, *Anat. Rec.,* 101, 81, 1948.
50. **Tiegs, O. W.,** Further remarks on the termination of the fibers in human teeth, *J. Anat.,* 84, 104, 1950.

51. **Brashear, A. D.,** Innervation of the teeth, *J. Am. Dent. Assoc.,* 23, 662, 1936.
52. **Narhi, M. V. O.,** Activation of Dental Pulp Nerves of the Cat and the Dog with Hydrostatic Pressure, Thesis, University of Kuopio, Finland, 1978.
53. **Frank, R. M.,** Etude autoradiographique de la dentinogenese en microscopie electronique al'aide de la proline tritiee chez le chat, *Arch. Oral Biol.,* 15, 583, 1970.
54. **Frank, R. M.,** Etude au microscope electronique de l'odontoblaste et du cannicule dentinaire human, *Arch. Oral Biol.,* 1, 179, 1966.
55. **Arwill, T.,** Studies on the ultrastructure of dentinal tissues. II. The predentine-pulpal border, *Odontol. Rev.,* 18(2), 192, 1967.
56. **Lilja, J.,** Innervation of different parts of the predentin and dentin in young human premolars, *Acta Odontol. Scand.,* 37, 339, 1979.
57. **Frank, R. M.,** Ultrastructural relationship between the odontoblasts, its process and the nerve fibre, in *Dentin and Pulp: Their Structure and Reactions,* Symons, N. B. D., Ed., Thomson, Dundee, Scotland, 1968, 115.
58. **Holland, G. R.,** Membrane junctions on cat odontoblasts, *Arch. Oral Biol.,* 20, 551, 1975.
59. **Cox, C. F., Avery, J. K., Lee, S. D., Tomaro, A. A., and Simmons, T. A.,** Ultrastructural characterization of junctional complexes between odontoblasts, *J. Dent. Res.,* 55 (Spec. Issue B), 86, Abstr. 102, February 1976.
60. **Byers, M. R.,** Large and small trigeminal nerve endings and their associations with odontoblasts in rat molar dentin and pulp, *Adv. Pain Res. Ther.,* 3, 265, 1979.
61. **Gunji, T.,** Morphological research on the sensitivity of dentin, *Arch. Histol. Jpn.,* 45(1), 45, 1982.
62. **Kolliker, A.,** *Handbuch der Gewelbelehre des Menschen,* Engelmann, Leipzig, 1852.
63. **Paul, F. T.,** *Trans. Odontol. Soc. G. B.,* 31, 121, 1898.
64. **Mummery, J. H.,** The nerve supply of the dentine, *Proc. R. Soc. Med. Odontol.,* 17, 35, 1924.
65. **Bernard, P. D.,** la cicatrisation neo-dentinaire des plaies pulpaires, *L'Odontologie,* 1, 1, 1949.
66. **Orban, B.,** *Oral Histology and Embryology,* C. V. Mosby, St. Louis, 1957, 97.
67. **Bradford, E. W.,** An investigation into the structure of the pulpo-dentinal junction, *Br. Dent. J.,* 3, 55, 1950.
68. **Watson, M. L. and Avery, J. K.,** The development of the hamster lower incisor as observed by electron microscopy, *Am. J. Anat.,* 95, 109, 1954.
69. **Quigley, M. B.,** Electron microscopy of the amelodentinal junction during early development of the molars of hamsters, *J. Dent. Res.,* 38(3), 558, 1959.
70. **Frank, R. M.,** Etude au microscope electronique de l'odontoblaste et du canalicule dentaire humain, *Arch. Oral Biol.,* 11, 179, 1966.
71. **Arwill, T.,** Studies on the ultrastructure of the pulpo-dentinal border zone, in *Dentine and Pulp: Their Structure and Reactions,* Symons, N. B. D., Ed., Thomson, Dundee, Scotland, 1968, 147.
72. **Garant, P., Szabo, G., and Nalbandian, J.,** The fine structure of the mouse odontoblasts, *Arch. Oral Biol.,* 13, 857, 1968.
73. **Jessen, H.,** The ultrastructure of odontoblasts in perfusion fixed, demineralized incisors of adult rats, *Acta Odontol. Scand.,* 25, 491, 1967.
74. **Reith, E. J.,** Ultrastructural aspects of dentinogenesis, in *Dentine and Pulp: Their Structure and Reactions,* Symons, N. B. D., Ed., Thomson, Dundee, Scotland, 1968, 19.
75. **Tsubo, Y.,** Electron microscopy of the fine structure and life cycle of the dentinogenic cells of the rat incisors, *Shika Gakuho.,* 68, 416, 1968.
76. **Takuma, S. and Nagai, N.,** Ultrastructure of rat odontoblasts in various stages of their development and maturation, *Arch. Oral Biol.,* 16, 993, 1971.
77. **Stockinger, V. L. and Pritz, W.,** Morphologische Aspekte der Schmerzempfindung im Zahn, *Dtsch. Zahnärztl. Z.,* 25, 557, 1970.
78. **Dahl, E. and Mjör, I. A.,** The structure and distribution of nerves in the pulp-dentin organ, *Acta Odontol. Scand.,* 31, 349, 1972.
79. **Holland, G. R.,** Membrane junctions on cat odontoblasts, *Arch. Oral Biol.,* 20, 551, 1975.
80. **Cox, C. F., Avery, J. K., Lee, S. D., Tomaro, A. A., and Simmons, T. A.,** Ultrastructural characterization of junctional complexes between odontoblasts, *J. Dent. Res.,* 55 (Spec. Issue B), 86, Abstr., 102, February 1976.
81. **Cohen, B. and Kramer, I. R. H.,** Contact specializations, in *Scientific Foundations in Dentistry,* William Heinemann Ltd., London, 1976, 70.
82. **McNutt, M. S. and Weinstein, R. S.,** Membrane ultrastructure of mammalian intercellular junctions, *Prog. Biophys. Mol. Biol.,* 26, 45, 1973.
83. **Larsen, W. J.,** Opaque deposits on gap junction membranes after glutaraldehyde-calcium fixation, *J. Cell Biol.,* 67, 801, 1975.

84. **Stella, A. and Fuentes, A.,** Inervacion dentindria intercanalicular su demonstracion por el metodo de la hematoxlina-ferrice de heidenhain, *Acta Fac. Odontol. (Montevideo),* 9, 157, 1963.
85. **Tsatsas, B. G. and Frank, R. M.,** Ultrastructure of the dentinal tubular substances near the dentino enamel junction, *Calcif. Tissue Res.,* 9, 238, 1972.
86. **Ogawa, K., Yamashita, Y., Ichijo, T., and Fusayama, T.,** The ultrastructure and hardness of the transparent layer of human carious dentin, *J. Dent. Res.,* in press.
87. **Byers, M. R. and Kish, S. J.,** Dilenination of somatic nerve endings in rat teeth by radioautography of axon-transported protein, *J. Dent. Res.,* 55, 419, 1976.
88. **Scott, D., Jr.,** Excitation of the dentinal-receptors in the tooth of the cat, in *Ciba Found. Symp. Touch, Heat, and Pain,* de Reuck, A. U. S. and Knight, J., Eds., Churchill, London, 1966, 261.
89. **Horiuchi, H. and Matthews, B.,** Evidence on the origin of impulses recorded from dentine in the cat, *J. Physiol.,* 243, 797, 1974.
90. **Matthews, B.,** Nerve impulses recorded from dentine in the cat, *Arch. Oral Biol.,* 15, 523, 1970.
91. **Horuchi, H. and Matthews, B.,** Neural responses evoked by stimulation of dentine, in *Oral Physiology,* Emmelin, N. and Zotterman, Y., Eds., Pergamon Press, Oxford, 1972, 291.
92. **Lilja, J., Nordenvall, K. J., and Brännström, M.,** Dentine sensitivity, odontoblasts and nerves under desiccated or infected experimental cavities, *J. Dent. Res.,* in press.
93. **Gysi, A.,** An attempt to explain the sensitiveness of dentin, *Br. J. Dent. Sci.,* 43, 865, 1900.
94. **Brännström, M.,** Observations on the exposed dentine and the corresponding pulp tissue, *Odontol. Rev.,* 13, 235, 1962.
95. **Brännström, M.,** Physiopathological aspects of dentinal and pulp responses to irritants, in *Dentine and Pulp: Their Structure and Function,* Symons, N. B. D., Ed., Thomson, Dundee, 1968, 231.
96. **Brännström, M. and Åström, A.,** The hydrodynamics of the dentine: its possible relationship to dentinal pain, *Int. Dent. J.,* 22, 219, 1972.
97. **Olgart, L.,** Excitation of intradental sensory units by pharmacological agents, *Acta Physiol. Scand.,* 92, 1, 1974.
98. **Hegerström, G.,** A Pharmacological Study on Intradentinal Sensory Endings in the Cat, Thesis, Karolinska Institute, Stockholm, 1976.
99. **Brännström, M., Johnson, G., and Nordenvall, K. V.,** Transmission and control of dentinal pain. Resin impregnation for the desensitization of dentin, *J. Am. Dent. Assoc.,* 99, 612, 1979.
100. **Horiuchi, H. and Matthews, B.,** In-vitro observations on fluid flow through human dentine caused by pain producing stimuli, *Arch. Oral Biol.,* 12, 275, 1973.
101. **Anderson, D. J. and Matthews, B.,** Osmotic stimulation of human dentine and the distribution of dental pain thresholds, *Arch. Oral Biol.,* 12, 417, 1967.
102. **Anderson, D. J. and Linden, R. W. A.,** Test of the hydrodynamic hypothesis for dentin sensitivity in man, *J. Dent. Res.,* 52, 963, 1973.
103. **Anderson, D. J. and Linden, R. W. A.,** Osmotic excitants of pain from human dentine, *J. Dent. Res.,* Abstr. 54 L141, 566, 1975.
104. **Horiuchi, H. and Matthews, B.,** Response of intradental nerves to chemical and osmotic stimulation of dentine in the cat, *Pain,* 2, 49, 1976.
105. **Horiuchi, H.,** A study of pulp-nerve excitation through a silver-wire electrode, *J. Dent. Res.,* 44, 1257, 1965.
106. **Dubner, R., Sessle, B., and Storey, A.,** Tooth pulp and dentine, in *The Neural Basis of Oral and Facial Function,* Plenum Press, New York, 1978, chap. 5.
107. **Avery, J. K.,** Possible ectodermal origin of the odontoblasts, *J. Dent. Res.,* 29(5), 663, 1950.
108. **Ross, R. B. and Johnson, M. C.,** *Cleft Lip and Palate,* Robert E. Krieger, Huntington, New York, 1978.
109. **Avery, J. K., Cox, C. F., Chiego, D. J., Jr., and Lee, S. D.,** The extent of the odontoblast process: an LM and Em survey, *J. Dent. Res.,* Abstr. 542, 403, 1980.
110. **Kelley, K. W., Bergenholtz, G., and Cox, C. F.,** The extent of the odontoblast process in rhesus monkeys (*Macaca mulatta*) as observed by scanning electron microscopy, *Arch. Oral Biol.,* 26, 893, 1981.
111. **Yamada, T., Nakamura, K., Iwaku, M., and Fusayams, T.,** The extent of the odontoblast process in normal and carious human dentin, *J. Dent. Res.,* in press.
112. **Kelley, K. W.,** The extent of the odontoblast process in human and rhesus monkey teeth: a light and scanning electron microscope analysis, *J. Dent. Res.,* submitted.
113. **Gunji, T., Wakita, M., and Kobayashi, S.,** SEM on nerve fibers of pulpo-dentinal region in human teeth, *J. Dent. Res.,* I.A.D.R. Abstr. 29, 1979.
114. **Yamada, M., Suzuta, K., and Teruki, K.,** A consideration on the excitation mechanisms of toothache caused by thermal stimulation, *Jpn. J. Physiol.,* 21, 133, 1971.
115. **Brännström, M. and Garberglio, A.,** The dentinal tubules and odontoblast processes. A scanning electron microscopic study, *Acta Odontol. Scand.,* 30, 291, 1972.
116. **Holland, G. R.,** An ultrastructural survey of cat dentinal tubules, *J. Anat. Br.,* 122, 1, 1976.

117. **Thomas, H.,** The effect of various fixatives of the odontoblast process, *J. Dent. Res.,* Abstr. 541, 403, 1980.
118. **Kroeger, D. C., Gonzales, F., and Krivoy, W.,** Transmembrane potentials of cultured mouse dentinal pulp cells, *Proc. Soc. Exp. Biol. Med.,* 108, 134, 1961.
119. **Winter, H. F., Bishop, J. G., and Dorman, H. L.,** Transmembrane potentials of odontoblasts, *J. Dent. Res.,* 42, 594, 1962.
120. **Yamada, M. K., Sagi, T., and Sheda, R.,** Mechanisms of excitation of nerve and tooth by thermal stimulation, in *Oral Facial Sensory and Motor Mechanisms,* Dubner, R. and Kawamura, Y., Eds., Appleton-Century-Crofts, New York, 1971, 73.
121. **Yamada, M., Kumano, T., and Suzuter, K.,** Neural response of oral tissues to mechanical and chemical stimuli, in *Oral Facial Sensory and Motor Mechanisms,* Dubner, R. and Kawamura, Y., Eds., Appleton-Century-Crofts, New York, 1971, 123.
122. **Dubner, R., Sessle, B. J., and Storey, A. T.,** *The Neural Basis of Oral Facial Function,* Plenum Press, New York, 1970, 118.
123. **Moss, M. L.,** An introduction to the neurobiology of oro-facial growth, *Acta Biotheor.,* 21(Abstr.), 236, 1972.
124. **Schwartz, J. H.,** Axonal transport: components, mechanisms and specificity, *Annu. Rev. Neurosci.,* 2, 467, 1979.
125. **Hendrickson, A. E.,** Electron microscopic radioautography: identification of origin of synaptic terminals in normal nervous tissue, *Science,* 165, 194, 1969.
126. **Hendrickson, A. E. and Cowan, W. M.,** Changes in the rate of axoplasmic transport during postnatal development of the rabbit's optic nerve and tract, *Exp. Neurol.,* 31, 403, 1971.
127. **Droz, B., Koenig, H. L., Biamberdino, L. et al.,** Axonal migration of protein and glycoprotein to nerve endings. I. Radioautographic analysis of the renewal of protein in nerve endings of chicken ciliary ganglion after intercerebral injection of ^{3}H lysine, *Brain Res.,* 60, 93, 1973.
128. **Byers, M.,** Structural correlates of rapid axonal transport: evidence that microtubules may not be directly involved, *Brain Res.,* 75, 97, 1974.
129. **Grafstein, B.,** Principles of anterograde, in *The Use of Axonal Transport for Studies of Neuronal Connectivity,* Cowan, W. and Cuenod, M., Eds., Elsevier, New York, 1975, 49.
130. **Graybel, A.,** Wallerian degeneration and anterograde tracing methods, in *The Use of Axonal Transport for Studies of Neuronal Connectivity,* Cowan, W. M. and Cuenod, M., Eds., Elsevier, New York, 1975, 173.
131. **Lasek, R., Joseph, B. S., and Whitlock, D. G.,** Evaluation of a radioautographic neuroanatomical tracing method, *Brain Res.,* 8, 319, 1968.
132. **Lasek, R. J.,** Protein transport in neurons, *Int. Rev. Neurobiol.,* 13, 89, 1970.
133. **Fink, R., Kish, S. J., and Byers, M. R.,** Rapid axonal transport in trigeminal nerve of rat, *Brain Res.,* 90, 85, 1975.
134. **Gutmann, E. and Zak, R.,** Nervous regulation of nucleic acid levels in cross-striated muscle. Changes in denervated muscle, *Physiol. Bohemoslov.,* 10, 493, 1961.
135. **Carlson, B. M.,** Studies on the mechanism of implant induced supernumerary limb formation in urodeles. I. The histology of supernumerary limb formation in the adult newt, *J. Exp. Zool.,* 164, 227, 1967.
136. **Guth, L.,** "Trophic" effects of vertebrate neurons, *Neurosci. Res. Prog. Bull.,* 7, 1, 1969.
137. **Oakley, B. and Benjamin, R. M.,** Neural mechanisms of taste, *Physiol. Rev.,* 46, 173, 1966.
138. **Chiego, D. J., Jr. and Singh, I. J.,** Evaluation of the effects of sensory denervation on osteoblasts by 3H-proline autoradiography, *Cell Tissue Res.,* 217, 569, 1981.
139. **Singh, I. J., Herskovits, M. S., Chiego, D. J., Jr., and Klein, R. M.,** Modulation of osteoblastic activity by sensory and autonomic innervation of bone, *Proc. Int. Conf. Factors and Mechanisms Influencing Bone Growth,* Dixon, A. D. and Sarnat, B. G., Eds., Alan R. Liss, New York, in press.
140. **Herskovits, M. S.,** The Effects of Sympathetic Denervation on Osteoblastic Activity in the White Rat, Ph.D., thesis, New York University, 1982.
141. **Taylor, A. C. and Butcher, E. D.,** The regulation of eruption rate in the incisor teeth of the white rat, *J. Exp. Zool.,* 17, 165, 1962.
142. **Brown, G. N., Kupfer, S. R., and Darlington, C. G.,** Effects of inferior alveolar nerve severance on the eruption rate of the mandibular incisor in the ten day old Wistar albino rat, *Oral Surg.,* 14, 1227, 1961.
143. **Devoto, R. H., Aries, N. H., and Perrotto, B. M.,** Growth of rats lower incisor teeth after unilateral section of alveolar nerve, *J. Dent. Res.,* 45, 1078, 1966.
144. **Butcher, E. D. and Taylor, A. C.,** The effects of denervation and ischemia upon the teeth of the monkey, *J. Dent. Res.,* 30, 265, 1951.
145. **Weatherred, J. G.,** Peripheral Nervous System Effects in the Dental Pulp of the Rat and Dog, Ph.D. thesis, The University of Texas, Austin, 1965.
146. **Rehak, J. R.,** Course and resection of the inferior alveolar nerve in the albino rat, *J. Dent. Res.,* 42, 1159, 1963.

147. **Avery, J. K., Cox, C. F., and Corpron, R. E.,** The effects of combined nerve resection and cavity preparation and restoration on response dentine formation in rabbit incisors, *Arch. Oral Biol.*, 19, 539, 1974.
148. **Chiego, D. J., Jr. and Singh, I. J.,** Effects of denervation on the growth and eruption of a continually growing incisor, *J. Dent. Res.*, 53, 74, 1974.
149. **Klein, R. M., Chiego, D. J. Jr., and Avery, J. K.,** Effects of chemical sympathectomy on cell proliferation in the progenerative compartment of the neonatal mouse incisor, *Arch. Oral Biol.*, 26, 319, 1981.
150. **Chiego, D. J., Jr., Klein, R. M., and Avery, J. K.,** Tritiated thymidine autoradiographic study of the effects of inferior alveolar nerve resection on the proliferative compartments of the mouse incisor formative tissues, *Arch Oral Biol.*, 26, 83, 1980.
151. **Chiego, D. J., Jr., Fisher, M. A., Avery, J. K., and Klein, R. M.,** Effects of denervation of 3H-fucose incorporation by odontoblasts on the mouse incisor, *Cell and Tissue Res.*, in press.
152. **Piminidis, M. Z. and Gianelly, A. A.,** Class III malocclusion produced by oral facial sensory deprivation in the rat, *Am. J. Orthodont.*, 71, 94, 1977.
153. **Ozeki, M.,** The effects of eugenol on the nerve and muscle in crayfish, *Comp. Biochem. Physiol.*, 50C, 183, 1975.
154. **Kozam, G.,** The effect of eugenol on nerve transmission, *Oral Surg.*, 44, 799, 1977.
155. **Trowbridge, H., Edwall, L., and Panopoulos, P.,** Effect of zinc oxide-eugenol and calcium hydroxide on intradental nerve activity, *J. Endodont.*, 8(9), 403, 1982.

Chapter 3

TOOTH MORPHOGENESIS AND DIFFERENTIATION

Jean-Victor Ruch

TABLE OF CONTENTS

I. INTRODUCTION

Teeth have been studied intensively for a long time by morphologists, comparative anatomists, and paleontologists[1-6] as well as biologists interested in mineralization.[7-10] Furthermore, the developing dentition offers a suitable model system for the study of developmental biology.[11] The crucial problem in this field is to determine the nature of controlling mechanisms which coordinate the expression of structural and regulatory genes. The molecular mechanisms involved have not yet been elucidated. However, for most organs, it is known that epigenetic (cell interaction-dependent) control mechanisms exist. Such a phenomenon exists according to Grobstein[12] when "two or more tissues of different history and properties become intimately associated and alteration of the developmental course of the interactants results."

Concerning teeth, as early as 1887, von Brunn[13] thought that the presence of the inner dental epithelium was essential to the differentiation of odontoblasts. Huggins et al.[14] demonstrated the fact that enamel will not form in the absence of dentin. In 1967, Kock,[15] analyzing transfilter associations between enamel organs and dental papillae, demonstrated that heterotypic cell interactions were necessary for morphological and functional differentiation.

The initial phases of tooth development are comparable in vertebrate embryos, but at later stages teeth display a great variety of forms, especially among the mammals, giving rise to specific dentitions.

At the histological level, *odontogenesis* begins during the early stages of craniofacial development. Dental primordial cells are provided by the epithelium and mesenchyme of the maxillary and mandibular processes. The developmental sequence integrates cell segregation, differential cell division, cell migration, and specific spatial distribution of overtly differentiated odontoblasts, thus secreting predentin and the overtly differentiated ameloblasts secreting enamel. All these developmental processes appear to be coordinated by continuous reciprocal heterotypic and homotypic cell interactions. According to Slavkin et al.,[16] "the morphogenetic phase of tooth development is precisely known, growth and differentiation occur at relatively different times in the cycle of odontogenesis." Morphologically, several stages may be distinguished: initiation, bud, and bell stages combining histogenetic and morphogenetic events, and terminal cytodifferentiations. It is apparently also justified to search independently for mechanisms controlling histogenesis, morphogenesis, cytodifferentiation, or cell kinetics. Nevertheless, odontogenesis is a continuous sequence of interdependent developmental phenomena. Terminal differentiation of odontoblasts (and ameloblasts) without morphogenesis is meaningless as far as tooth function is concerned. Physiological terminal differentiation appears to be the happy ending of a many generations old cell saga.

II. MORPHOLOGICAL ASPECTS OF DEVELOPING DENTITION

The progressive development of teeth involving oral epithelium and mesenchyme has been subdivided into several successive stages: dental lamina, bud, cap, and bell stages. Figures 1 and 2 summarize some of the morphological aspects. The embryological origin of most dental cells has been established precisely in amphibia;[17-20] tooth formation requires the neural crest, the presumptive mouth ectoderm, and entoderm. In mammals, the participation of the neural crest with the dental papilla is generally admitted. Milaire[21] and Pourtois[22] presented histochemical data supporting this very strong probability. In a more dynamic approach, odontogenesis includes initiating events, cell proliferation and growth, histo- and morphodifferentiation, as well as specific functional differentiation mainly of odontoblasts and ameloblasts. These cells secrete dentin and enamel, respectively. These extracellular matrices mineralize. Later the teeth erupt and present the phenomenon of functional attrition.

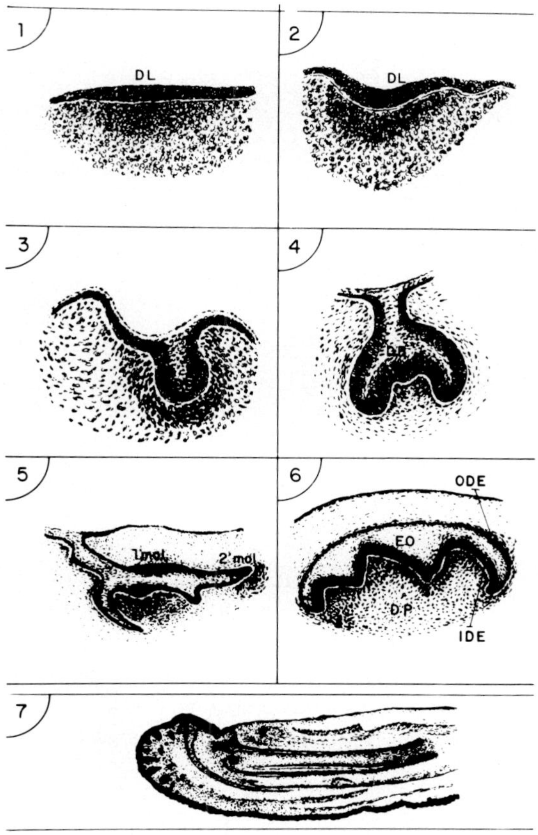

FIGURE 1. Diagrams depicting successive stages of mouse odontogenesis: 1, 2: dental lamina (DL); 3: dental bud; 4, 5, 6: bell stages; ODE: outer dental epithelium; IDE: inner dental epithelium; EO: enamel organ; DP: dental papilla. Drawings of sagittal sections (5, 6) illustrate the appearing of the second molar (5) and the typical cusp pattern of the first lower molar (6). Drawing 7 illustrates a sagittal section of an incisor (compare with Figure 2B).

During the early cap stage, histogenesis is initiated. The epithelial *enamel organ* differentiates progressively into four compartments: the *inner dental epithelium* formed by tall columnar cells giving rise to the *ameloblasts,* the *outer dental epithelium* formed by cuboidal cells, the *stratum intermedium,* and the *stellate reticulum.* Terminal cytodifferentiation of odontoblasts and ameloblasts intervene in each tooth according to a specific timing and spatial pattern. The terminal differentiation of odontoblasts always precedes that of ameloblasts. For detailed cytological descriptions see References 23 to 28. Nearly all mammals are distinguished from most other vertebrates by the possession of a heterodont dentition. These teeth are divisible into four classes: the *incisors, canines, premolars,* and *molars.* Within each class, the teeth differ one from the other. The four classes do not always coexist. For evolutionary and comparative anatomical aspects see References 3 and 4.

Table 1 shows an example of mammalian odontogenesis. Table 2 gives the highlights of human embryonic and fetal development according to Slavkin et al.[16]

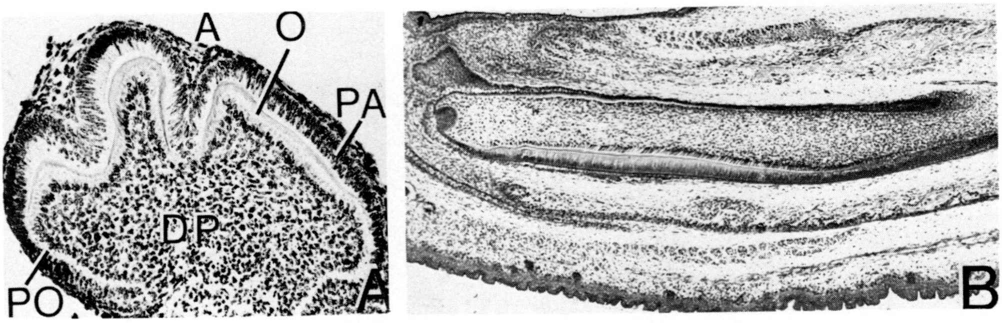

FIGURE 2. Sagittal section of a lower first embryonic mouse molar (A: magnification × 120) and an incisor (B: magnification × 80). The molar was dissected free on day 18 of gestation and cultured in vitro for 3 days. The patterns of progressive terminal differentiation of odontoblasts and ameloblasts can be observed. A: ameloblasts; O: odontoblasts; PA: preameloblasts; PO: preodontoblasts; DP: dental papilla. The sagittal section of a 17-day-old embryonic mouse molar illustrates the anterior-posterior gradient of terminal differentiation of odontoblasts and ameloblasts.

III. PATTERN FORMATION: FIELDS VS. CLONES

Since teeth are serially homologous structures, the developmental biologist may be interested in the progression of one given specific tooth or by the determinism of the development of the whole dentition. This second, global approach is supported by two theories, the field or gradient theory and the cell lineage theory. Lumsden[29] discussed these concepts in detail.

A. Regional Field Theory and Prepattern Gradient Model

In both the regional field theory[30,31] and the prepattern gradient model,[32] it is assumed that the morphological gradient of adult dentition results from the activities of a *morphogenetic gradient* in the embryo. The teeth primordia are considered to be equivalent. The field corresponds to those unknown factors that control the regional differentiation of dental mesenchyme.[33] Wolpert's positional information theory,[34] Crick's source-sink diffusion theory,[35] and Summerbell's theory of the progress zone[36] were also discussed by Lumsden[29] in function of odontogenesis.

B. The Cell Lineage Theory

The cell lineage theory describes odontogenesis in terms of cell clones.[37] Homogeneous cells were assumed to have the ability to grow, differentiate, and realize morphogenesis without any supracellular control. Osborn[37] predicted three *dental clones,* one each for the incisors, canines, and all the molars. Taking the mouse dentition as an example, he postulates that the interactions between oral ectomesenchyme and oral epithelium establish the molar and incisor clones.

The evolution of the molar clone, for example, is the following. After a certain number of cell divisions, the cell mass gives rise to the first molar primordium which generates transitory inhibitory action on adjacent tissues which prevents the formation of the second molar primordium until the growing margin of the clone has proliferated beyond the edge. Furthermore, the clones give rise to different "clades". According to Holtzer's hypothesis,[38] the cells of the clone have never more than two options for entering a new differentiation compartment and the segregation takes place during "quantal cell cycles".

C. Experimental Data

Glasstone[39] cultured anterior and posterior parts of 11- to 12-day-old mouse embryos'

Table 1
CHRONOLOGY OF ODONTOGENESIS IN MOUSE EMBRYO

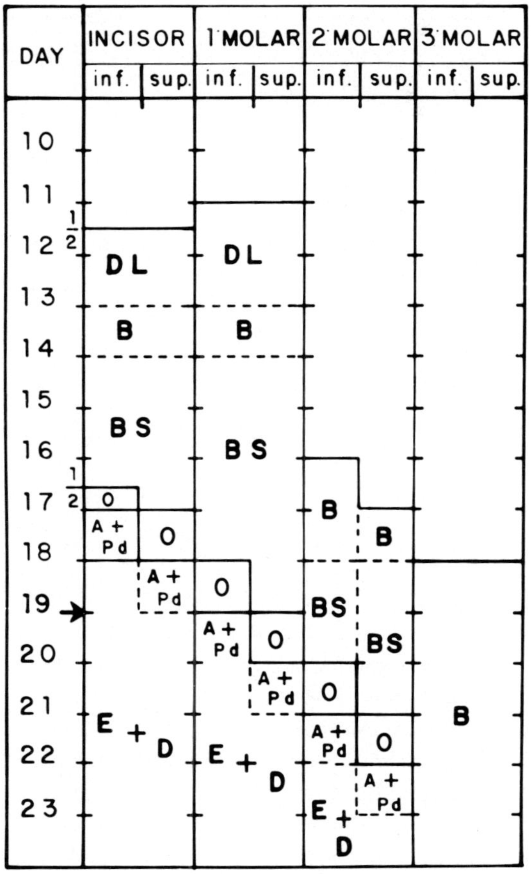

Note: DL: dental lamina; B: bud stage; BS: bell stage; O: odontoblasts; A: ameloblasts; Pd: predentin; E: enamel; D: dentin.

Table 2
HUMAN EMBRYONIC TOOTH DEVELOPMENT

Age	Developmental characteristics
44 to 48 days	Dental lamina formation
55 to 56 days	Bud stage for deciduous incisors, canines, and molars
14 weeks	Bell stage for deciduous tooth organs; terminal differentiation of odontoblasts begin; bud stage for permanent teeth
18 weeks	Dentin and functional ameloblasts exist in deciduous teeth
32 weeks	Dentin and functional ameloblasts exist in permanent first molars

lower jaws separately. Glasstone observed incisor differentiation from the arterior part and molar differentiation from the posterior half and concluded that a morphogenetic field could

Table 3
EVOLUTION IN VITRO OF EMBRYONIC MOUSE MOLAR RUDIMENTS

		Duration of culture (days)								No. and stages of 1st, 2nd, 3rd molars		
Stage of rudiments	**No. of rudiments**	**4**	**6**	**8**	**10**	**12**	**14**	**16**	**18**	**1st**	**2nd**	**3rd**
Day 13	27	3								3	1 + 2L	—
			1							1	1	—
				2						2	2	2B
					4					4	2	1L
						4				4	2	1B
							2			2	1	1B
								—	11	11	5	2B
Day 14	13	6								6	1C + 3B	—
			—	1						1	1	1B
					—	1				1	1	1B
							—	—	5	5	2	1B + 1L
Day 15	65	2								2	2	1L
			3							3	3	2B
				3						3	3	3B
					1					1	1	—
						3				3	3	—
							13			12	11	4C + 4B
								40	—	39	39	4 + 19C + 4B

Note: L: dental lamina; B: bud stage; C: bell stage.

be present. Hay[40] found that first and second molars developed in cultures of 14 to 15 day mouse first molar germs. Lumsden[29] dissected the developing molar tissues from 10- to 16-day-mouse embryos and grafted these tissues in the anterior eye chambers of homologous adult mice. From the 12th day, the entire molar dentition developed. Lumsden interpreted his interesting results according to the cell lineage theory; shape and size of the cheek teeth seem to be expressions of intrinsic time-dependent modifications in a growing cell population. Developing molar tissues of lower jaws from 13-, 14-, and 15-day-old mouse embryos were grown in vitro in our laboratory.[41] Complete molar dentition differentiated (Table 3, Figure 3). We concluded that the realization of the normal pattern of molars probably does not require the presence of an extradental morphogen.

Lumsden also explored the regulative capacity of the growing odontogenic tissue. He performed heterochronal recombinations and showed mosaic properties. Nevertheless, at the level of individual teeth, regulation was observed.[42,43]

IV. CELL KINETICS DURING ODONTOGENESIS

Differential mitotic activities exist during odontogenesis. Gaunt[44] suggested that dental lamina formation resulted from locally increased mitotic activity. Butler[45] thought that differential mitotic activity could explain specific morphogenesis. More systematic analyses were performed by way of establishing the mitotic index on serial sections and radioautographic data.[46-48]

A. Dental Lamina Formation

Dental lamina formation does not result from differential mitotic activities (Figure 4), but is at least partially explained by modification in orientation of the spindle of epithelial cells. Before dental lamina formation, the preferential orientation is parallel to the surface of the

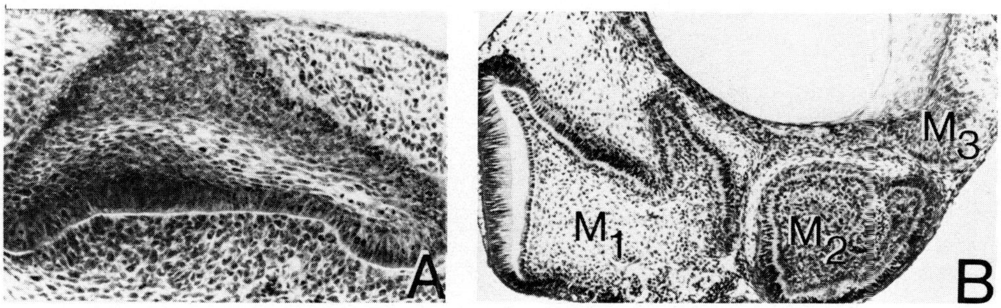

FIGURE 3. In vitro evolution of embryonic mouse molar rudiment. (A) The anlage isolated on day 15 of gestation (magnification × 160); (B) first (M_1), second (M_2), and third (M_3) molars differentiate after 6 days in culture (magnification × 120).

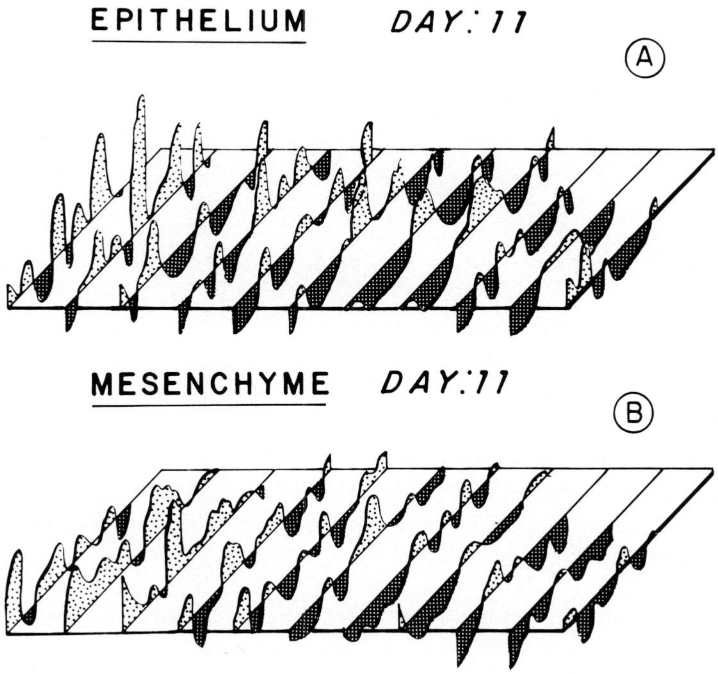

FIGURE 4. Regional variations of mitotic indexes of oral epithelium (A) and ectomesenchyme (B) during dental lamina formation. Serial frontal sections of 11-day-old embryonic mouse mandibular arches were analyzed. No differential mitotic activity corresponds to the appearing dental lamina (for details see Reference 46).

oral epithelium. Later, the spindle becomes perpendicular and the daughter cells are superposed (Figure 5). During lamina formation, the mitotic index (MI), the labeling index (LI), and the growth fraction (P) of epithelial cells are significantly lower than those of mesenchymal cells (Tables 4 and 5). The duration of cell cycle (TC) for epithelial and mesenchymal cells is 8 and 9 hr, respectively (Tables 6 and 7).

B. Late Bud, Cap, and Bell Stages (Histogenesis and Morphogenesis)

The analysis of serial frontal sections of lower mandibular arches of 14- to 18-day-old mice embryos demonstrates: (1) a very clear dissociation between the values of mitotic

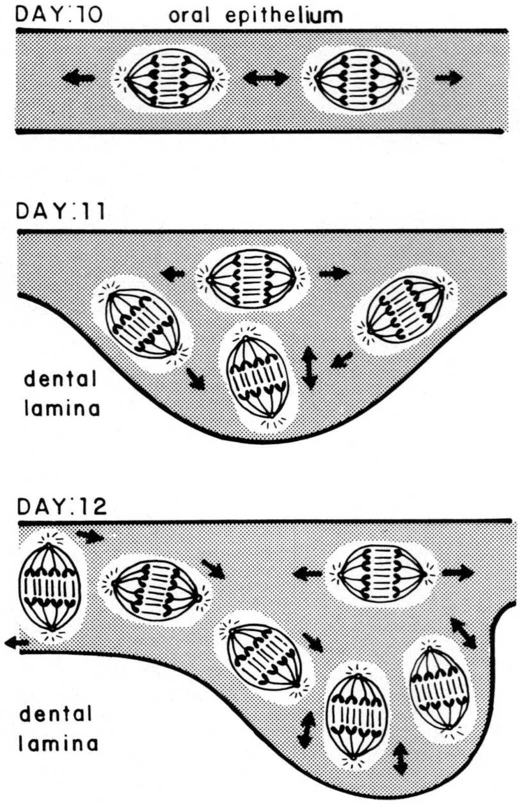

FIGURE 5. Diagrams depicting the orientation of spindles in epithelial cells during dental lamina formation.

indexes of inner and outer dental epithelium. The values of the outer epithelium decrease rapidly while the values of the inner dental epithelium and of the cervical loop, remain increased (Table 4); (2) specific distribution patterns of mitosis in incisors and molars (Figure 6). The incisor appears to be rapidly subdivided into three zones:

- An anterior one, where the mitotic activity of mesenchymal and epithelial cells is low. Progressively, postmitotic odontoblasts and ameloblasts appear. The extension of this zone increases with time (Figure 6).
- A transition zone where the mitotic indexes increase apically.
- An apical zone where the mitotic activities are high, nevertheless demonstrating significant differences in function of the different histological compartments. This apical zone of probably constant dimension corresponds to the compartment of proliferation.

Progressively, the cell kinetics of the embryonic incisor become comparable to that of continuously growing rodent incisors where cell kinetic parameters have been carefully analyzed.[49-52] In molars, regional variations of mitotic activities in the inner dental epithelium seem to be correlated with cusp formation. Between days 14 and 18, TC increases mainly by a lengthening of the phase G_1. TC, LI, and P are different in the various histological compartments (Figure 7, Tables 5 to 7). The appearance of the second lower molar, at the apical ridge of the first molar, is accompanied by a significant increase of the MI of epithelium and mesenchyme. On day 16 (bud stage), the TC of the dental epithelium and dental mesenchyme are 13.8 and 14 hr, respectively. These values are nearly the same as those of the first lower molar of day 16 (bell stage).

Table 4
MEAN MITOTIC INDEX (%) OF TOOTH COMPONENTS IN THE LOWER JAWS OF MOUSE EMBRYO FROM DAY 11 TO 18 OF GESTATION

		Epithelium		Mesenchyme (dental papilla)	
Day	Tissue components	Molar	Incisor	Molar	Incisor
11	Dental lamina	3.8		5.5	
12	Dental bud	4.0	4.2	6.0	5.6
13	Dental bud	5.7	6.3	6.7	6.2
14	Enamel organ	7.2	7.2	5.4	6.4
15	Cervical loop	8.7	6.3	5.3	7.1
	IDE	3.3	9.1		
	ODE	4.1	4.2		
16	Cervical loop	7.9	6.7	4.5	6.1
	IDE	4.6	9.7		
	ODE	4.2	2.8		
17	Cervical loop	6.7	6.5	4.9	6
	IDE	5.5	7.3		
	ODE	2.1	1.3		
18	Cervical loop	4.8	6.6	2.5	5.4
	IDE	3.9	6.0		
	ODE	0.7	0.8		

Note: IDE: inner dental epithelium; ODE: outer dental epithelium.

Table 5
LABELING INDEX (LI) AND GROWTH FRACTION (P), %, OF TOOTH COMPONENTS IN THE LOWER JAW OF THE MOUSE EMBRYO (DAYS 11, 14, AND 16)

Day	Epithelium			Mesenchyme		
		LI	P	P	LI	
11	Dental lamina	31	50	81	45	
14	First molar	33	55	44	28	
	(Enamel organ)					Dental papilla
	Incisor	27	45	53	35	
16	*First molar*					
	Cervical loop	44	82	69	40	
	IDE	28	51			
	ODE	17	33			Dental papilla
	Incisor					
	Cervical loop	33	64	65	37	
	IDE	39	79			
	ODE	14	28			

Note: IDE: inner dental epithelium; ODE: outer dental epithelium.

C. Cytodifferentiation

Terminal differentiation of odontoblasts and ameloblasts occurs according to a specific timing and spatial pattern. Odontoblasts and ameloblasts are postmitotic cells. During the last cell division, the spindle of the preodontoblasts is orientated perpendicularly to the epithelio-mesenchymal junction. The two daughter cells are superposed and only the cell in relation with the basement membrane differentiates into a functional odontoblast. It is gen-

Table 6
DURATION (HOURS) OF CELL CYCLE PHASES OF MESENCHYMAL CELLS DURING EMBRYONIC MOUSE ODONTOGENESIS

Day	Tissues	TC	Ts	T (G_2 + $^1/_2$M)	T (G_1 + G_2 + M)	T_M	TG_2	TG_1
11	Mesenchyme in relation with the dental lamina	8.9	4.9	1.6	4.0	0.6	1.3	2.1
14	Presumptive dental papilla							
	First molar	11.8	7.5	1.5	4.3	0.8	1.1	2.4
	Incisor	10.7	7.0	1.5	3.7	0.8	1.1	1.8
16	Dental papilla							
	First molar	13.9	8.0	1.5	5.9	0.8	1.1	4.0
	Incisor	12.2	6.9	1.5	5.3	0.9	1.0	4.2

Table 7
DURATION (HOURS) OF CELL CYCLE PHASES OF EPITHELIAL CELLS DURING EMBRYONIC MOUSE ODONTOGENESIS

Day	Tissues	TC	Ts	T (G_2 + $^1/_2$M)	T (G_1 + G_2 + M)	T_M	TG_2	TG_1
11	Dental lamina	10.0	6.1	2.4	3.9	0.5	2.1	1.2
14	Enamel organ							
	First molar	12.3	7.3	1.5	5.0	1.1	0.9	2.9
	Incisors	11.1	6.8	1.5	4.3	1.0	1.0	2.3
16	*First molar*							
	Cervical loop	12.6	6.7	1.5	5.9	1.2	0.9	3.8
	IDE	13.9	7.5	1.5	6.4	1.0	1.0	4.4
	ODE	14.2	7.3	1.5	6.9	0.7	1.1	5.0
	Incisor							
	Cervical loop	13	6.7	1.5	6.3	1.1	0.9	4.2
	IDE	11.2	6.0	1.5	5.2	1.3	0.8	3.0
	ODE	13.7	6.9	1.5	6.8	0.5	1.2	5.0

Note: IDE: inner dental epithelium; ODE: outer dental epithelium.

erally assumed that odontoblasts and ameloblasts are diploid cells. However, Starkey[53] suggested that these cells might be tetraploid. Radioautographic and cytophotometric data[54] confirm that the DNA content of these cells is close to tetraploid values.

D. Cell Kinetics in Vitro

Detailed analysis of cell kinetics of cultured tooth germs has not been performed. Nevertheless, it was shown[55] that such teeth did not demonstrate TC lengthening which takes place during evolution in vivo. Furthermore, the P values were different. Despite these discrepancies in vitro, culture of tooth germs provide normal-looking morphogenesis and cytodifferentiations. In fact, culture in vitro gives rise to mini-teeth. Systematic comparison of cell kinetics in vivo and in vitro should permit a better understanding of the implications of kinetics in morphogenesis and differentiation. In a review, Snow et al.[56] provided further information on the control and regulation of size in mammalian embryos.

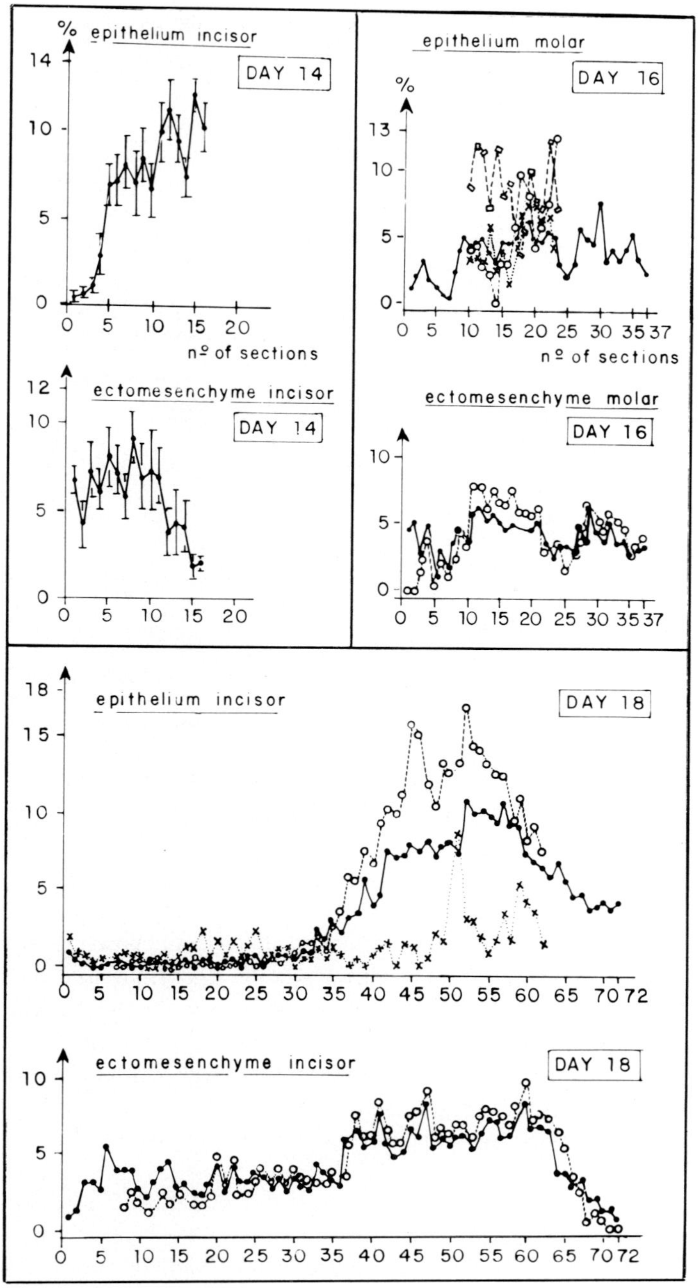

FIGURE 6. Sagittal projections of the mean values of mitotic indexes in embryonic mouse incisors and molars. For the incisors (days 14 and 18) clear anterior-posterior gradients exist. O: inner dental epithelium or preodontoblasts; X: outer dental epithelium; ●: mean values for the whole enamel organ or dental papilla. For the molar (day 16) the values of the inner dental epithelium (○) are significantly higher than those of the outer dental epithelium (X). ●: mean values for the whole enamel organ or dental papilla (for details see Reference 47).

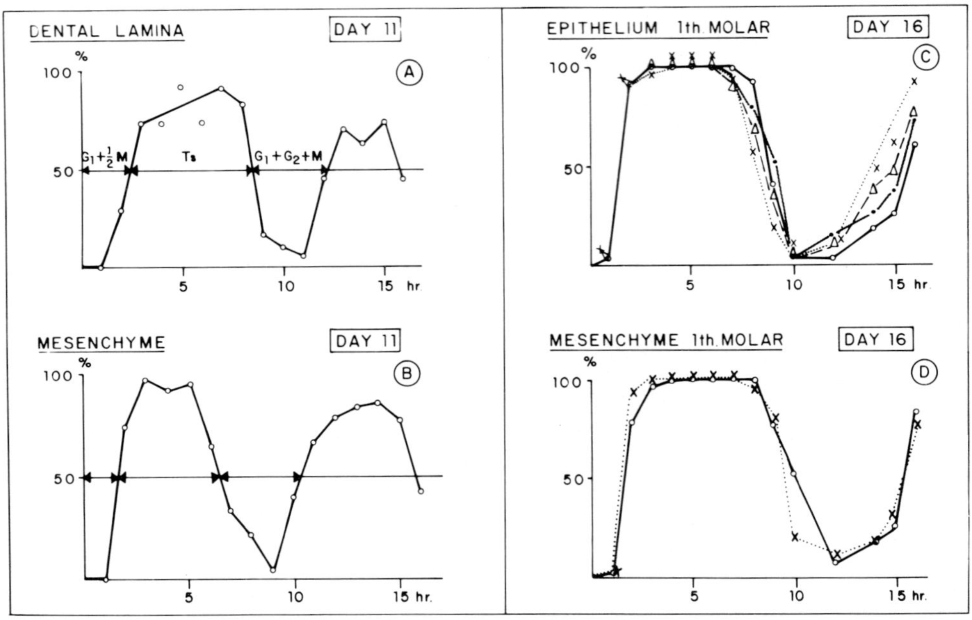

FIGURE 7. Labeled mitosis curves of embryonic mouse dental cells. The progressive lengthening of the cell cycle is obvious. (C) x: cervical loop, △: inner dental epithelium, ○: outer dental epithelium, ●: mean results for whole enamel organs; (D) x: dental papilla, ○: peridental mesenchyme (for details see Reference 48).

V. ROLE AND MECHANISM OF CELL INTERACTIONS DURING ODONTOGENESIS

Morphogenesis and cytodifferentiations are genetically determined. However, neither the nature of genes intervening during specific morphogenesis, nor the nature of control mechanisms allowing time and space dependent differential gene expression, nor why specific gene products corresponding to terminal differentiation are synthesized by particular cells are known. It is believed that within the genotype, there is probably a program that governs or at least allows the developmental and postdevelopmental life cycle. For rather phenomenological, classical, experimental embryology most developmental biologists think that differentiation in a broad sense is epigenetically controlled by changing the local environment. Holtzer,[57] however, suggested a possible self-programming, step-wise evolution during quantal cell cycle.

How might epigenetic processes mediate the sequential gene expression? Diffusion of signal substances, matrix-mediated, or cell-mediated interactions have been documented (see Reference 58 for review). Furthermore, these interactions could be directive or permissive,[58] the first allowing commitment of phenotypic pathways, the second modulating activities of committed cells. In Holtzer's hypothesis, the epigenetic factors would only work at a permissive level. Developmental biologists interested in odontogenesis, admit that tooth development is dependent on a continuous sequence of epithelial-mesenchymal interactions. When tooth epithelium and mesenchyme are separated, neither of the components is able to differentiate normally. For didactic reasons, the possible epigenetic control mechanisms for dental lamina formation, morphogenetic events, and cytodifferentiations are summarized.

A. Dental Lamina Formation

During odontogenesis initiating events occur very early to establish epithelial and mesenchymal sites of toothness. There is a complex spatial patterning of functional subunits.

Miller[59] admits that in mouse embryo, the presumptive molar region is established by 10 days and that of the incisor by day 10.5. The molar dental lamina appears at day 11, the incisor lamina at day 12.[60] The appearance and spatial behavior of dental lamina of mouse embryos has been documented.[60] In species without a diastema, the lamina appears as a continuous band of thickened oral epithelium. The premaxillary and maxillary portion may arise separately and later unite.[61] The mesenchymal condensation appears during dental bud formation. The determinism of the localization of the dental lamina is not known. It has been suggested[62,63] that the innervation of the early mandibular and maxillary processes influences the patterning of presumptive tooth anlagen.

Gerber et al.[60] dissected developing lower jaws from 9-day-mouse embryos and cultured them for periods of up to 24 days in testis of homologous adult hosts. In 15 grafts, 27 teeth developed, i.e., 17 incisors, 6 molars, and 4 nonidentified bell stages. The higher frequency of incisors might be explained by a time-spatial segregation of incisor and molar neural crest-derived dental cells. In any case, these observations illustrate that in mouse embryos by the ninth day, specific "dental cells" exist in the lower jaw.

Ruch et al.[64] isolated lower jaws of 11-day-mouse embryos. After trypsin dissociation, they performed associations between mandibular mesenchyme and either oral epithelium or epithelium from the developing foot, and associations between oral epithelium and nonoral mesenchyme. Teeth developed only in cultured associations containing oral (dental) mesenchyme. Thus, it was assumed that oral ectomesenchymal cells bearing tooth specificity, after specific distribution in the developing maxillary and mandibular processes, interact with the oral epithelium and control DL formation. It was suggested as a working hypothesis that the mesenchymal cells modify the structure and/or composition of the epithelially derived basal lamina and that these modifications influence the orientation of the spindle of the epithelial cells by a transmembranous mechanism, allowing the localized thickening (Figure 5). It is not yet known whether the neural crest-derived ectomesenchymal cells are already committed before they reach the mandibular arches (interaction with pharyngeal endoderm might play a role[19]), or if commitment occurs in the arches.

B. Morphogenetic and Histogenetic Processes

1. Morphogenesis

Preliminary data[59-65] suggested that the ectodermal (epithelial) component determined the tooth type. These authors dissected the developing jaws of embryonic mice (9 to 12 days postconception) and the presumptive tooth bearing areas were separated into mesodermal and ectodermal portions. Recombinations were grown on chick chorioallantois. Heritier and Deminatti,[66] also using very young presumptive tooth components, concluded that the mesenchyme directs molar or incisor morphogenesis. Kollar and Baird[67] using 13- to 17-day-old embryonic tooth component reassociations demonstrated the directive role of dental papilla during crown morphogenesis. Kollar and Baird[68,69] further documented that the dental papilla can initiate tooth development from nondental epithelium. Heterospecific associations between enamel organs and dental papillae from mouse and rabbit incisors or molars were also performed.[70] In associations of early bell stage tooth components, the crown pattern effectuated was in conformity with the prospective fate of the dental papilla. In associations of late bell stage components, the enamel organs demonstrated relative morphogenetic independence (Figure 8).

Grobstein and Cohen[71] showed that the disruption of collagen in the extracellular matrix by collagenase prevents salivary gland morphogenesis. Since this observation, a morphogenetic role of the extracellular matrix has been documented in several cases (for review see Reference 72). If collagenase is administered to cultures of embryonic tooth germs, morphogenesis is also disturbed.[15] Several drugs affecting synthesis and/or excretion of extracellular matrix components, such as collagens, glycoproteins, glycosaminoglycans, prevent tooth morphogenesis, α,α′-dipyridyl, L-azetidine carboxylic acid, β-amino propionitrile, tetracycline, hadacidin, diazo-oxo-norleucine, and tunicamycin.[73-78] Kollar[79] showed that the action of tetracycline may be partially circumvented by the introduction of procollagen in the culture medium.

The correct interpretation of the effects of drugs with known and unknown side effects is difficult and these studies have not provided "insights into the rate-limiting steps associated with morphogenesis".[80] Furthermore, there are no objective data demonstrating incisor- or molar-specific extracellular matrix. Hypervitaminosis A as well as hypovitaminosis A were shown to impair tooth morphogenesis.[81] Ascorbic acid deficiency, producing the synthesis of underhydroxylated collagens, also leads to abnormal teeth.[82] In connection with hormones, teeth eruption rate has been mainly focused on.[83] Thyroxin hastens tooth replacement in amphibians[84] and increases dentin production.[85] For dental sexual dismorphism see Reference 86.

Mitostatic drugs also disturb tooth morphogenesis[87] and differentiation.[87,88] The cell kinetic analysis[44-48] summarized above, suggests that tooth morphogenesis is correlated with differential mitotic activity. These results support Osborn's theory[89] which relates cusp formation to differential growth rates between preodontoblasts and inner dental epithelium. It would be important to elucidate the role of extracellular matrix in the control of cell kinetics.

2. Root Formation — Hertwig's Epithelial Sheath

The fact that the inner and outer dental epithelia proliferate at the margins of the bell-shape enamel organ and give rise to *Hertwig's epithelial root sheath,* is generally accepted. This sheath outlines the dentino-cemental junction and "acts as a blueprint pattern for the shape, size, and length of the future root or roots."[1] For morphological reasons, it has been suggested that the epithelial sheath initiates the differentiation of the *cementoblasts*. The problem of root formation requires further experimental approaches.

3. Histogenesis of the Enamel Organ

In cultured heterotopic associations between outer dental epithelium and dental papilla, the outer dental epithelium acquires the histogenic specificity of an inner dental epithelium and gives rise to ameloblasts. These cytological modifications are accompanied by a significant increase of the labeling and mitotic indexes.[91] The specific histological and cytological outcome of the inner dental epithelium seems to be coordinated with specific cell kinetics, the whole developmental process being controlled by interactions with the preodontoblasts.[91] The possible role of the basal lamina in the control of the cell kinetics of dental epithelium has been discussed.[91] Tooth histogenic properties are conserved by isolated cells. Slavkin et al.[92] demonstrated that when isolated epithelial and mesenchymal cells from the cervical loop of embryonic rabbit incisors were mixed and suspended on the chorioallantoic membrane, these cells were capable of cell-cell recognition and initiation of dental histogenesis. Orams et al.,[93] however, could not confirm these observations. Kollar[94] cultured dental papillae cells as monolayers. Such cells lose their cytological characteristics. If they are sedimented by centrifugation and combined with fresh epithelium, teeth were formed. It was also shown that dental epithelial cells, grown as a monolayer for several days and then pelleted and associated with dental papillae, give rise to enamel organs with the usual appearance.[70]

C. Terminal Cytodifferentiations

The final events in odontogenesis are the deposition of mineralizing extracellular matrices by odontoblasts and ameloblasts, cells which are no longer dividing.

1. Odontoblasts

Characterization of odontoblast terminal differentiation — The terminal differentiation of odontoblasts occurs for each tooth in a specific temporo-spatial pattern. For example, in the first mandibular mouse molar (laboratory-raised Swiss mice, vaginal plug = day 0) the first overtly differentiated odontoblasts are found at day 18 at the top of the principal cusps. Progressively, more odontoblasts appear toward the basal parts of the cusps. As stated above, the preodontoblasts appear to be committed very early during development, but there is no precise information about the mechanisms involved. The terminal differentiation is characterized by the following steps: odontoblasts become postmitotic, assume an epithelial arrangement, and polarize. Polarization implies important cytological modifications. The cell becomes larger, the nucleus takes up an excentric position, cisternae of the granular cytoplasmic reticulum multiply, flatten, and become parallel with the long axis of the cell (Figure 9). The apical part of the cell forms the odontoblast cell process which is devoid of major cytoplasmic organelles but contains coated vesicles. The cells begin to secrete the initial (mantle) predentin. This phase of terminal differentiation lasts a few hours (for a detailed cytological description, see References 95 to 97). The functional aspects of odontoblast terminal differentiation are not completely known. The preodontoblasts synthesize collagen Type I, Type I trimer, Type III,[98-101] fibronectin,[102,103] and glycosaminoglycans.[104,105] Functional differentiation of odontoblasts implies amplifications of collagen Type I and Type I trimer synthesis and suppression of collagen Type III synthesis.[99-102] Fully differentiated odontoblasts also synthesize a phosphoprotein.[106,107] It is not yet clear if preodontoblasts and odontoblasts synthesize different glycosaminoglycans.[108,109] The identification of odontoblasts combining cytological and functional criteria is easy in the intact tooth but is still very difficult for isolated cells growing in vitro. It would be important to find out the exact biochemical phenotype of odontoblast.

Terminal differentiation of odontoblasts requires structural integrity of the cytoskeleton — The cytoskeleton consists of various structural components: intermediate filaments, microfilaments, and microtubules. Using immunofluorescence methods,[110-113] the organization and distribution of these components have been analyzed in several different tissues and cell types. The molecular composition of these components has also been extensively investigated.[112,114,115] Vimentin (intermediate filament) and actin have been localized in the dental papilla. A change in the distribution of vimentin was observed during odontoblast polarization. This protein was uniformly localized within the cytoplasm of preodontoblasts while it accumulated in the apical poles of polarized odontoblasts.[116] The cytoskeleton (microtubules and filaments) of polarized odontoblasts has been well documented.[117] Colchicine, as well as cytocholasin B was found to inhibit the polarization of odontoblasts.[118] Colchicine also inhibited the secretion of predentin.

Cell kinetics during terminal differentation of odontoblasts — Functional odontoblasts are postmitotic cells. It is generally believed that these cells are diploid. Nevertheless, Starkey,[53] using radioautographic data, stressed the possibility that these cells could be tetraploid. Cytophotometric DNA quantification and radioautographic data demonstrate gene amplification in postmitotic odontoblasts.[54] During the last division of preodontoblasts, the spindle is always oriented perpendicularly to the basal lamina underlying the inner dental epithelium. The two daughter cells are superposed and only the cell closest to the basement membrane gives rise to a functional odontoblast.[47]

From the early stage of odontogenesis (day 11) to the terminal differentiation of odontoblasts of first mandibular molars, a maximum of 14 to 15 cell generations may exist. Experimental data, summarized below, suggest that odontoblast terminal differentiation can be achieved only after a minimum number of cell cycles. Supplementary cell cycles can be added.[119] Replicating preodontoblasts, held in the G_1-S interface by fluorodeoxyuridine (FudR), did not polarize. This effect was reversible. FudR had no marked effect on post-

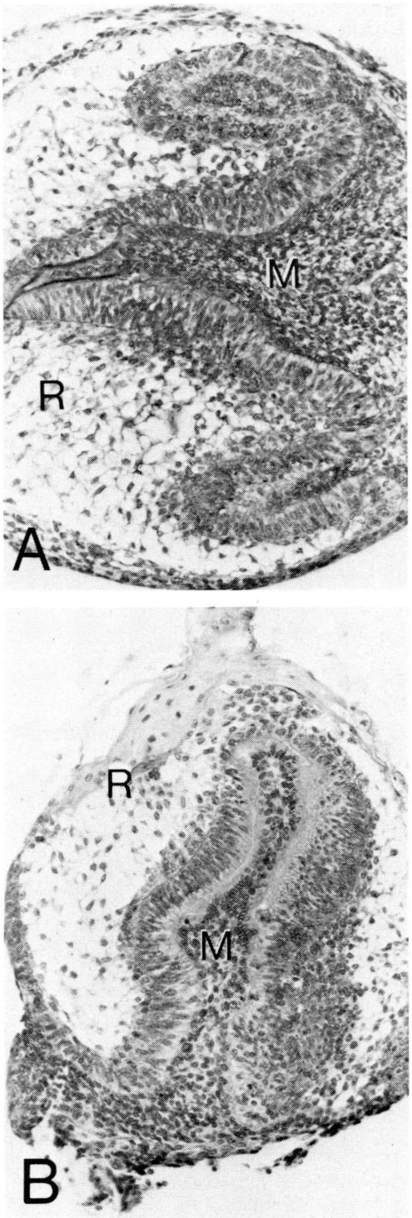

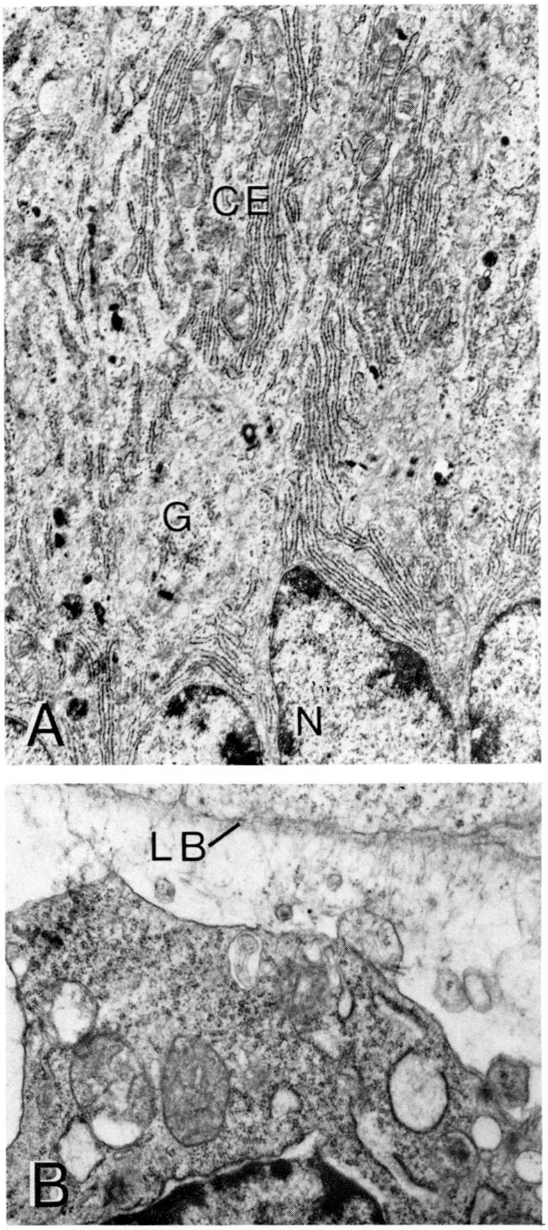

FIGURE 8 (left). Sections of heterospecific, cultured reassociations between dental papillae and enamel organs of early (A) and late (B) bell stages (magnification × 190). (A) Mouse molar papilla (M) associated with rabbit incisor enamel organ (R), a molar has differentiated; (B) mouse molar papilla (M) associated with rabbit molar enamel organ (R), an incisor-like tooth has differentiated. FIGURE 9 (right). Electron micrograph showing polarized odontoblasts (A; magnification × 10,700) and a depolarized odontoblast; assuming the typical structure of a preodontoblast (B; magnification × 12,500). CE: cisternae of endoplasmic reticulum; G: Golgi zone; N: nucleus; LB: basal lamina. (From Ruch et al., *Differentiation,* 5, 165, 1976. With permission.)

mitotic odontoblasts. In the presence of FudR, uridine, and thymidine, the preodontoblasts undertook normal terminal differentiation.[87] The last cell cycle seems important for functional differentiation under physiological conditions.[119]

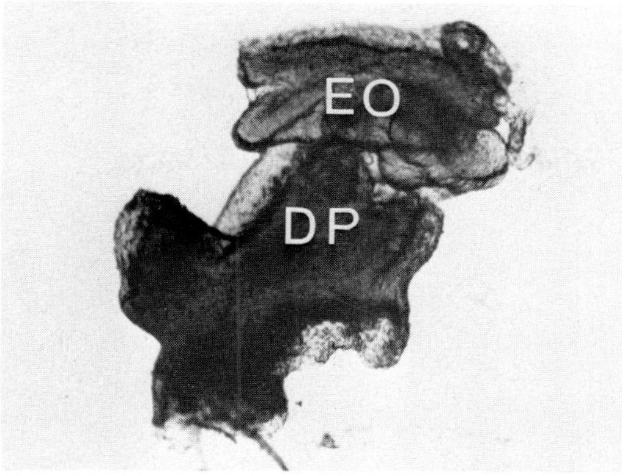

FIGURE 10. Heterochronal association between inner dental epithelium of a 16-day-old embryonic mouse molar enamel organ (EO) and a principal cusp of a 18-day-old embryonic mouse molar papilla (DP). (Magnification × 100.)

The inner dental epithelium intervenes in terminal differentiation of odontoblasts — Preodontoblasts of dental papillae, isolated by treatment with proteolytic enzymes, cultured in vitro[15,67,120] or in vivo,[14] never become functional. Polarized odontoblasts existing in teeth at the moment of papilla isolation depolarize and never become functional, even after 6 to 8 days in culture.[119] Predentin or dentin stabilizes the functional state of odontoblasts.[121] Iso- or heterochronal associations between dental papillae and inner dental epithelia (Figure 10) cultured in vitro[119,120] were shown to demonstrate the following points:

- Reassociation between polarized odontoblasts and isochronal inner dental epithelium allowed maintenance and functional differentiation of odontoblasts.
- In association between polarized odontoblasts and younger inner dental epithelium, the odontoblasts depolarized (Figure 9B) and were able to incorporate ^{3}H-thymidine and to divide. Later, daughter cells became postmitotic, polarized again, and secreted predentin.
- Association between preodontoblasts and older inner dental epithelium, previously in contact with postmitotic odontoblasts, did not allow anticipated terminal differentiation of odontoblasts.

Heterotopic, homospecific associations between dental papillae and nondental epithelia have been shown to allow functional differentiation of odontoblasts.[64,68,69] In such associations, the dental papilla first conditions the transformation of the nondental epithelium into inner dental epithelium. Later, this inner dental epithelium is able to initiate the differentiation of odontoblasts. Bromodeoxyuridine (BrdU) inhibits odontoblast terminal differentiation.[122-124]

Cultivated associations between either control or BrdU-treated dental papillae with either control or BrdU-treated enamel organs have been analyzed. The primary effect of BrdU on odontoblast cytodifferentiation results in its incorporation in the preameloblasts which are no longer able to interact normally with competent preodontoblasts.[123]

Odontoblast differentiation may be triggered by contact between preodontoblasts and the basement membrane — The extracellular matrix interposed between the inner dental epithelium and the preodontoblasts, and odontoblasts before secretion of predentin, is formed by a basement membrane (a basal lamina and associated microfibrils) (Figure 11). Separation of dental papilla from dental epithelium by trypsin results in removal of the

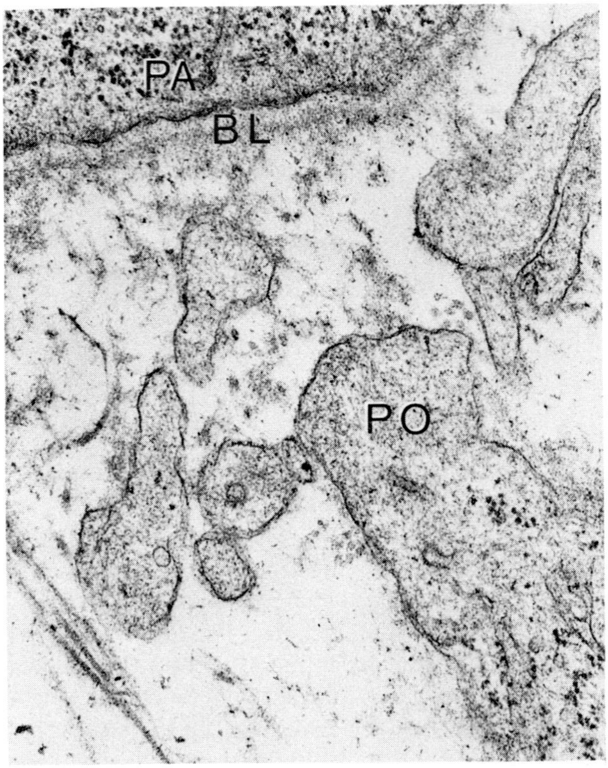

FIGURE 11. Epithelial-mesenchymal junction between the inner dental epithelium, preameloblasts (PA), and preodontoblasts (PO). BL: basal lamina. (Magnification × 32,000.)

basement membrane. Culture of dental papillae and epithelia with interposed filters resulted in basement membrane redeposition if the filter pores (0.6 μm) allowed penetration of cytoplasmic processes. Differentiation of odontoblasts occurred only in explants in which a new basement membrane was formed.[125] Basement membrane reconstitution and terminal differentiation of odontoblasts have also been analyzed in isochronal and heterochronal direct associations of dental papillae and inner dental epithelia.[126] Postmitotic odontoblasts were associated with isochronal or younger inner dental epithelium. In both cases, a typical basement membrane, i.e., a basal lamina and associated fibrillar and granular material, was restored within 6 to 18 hr. In isochronal associations, polarized odontoblasts were always present and these cells were functional after 24 hr. In heterochronal associations polarized odontoblasts were observed only 2 to 3 days after the reconstitution of the basement membrane.

If the basement membrane is secreted by the epithelial cells and plays a specific role during odontoblast terminal differentiation, then one must assume that the membranes deposited in iso- and heterochronal associations do not have the same composition or structure, even if the cytological aspects are similar. So far, attempts to induce odontoblast differentiation with gels of collagen Type I, Type II, and Type III, as well as with collagen gels substituted with proteoglycans, have not been successful.[125]

The dental basement membrane is at least partially epithelially derived — Trypsin-isolated dental epithelia, cultured in vitro or on chick chorioallantoic membrane[127,128] restored a basal lamina with associated fibrillar and granular material. [^{3}H]proline and [^{3}H]glucosamine allowed radioautographic labeling of this basement membrane (Figure 12).[129,130]

The basement membrane and odontoblasts of EDTA-isolated dental papillae — EDTA-

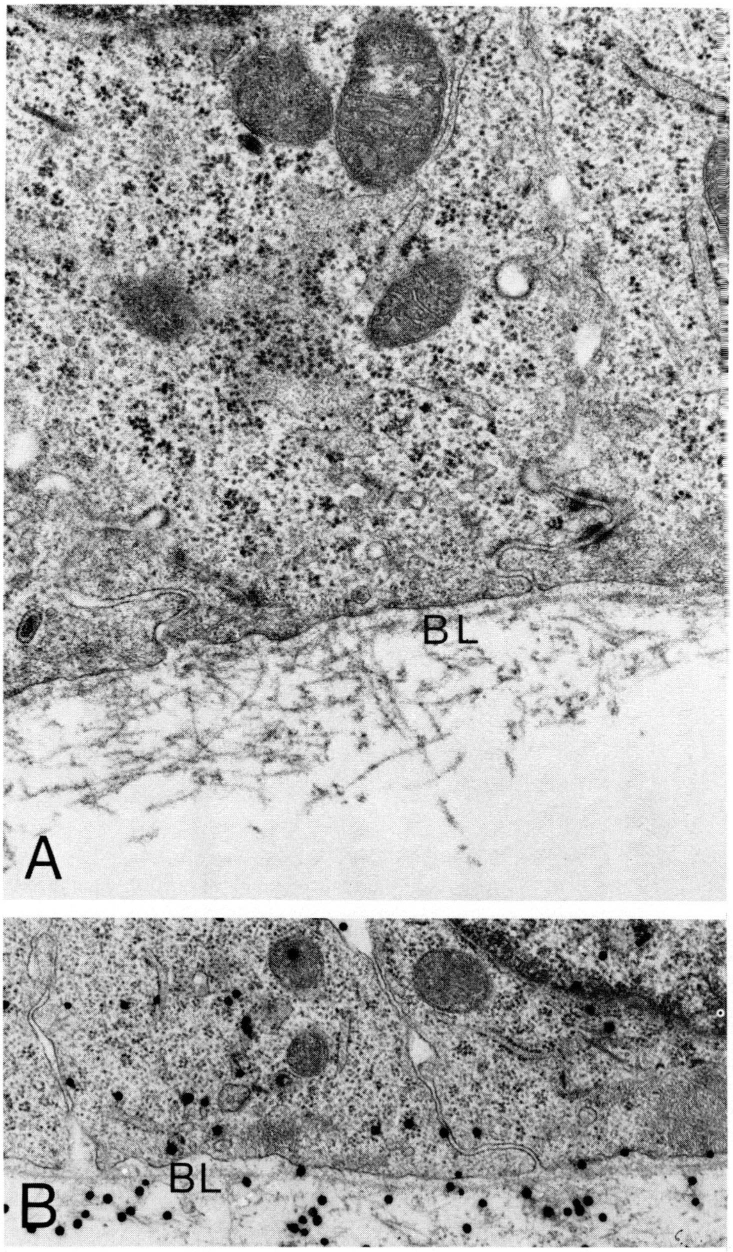

FIGURE 12. (A) Reconstruction of a basement membrane (BL: basal lamina and associated material) by trypsin-isolated in vitro cultured enamel organ. (Magnification × 40,000.) (B) This basement membrane can be labeled with [^{3}H] glucosamine. (Magnification × 21,000.)

dissociation of embryonic mouse mandibular molars was demonstrated to remove the basement membrane from the basal surface of epithelium but left it in association with the dental papilla[131] (Figure 13). In short-term culture, EDTA-isolated dental papillae remained covered by basement membrane for 15 to 18 hr. During this time the postmitotic odontoblasts, present at the onset of culture, but not the preodontoblasts, polarized and secreted predentin. Such a result has never been observed after trypsin dissociation. Nevertheless, when EDTA-

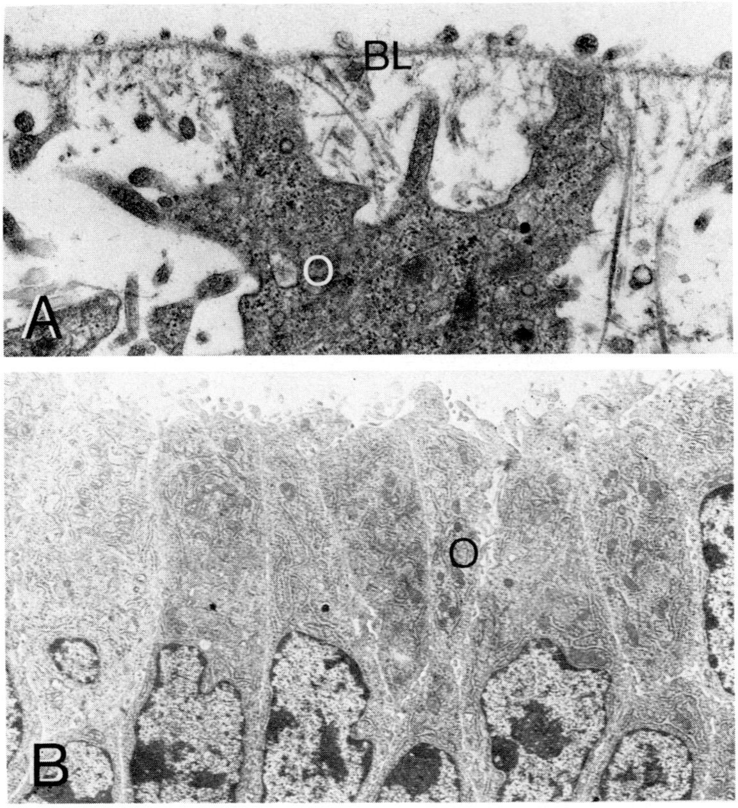

FIGURE 13. EDTA- and trypsin-isolated 18-day-old embryonic mouse molar papillae. (A) After EDTA-dissociation an intact basement membrane (BL: basal lamina and associated material) remains associated with the odontoblasts (O). (Magnification × 16,000.) (B) After trypsin dissociation the basement membrane has disappeared. Odontoblasts (O) demonstrate blebbing. (Magnification × 5000.)

dissociated dental papillae were cultured, the odontoblasts did not demonstrate the normal temporal and spatial patterns of terminal differentiaton occurring in intact teeth. This was attributed to the absence of renewal of the basement membrane in EDTA-isolated dental papillae. These observations led to the hypothesis that the physiological pattern of odontoblast terminal differentiation was correlated with a specific temporal, spatial, compositional, and structural pattern of the dental basement membrane.[131]

Modifications of the basement membrane and terminal differentiation of odontoblasts — Embryonic basement membranes contain glycosaminoglycans (GAG), collagens, and glycoproteins.[132] By means of indirect immunofluorescence, collagen Types I, III, IV, laminin, fibronectin, and proteoglycan were localized in the basement membrane.[102,103,133] The main phenomenon observed by indirect immunofluorescence during the terminal differentiation of odontoblasts was the disappearance of collagen Type III at the epithelial-mesenchymal junction[102] and a redistribution of fibronectin.[102,103] The latter completely surrounded the preodontoblasts but was confined to the epithelial-mesenchymal junction when odontoblasts polarized.

[^{3}H]glucosamine radioautography was performed to analyze the labeling of mouse embryonic dental basement membrane (basal lamina and associated material) before and during odontoblast terminal differentiation. Intact molars and trypsin-isolated dental epithelia were used.[130] After 6 hr of labeling, the epithelial mesenchymal junction was heavily labeled and the isolated epithelia accumulated substantial amounts of surface label. Before odontoblast terminal differentiation, the labels always had a uniform distribution and decreased during chase without any redistribution. During terminal differentiation, the label accumulated in a unique pattern; much more label was seen at the epithelial surface corresponding to the top of the cusps than in the inferior parts. During the chase, and only in intact tooth germs, epithelial surfaces which were poorly labeled during the pulse became labeled, but those heavily labeled during the pulse lost label. This pattern existed only in presence of mesenchyme; the mesenchyme thus seems to control the synthesis and/or the degradation of epithelially derived [^{3}H] glucosamine-labeled material (Figure 14).

Ruthenium red (RR) staining and tannic acid fixation were used to analyze the ultrastructure of embryonic mouse dental basement membrane in intact teeth or in EDTA-isolated dental papillae[134] (Figure 15). The inner leaflet of the preameloblast plasmalemma (inner dental epithelium) exhibited irregularly distributed RR positive material which was connected to intracellular tonofilaments. RR positive granules assumed a highly ordered symmetrical array in the internal and external lamina rara. This distribution pattern was particularly clear after EDTA-dissociation. The frequency of RR positive granules observed in the basal lamina was higher in the regions of dividing preodontoblasts than in the region of polarized postmitotic odontoblasts. Tannic acid fixation allowed detection within the lamina lucida of filaments connecting the lamina densa with the plasma membrane of preameloblasts. It is possible that such filaments and RR positive granules are structurally related.[135]

Adenylate cyclase activity and terminal differentiation of odontoblasts — The cytochemical methods of Howell and Whitfield[136] and Kempen et al.[137] have been used to investigate the localization of adenylate cyclase activity in tooth germs.[138] Increased adenylate cyclase activity was observed in preameloblasts and odontoblasts localized in the area where preodontoblasts become postmitotic (Figure 16). It is worth noting that, according to Kelly et al.,[139] glycosaminoglycans in the external cell surface of fibroblasts interact with receptor components of the adenylate cyclase system. Reduction of glycosaminoglycan at the periphery of a cell can increase the relative activity of adenylate cyclase.[139]

Experimental modifications of dental basement membrane — Hurmerinta et al.[77] showed that diazo-nor-leucine (DON), which causes a decrease of the synthesis of glycosaminoglycans and glycoproteins, inhibited the differentiation of odontoblasts. However we have shown[140] that DON decreased the mitotic activity. This effect per se may explain the inhibition of odontoblast differentiation. Hurmerinta et al.[81] also demonstrated that an excess of vitamin A prevented odontoblast differentiation. Vitamin A also inhibited the reformation of basement membrane between dental epithelium and dental papilla, recombined after trypsin-pancreatin separation. Tunicamycin, which inhibits glycosylation, prevented the differentation of odontoblasts.[78,141] After tunicamycin treatment, the dental basement membrane was discontinuous and fibronectin was drastically reduced.

Differentiation of odontoblasts in heterospecific associations — Kollar[94] combined the mandibular epithelium from 4- or 5-day-chick embryos with the dental papilla from 15- or 16-day-mouse tooth germs. After 1 week of growth on the chorioallantoic membrane (embryonated chick eggs), odontoblasts differentiated in some cases. On the other hand, Karcher-Djuricic and Ruch[142] failed to show any odontoblast differentiation in culture associations between 11-day-old embryonic mouse oral tissues and 5-day-old chicken embryonic tissues. Kollar and Fischer[143] observed ameloblast differentiation in some cases. Slavkin et al.[144,145] performed tissue-recombinations between mouse molar mesenchyme and quail mandibular epithelium and observed dentin formation but no amelogenesis. Knowing that mesenchyme may control structural and compositional aspects of the basal lamina,[130,146] it is important to determine whether the redeposited, epithelially derived basal lamina of heterospecific associations displays some dental specificity. It is important to note that the ultrastructural organization of the basal lamina might result from supramolecular interactions between

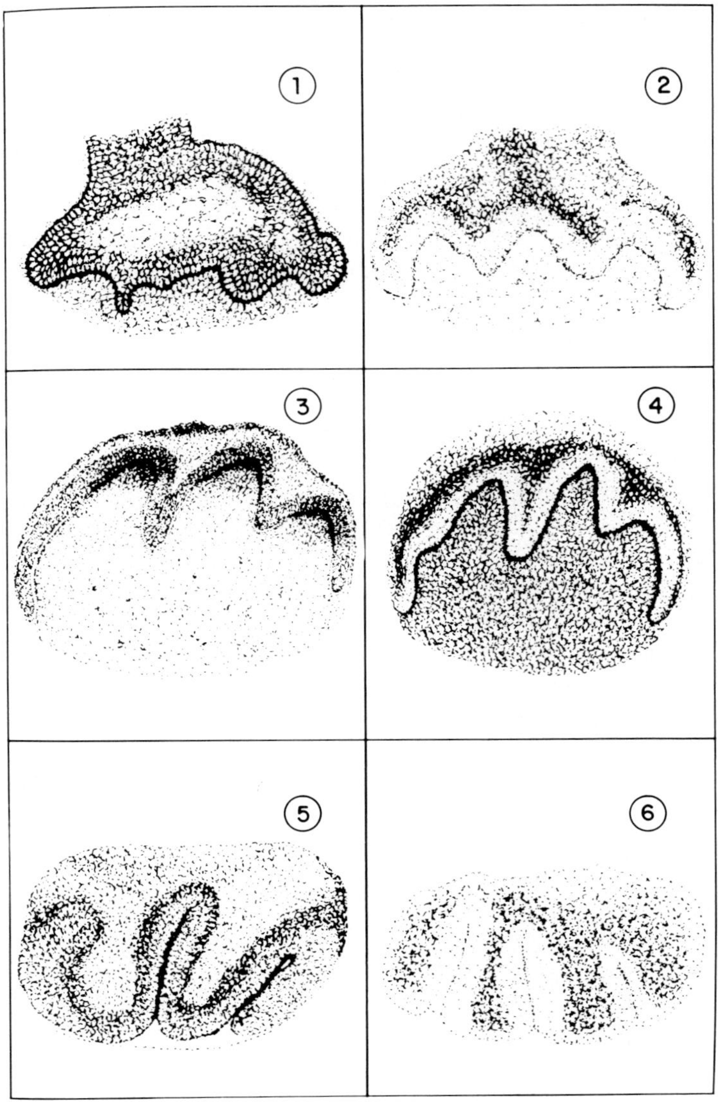

FIGURE 14. Drawings of [^{3}H] glucosamine radioautographs.[120] (1) 16-day-old first lower embryonic mouse molar after 6 hr labeling. The epithelial-mesenchymal junction is heavily labeled. (2) Localization of label after labeling as in (1) and chasing for 6 hr. The label of the epithelial-mesenchymal interface decreases without redistribution. (3) 18-day-old first lower embryonic mouse molar after 6 hr labeling. Substantial amounts of label are at the epithelial-mesenchymal interface of the tip of the cusps. (4) Localization of label after labeling as in (3) and chasing for 24 hr. During chase the epithelial-mesenchymal interface, poorly or not at all labeled during the pulse, becomes labeled. (5) Trypsin-isolated 18-day-old molar enamel organ labeled for 6 hr. The inner dental epithelium, corresponding to the tip of the cusps, accumulated surface label (compare with 3). (6) Localization of label after labeling as in (5) and chasing for 6 hr. The surface label progressively decreases without any redistribution.

epithelially derived macromolecules with mesenchymally derived cell surface fibronectin.[147]

Hypotheses concerning the control of physiological odontoblast terminal differentiation — Epigenetic controls are required for the progressive realization of the genetically

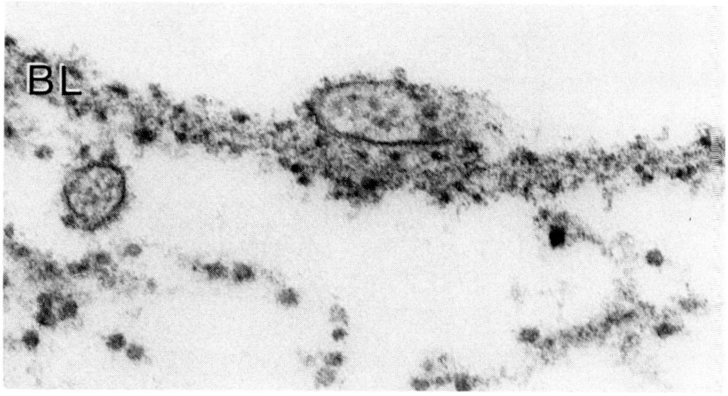

FIGURE 15. Basal lamina (BL) of EDTA-isolated 18-day-old embryonic mouse molar papilla. Ruthenium red-positive granules coat the basal lamina and the associated microfibrils. (Magnification × 57,000.)

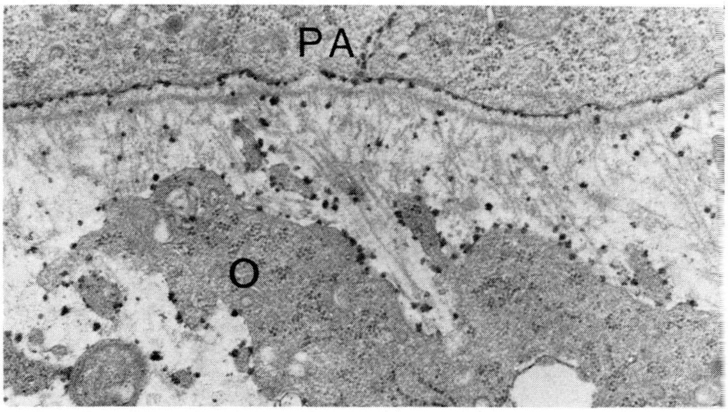

FIGURE 16. Cytochemical localization of adenylate cyclase. Membrane-bound precipitates in preameloblasts (PA) and odontoblasts (O). (Magnification × 16,000.)

determined phenotype of the odontoblast. The terminal differentiation of odontoblasts is characterized by:

- Withdrawal from the cell cycle
- Cytological and functional polarization
- Transcriptional and/or posttranscriptional modifications

The last two phenomena lead to predentin secretion. Our hypotheses[148] concerning the control of odontoblast differentiation are summarized in Figure 17.

The preodontoblasts (PO) probably undergo progressive maturation. Their terminal differentiation cannot be anticipated but can be delayed. The progressive lengthening of T_{G1} allows transcriptional modifications. After a minimum number of cell cycles, the preodontoblasts become potentially mature preodontoblasts (MPO). During the last preodontoblast cell division, the spindle is perpendicular to the basement membrane. There is no available evidence for the role of extracellular matrix in spindle orientation so far. The overt differentiation of mature preodontoblasts occurs only in contact with stage-specific basement membrane.

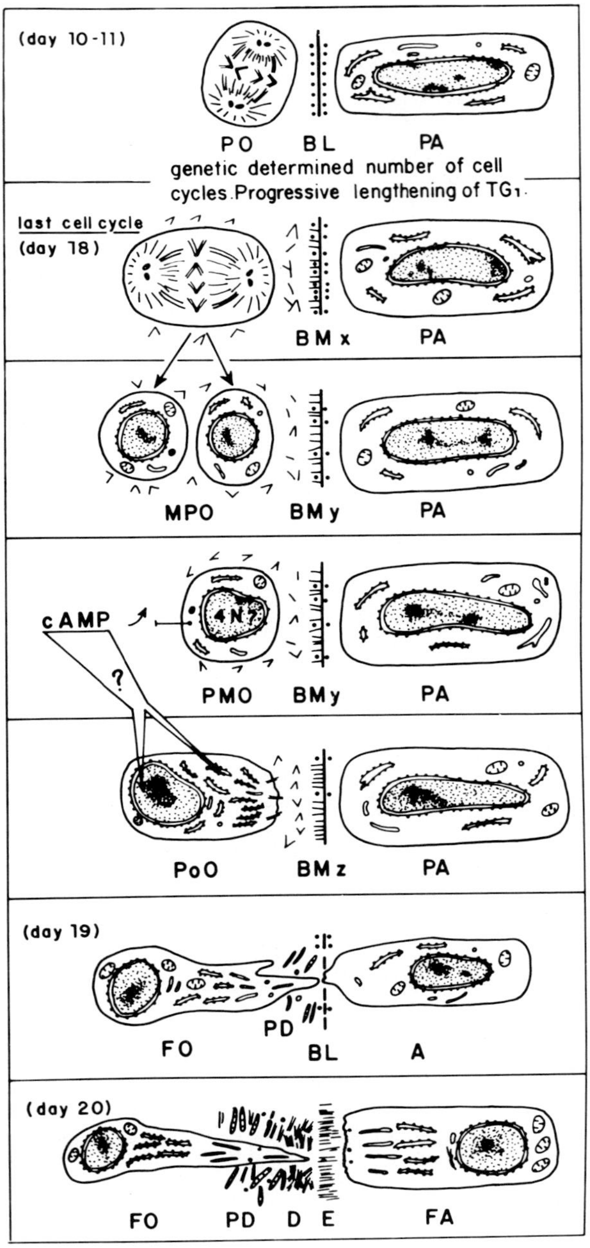

- Initiation of dental lamina formation by the preodontoblasts (PO).
- Progressive addition of collagens, glycoproteins, and proteoglycans to the basal lamina (BL) gives rise to stage specific basement membranes (BM).
- BMx might control the orientation of PO spindle. The daughter cells become potential mature preodontoblasts (MPO). The MPO in relation with the BM will overtly differentiate.
- MPO control the turnover of glycosaminoglycans (GAG) synthesized by the preameloblasts (PA). BMx becomes BMy.
- GAG (modifications might increase the adenylate cyclase activity of MPO which become postmitotic odontoblasts (PME). Gene amplification might occur. These cells no longer synthesize collagen Type III. Fibronectin is redistributed. BMy becomes BMz.
- BMz modifies the activity of the cytoskeleton: PMO become polarized odontoblasts (PoO). PoO present amplification of collagen Type I and Type I trimer synthesis.
- The predentin (PD) secreted by functional odontoblasts (FO) maintain their functional state. The BL disappears, heterotypic cell contacts exist between FO and postmitotic ameloblasts (PMA). Predentin and/or cell contacts mediate the functional differentiation of ambloblasts (A).
- The ameloblasts secrete enamel.

FIGURE 17. Hypotheses concerning the control of odontoblast and ameloblast differentiation (stages corresponding to the first mandibular molar of Swiss mouse embryos).

The basement membrane components have different origins; laminin, collagen Type IV, and, at least some glycosaminoglycans, covalently bound to protein to form proteoglycan, are epithelially derived. Collagen Type I trimer and Type III, as well as fibronectin, are produced by the dental papilla. The basement membrane presents compositional and structural modifications during the terminal differentiation such as mesenchyme-dependent modifications of glycosaminoglycan turnover, disappearance of collagen Type III, and redistribution of fibronectin. Glycosaminoglycan modifications might increase the adenylate cyclase activity of the mature preodontoblasts. The increased intracellular level of cAMP could transform these cells into postmitotic odontoblasts (PMO).

Ruch and Karcher-Djuricic[149] postulated that the polarization of postmitotic odontoblasts is controlled by cell membrane-bound receptors which could modulate the activity of the cytoskeleton. The distribution of concanavalin A surface receptors of odontoblasts was examined. Fixed preodontoblasts and odontoblasts demonstrated uniform distribution of concanavalin A. If unfixed odontoblasts were reacted with concanavalin A, redistribution occurred. These observations showed that membrane changes accompanied polarization of odontoblasts.[150] The activity or topographical distribution of cell membrane-bound receptors could be controlled by the extracellular matrix. It was shown that the postmitotic odontoblasts no longer synthesize collagen Type III. Furthermore, fibronectin which surrounds preodontoblasts becomes confined to the apical part of odontoblasts. This leads to modifications of the interactions between matrix components. It is also known that some of these components, at least fibronectin, could interact with the cytoskeleton.[151-153] cAMP could also play a role in polarization and functional differentiation of odontoblasts; cAMP promotes polymerization of platelet tubulin[154] and, in heart muscle cells, a relationship between dibutyryl-cAMP and microtubule organization has been documented.[155]

Odontoblast polarization is followed rapidly by predentin secretion. Polarized nonfunctional odontoblasts are not observed. The relationship between cytological and functional differentiation is not clear. It is not known if specific activities of the cytoskeleton per se can control transcriptional and/or posttranscriptional modifications. This possibility has been stressed in other models. Functional odontoblasts (FO) secrete predentin. This predentin stabilizes these cells by a feedback mechanism.[121]

2. *Ameloblasts*

Enamel will not form in the absence of odontoblasts or dentin. Transplanted ameloblasts lose their cylindrical character and fail to form enamel, unless odontoblasts accompany the transplant.

Characterization of ameloblast terminal differentiation — The terminal differentiation of ameloblasts occurs for each tooth according to the same spatial pattern as for odontoblasts but is delayed for 24 to 36 hr. These cells withdraw from the cell cycle and slowly polarize (Figure 18). The phenotype markers for ameloblast functional differentiation are several proteins: enamelins of about 72,000 daltons and amelogenins of approximately 25,000 to 30,000 daltons (for review see Reference 16).

Terminal differentiation of ameloblasts requires the structural integrity of cytoskeleton — Colchicine, as well as cytochalasin B, inhibits polarization of ameloblasts and interferes with pre-enamel secretion.[118,156] The use of specific antibodies and observations made by indirect immunofluorescence demonstrated a redistribution (apical accumulation) of actin and prekeratin during polarization.[116]

The predentin-dentin layer intervenes in terminal differentiation — Bacterial collagenase was shown to inhibit ameloblast polarization in a reversible manner.[121] The action of L-azetidine 2-carboxylic acid, a proline analogue, on the cytodifferentiation of ameloblasts was also analyzed.[75] The results of morphological, cytological, and functional investigations suggest that the polarization and functional differentiation of these cells are at least partially conditioned by collagen and/or associated glycosaminoglycans of predentin. Wolters[157] also suggested that collagen could have a stabilizing influence on the differentiation of ameloblasts.

Correlation between transfilter recombination experiments and electron microscopic observations suggest that odontoblast cell processes and/or extracellular matrix vesicles in predentin were involved in the programming of preameloblasts to synthesize enamel protein.[158] Using similar techniques, Wolters and Van Mullem[159] concluded that matrix vesicles were not responsible for initiation of ameloblast differentiation. The possible role of direct heterotypic odontoblast-preameloblast cell contacts was also discussed.[160] Kallenbach and Piesco[161] analyzed the changing morphology of epithelium-mesenchyme interface in teeth

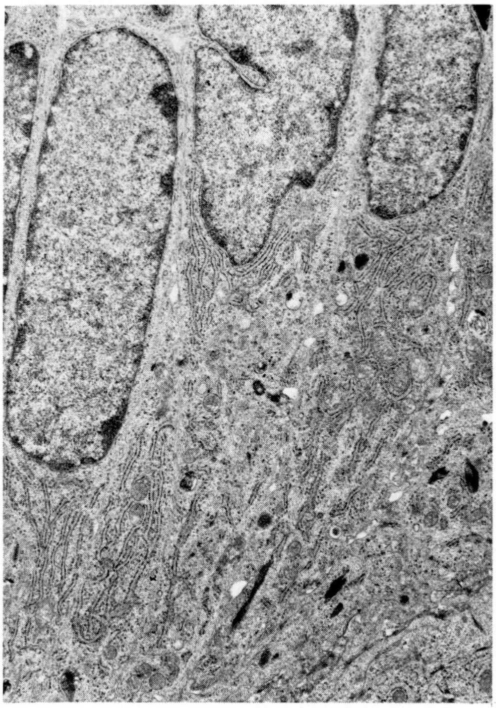

FIGURE 18. Polarizing ameloblasts. (Magnification × 9000.)

from selected vertebrates. After predentin secretion is initiated, preameloblast processes grow through the basal lamina which is progressively eliminated in mammals but not in shark. Dental mesenchymal cells may mediate the degradation of basal lamina by particulate enzymatic activity associated either with matrix vesicles or odontoblast cell processes.[162] It was suggested that heterotypic cell contacts exist at the time when preameloblasts withdraw from the cell cycle.[163]

Enamel-free areas in some molars and asymmetrical enamel secretion in incisors remain to be explained. Recent experiments[143] indicate that mouse molar mesenchyme is able to induce ameloblast differentiation in chick epithelium. Kollar and Fischer[143] suggested that the absence of enamel synthesis in birds is due to alterations in the interactions required for odontogenesis and not to a loss of genetic information. This observation has not been confirmed.[144]

Cell kinetics during terminal differentiation of ameloblasts — Some experimental data suggest that ameloblast terminal differentiation can be achieved only after a minimum number of cell cycles; iso- and heterochronal associations between dental papilla and inner dental epithelium were performed. The terminal differentiation of preameloblasts, associated with polarizing nonfunctional odontoblasts or with predentin, occurred with the same timing. The terminal differentiation of ameloblasts could not be anticipated.[121] As for odontoblasts, it is possible that the genetic program of ameloblasts determines cell kinetic-dependent maturation and sensitivity to epigenetic factors.

VI. CONCLUSION

Complex tissue interactions control tooth morphogenesis and differentiations (see also Reference 164). Odontogenesis results from integration of many different developmental processes. The evolution of each component is influenced by the behavior of the others. Heterotypic and isotypic, direct- and matrix-mediated cell communications exist, allowing each cell to appreciate the functional state and the developmental stage of the others and then to modulate its own state.

The molecular mechanisms involved are still unknown. It seems, however, that the extracellular environment and particularly the basement membrane, i.e., the basal lamina and associated material, influences the specific phenotypic aspects. In several organ systems, it was shown that epithelial-mesenchymal interactions control the composition and structure of the basement membrane, which seem specific for different developmental stages within a particular organ. The changing asymmetric basement membrane may assume multiple developmental functions (for review see Reference 165). During odontogenesis, the basal lamina probably directs cell migration and the basement membrane might control cell kinetics and affect tooth morphogenesis and histogenesis. Terminal differentiation of odontoblasts seems to be triggered by interactions with the basement membrane. Figure 17 summarizes some facts and hypotheses which are in partial agreement with the "membrane impression and gene expression" concept.[166]

It must be emphasized that many of the inferred developmental functions of the basement membrane may be more imaginative than facts. It should be obvious that, although different tooth matrix components have been defined, total macromolecular composition cannot yet be described. Detailed analysis of structural and compositional modifications accompanying odontogenesis have to be performed. The cell surface macromolecules, which are supposed to interact with the extracellular matrix components and the cytoskeleton constituents, will have to be identified. Possible time- and cell kinetic-dependent modifications of these receptors might be correlated with phenotypic cytoskeleton-dependent modifications. The biochemical phenotype of preodontoblasts and odontoblasts, as well as preameloblasts and ameloblasts, should be further elucidated. A great amount of work has to be carried out in order to know how the extracellular matrix controls transcription and translation, and to understand the relationship between histogenesis, morphogenesis, and cytodifferentiation under physiological conditions.

For practical, conceptual, and phylogenetic reasons, the developing tooth provides an accurate tool for analysis of the various aspects of differentiation. Furthermore, several genetic disorders affect odontogenesis.[16,167] Detailed investigations using selected strains should provide interesting information. The author hopes that reading of this incomplete review will encourage young biologists to choose the tooth model.

ACKNOWLEDGMENTS

I thank Dr. V. Karcher-Djuricic, Dr. H. Lesot, Dr.J. M. Meyer, Dr. A. Osman, and Dr. M. Osman, as well as A. Staubli, A. Roux, and N. Stoeffler. The original work reported in this paper was mainly supported by CNRS, INSERM, DGRST, and la Fondation pour la Recherche Médicale Française.

REFERENCES

1. **Schour, I.,** Teeth, in *Analysis of Development,* Willier, Weiss, and Hamburger, Eds., W. B. Saunders, Philadelphia, 1955, 7.
2. **Gaunt, W. A. and Miles, A. E. W.,** Fundamental aspects of tooth morphogenesis, in *Structural and Chemical Organization of Teeth,* Miles, A. E. W., Ed., Academic Press, New York, 1967.
3. **Lavelle, C. L. B., Shellis, R. P., and Poole, D. F. G.,** *Evolutionary Changes to the Primate Skull and Dentition,* Charles C Thomas, Springfield, Ill., 1977.
4. **Butler, P. M. and Joysey, K. A., Eds.,** *Development, Function and Evolution of Teeth,* Academic Press, New York, 1978.
5. **Baume, L. J.,** *The Biology of Pulp and Dentine,* Monographs in Oral Science, S. Karger, Basel, 1980.
6. **Van der Linden, F. P. G. M. and Duterloo, H. S.,** *Development of the Human Dentition, An Atlas,* Harper & Row, New York, 1976.
7. **Hall, B. K.,** *Developmental and Cellular Skeletal Biology,* Academic Press, New York, 1978.
8. **Frank, R. M.,** Electron microscope autoradiography of calcified tissues, *Int. Rev. Cytol.,* 56, 183, 1979.
9. **Linde, A., Bhown, M., and Butler, W. T.,** Non collagenous proteins of dentin, *J. Biol. Chem.,* 255, 5931, 1980.
10. **Lee, S. L. and Veis, A.,** Studies on the structure and chemistry of dentin collagen-phosphophoryn covalent complexes, *Calcif. Tissue Int.,* 31, 123, 1980.
11. **Slavkin, H. C.,** *Embryonic Tooth Formation. A Tool for Developmental Biology,* Oral Sciences Reviews, Melcher, A. H. and Zarb, G. A., Eds., Munksgaard, Copenhagen, 1974.
12. **Grobstein, C.,** Inductive tissue interactions in development, *Adv. Cancer Res.,*4,.187, 1956.
13. **Von Brunn, A.,** Ueber die Ausdehnung des Schmelzorgans und seine Bedeutung fur die Zahnbildung, *Arch. F. Mikr. Anat.,* 29, 367, 1887.
14. **Huggins, C. B., McCarroll, H. R., and Dahlberg, A. A.,** Transplantation of tooth germ elements and the experimental heterotopic formation of dentin and enamel, *J. Exp. Med.,* 60, 199, 1934.
15. **Koch, W.,** In vitro differentiation of tooth rudiments of embryonic mice. I. Transfilter interaction of embryonic tissues, *J. Exp. Zool.,* 165, 155, 1967.
16. **Slavkin, H., Zeichner-David, M., and Siddiqui, M. A. Q.,** Molecular aspects of tooth morphogenesis and differentiation, in *Molecular Aspects Med.,* 4, 125, 1981.
17. **Stone, L. S.,** Further experiments on the extirpation and transplantation of mesectoderm in Amblystoma punctotum, *J. Exp. Zool.,* 44, 95, 1926.
18. **Raven, C. P.,** Zur Entwicklung der Ganglienleiste. I. Die Kinematik der Ganglienleisteentwicklung bei den Urodelen, *Arch. Entwicklungsmech. Org.,* 125, 210, 1932.
19. **Sellman, S.,** Some experiments on the determination of the larval teeth in Amblystoma mexicanum, *Odontol. Tidskr.,* 54, 1, 1946.
20. **Chibon, P.,** Analyse expérimentale de la régionalisation et des capacités morphogénétiques de la crète neurale chez l'amphibien urodèle Pleurodeles Waltlii Michah, *Mem. Soc. Zool. (France),* 36, 1, 1966.
21. **Milaire, J.,** Predifferenciation cytochimique de diverses ébauches céphaliques chez l'embryon de souris, *Arch. Biol. (Liège),* 70, 587, 1959.
22. **Pourtois, M.,** Contribution à l'étude des bourgeons dentaires chez la souris. I. Periodes d'induction et de morphodifférenciation, *Arch. Biol. (Liège),* 72, 17, 1961.
23. **Garant, P. R., Szabo, G., and Nalbandian, J.,** The fine structure of mouse odontoblast, *Arch. Oral. Biol.,* 13, 857, 1968.
24. **Frank, R. M. and Nalbandian, J.,** Ultrastructure of amelogenesis, in *Structural and Chemical Organization of Teeth,* Vol. 1, Miles, A. E. W., Ed., Academic Press, New York, 1967, chap. 10.
25. **Reith, E. J.,** The stages of amelogenesis as observed in molar teeth of young rats, *J. Ultrastruct. Res.,* 30, 111, 1970.
26. **Holland, G. R.,** An ultrastructural survey of cat dentinal tubules, *J. Anat.,* 122, 1, 1976.
27. **Kallenbach, E.,** Fine structure of secretory ameloblasts in the kitten, *Am. J. Anat.,* 148, 479, 1977.
28. **Leblond, C. P. and Warshawsky, A.,** Dynamics of enamel formation in the rat incisor, *J. Dent. Res.,* Spec. issue B, 950, 1979.
29. **Lumsden, A. G. S.,** Pattern formation in the molar dentition of the mouse, *J. Biol. Buccale,* 7, 77, 1979.
30. **Butler, P. M.,** Studies of the mammalian dentition. Differentiation of the post-canine dentition, *Proc. Zool. Soc. Lond.,* B109, 1, 1939.
31. **Butler, P. M.,** Dental merism and tooth development, *J. Dent. Res.,* 46, 845, 1967.
32. **Van Valen, L.,** An analysis of developmental fields, *Dev. Biol.,* 23, 456, 1970.
33. **Butler, P. M.,** The ontogeny of mammalian heterodonty, *J. Biol. Buccale,* 6, 217, 1978.
34. **Wolpert, L.,** Positional information and the spatial pattern of cellular differentiation, *J. Theor. Biol.,* 25, 1, 1969.
35. **Crick, F. H. C.,** Diffusion in embryogenesis, *Nature (London),* 225, 420, 1970.

36. **Summerbell, D., Lewis, J. H., and Wolpert, L.,** Positional information in chick limb morphogenesis, *Nature (London),* 244, 492, 1973.
37. **Osborn, J. W.,** A cladistic interpretation of morphogenesis, *J. Biol. Buccale,* 6, 327, 1978.
38. **Dienstmann, S. R. and Holtzer, H.,** Myogenesis: a cell lineage interpretation, in *Results and Problems in Cell Differentiation,* Vol. 7, Reinert, J. and Holtzer, H., Eds., Springer-Verlag, Berlin, 1977, chap. 1.
39. **Glasstone, S.,** Morphodifferentiation of teeth in embryonic mandibular segments in tissue culture, *J. Dent. Res.,* 46, 611, 1967.
40. **Hay, M. F.,** The development in vivo and in vitro of the lower incisor and molars of the mouse, *Arch. Oral Biol.,* 3, 86, 1961.
41. **Osman, M., Karcher-Djuricic, V., and Ruch, J. V.,** Différenciation in vitro du matériel molaire présomptif de l'embryon de souris, *C. R. Acad. Sci. (Paris),* 289, 149, 1979.
42. **Glasstone, S.,** The development of halved tooth germs. A study in experimental embryology, *J. Anat. (London),* 86, 12, 1952.
43. **Fisher, A. R.,** Morphological development in vitro of the whole and halved lower molar tooth germ of the mouse, *Arch. Oral Biol.,* 16, 1481, 1971.
44. **Gaunt, W. A.,** The development of enamel and dentine of the molar of the mouse with an account of the enamel free areas, *Acta Anat.* 28, 111, 1956.
45. **Butler, P. H.,** The ontogeny of molar pattern, *Biol. Rev.,* 31, 30, 1956.
46. **Osman, A. and Ruch, J. V.,** Répartition topographique des mitoses dans les territoires odontogènes de la mâchoire inférieure de l'embryon de souris, *J. Biol. Buccale,* 3, 117, 1975.
47. **Osman, A. and Ruch, J. V.,** Répartition topographique des mitoses dans l'incisive et la lère molaire inférieures de l'embryon de souris, *J. Biol. Buccale,* 4, 331, 1976.
48. **Osman, A. and Ruch, J. V.,** Contribution à l'étude des paramètres du cycle cellulaire au cours de l'odontogenèse chez la souris, *J. Biol. Buccale,* 6, 43, 1978.
49. **Zajicek, G. and Bar-Lev, M.,** Kinetics of the inner enamel epithelium in the rat incisor. Ic. Experimental results, *Cell Tissue Kinet.,* 4, 163, 1971.
50. **Zajicek, G.,** The rodent incisor tooth proliferon, *Cell Tissue Kinet.,* 9, 207, 1976.
51. **Smith, C. E. and Warshawsky, H.,** Cellular renewal in the enamel organ and the odontoblast layer of the rat incisor as followed by radioautography using ^{3}H-thymidine, *Anat. Rec.,* 183, 523, 1975.
52. **Smith, C. E. and Warshawsky, H.,** Movement of entire cell population during renewal of the rat incisor as shown by radioautography after labelling with ^{3}H-thymidine, *Am. J. Anat.,* 145, 225, 1976.
53. **Starkey, W. E.,** The migration and renewal of tritum-labelled cells in the developing enamel organ of rabbits, *Br. Dent. J.,* 125, 143, 1963.
54. **Olive, M. and Ruch, J. V.,** La différenciation fonctionnelle des odontoblastes d'embryon de Souris implique une synthèse d'ADN sans division cellulaire, *C. R. Acad. Sci. (Paris),* 295, 93, 1982.
55. **Osman, A., and Ruch, J. V.,** Paramètres de la cinétique cellulaire de la première molaire inférieure de l'embryon de souris cultivée in vitro, *C. R. Acad. Sci. (Paris),* 289, 359, 1979.
56. **Snow, M. H. L., Tam, P. P. L., and McLaren, A.,** On the control and regulation of size and morphogenesis in mammalian embryos, in *Levels of Genetic Control in Development,* Subtenly, S. and Abbott, U. K., Eds., A. R. Liss, New York, 1980.
57. **Holtzer, H.,** Discussion, in *Extracellular Matrix Influences on Gene Expression,* Slavkin, H. C. and Greulich, R. C., Eds., Academic Press, New York, 1975, 570.
58. **Saxen, L., Karkinen-Jaaskelainen, M., Lehtonen, E., Nordling, S., and Wartiovaara, J.,** Inductive tissue interactions, in *The Cell Surface in Animal Embryogenesis and Development,* Poste, G and Nicolson, G. L., Eds., North-Holland, Amsterdam, 1976.
59. **Miller, W. A.,** Inductive changes in early tooth development. I. A study of mouse tooth development on the chick chorioallantois, *J. Dent. Res.,* (Suppl. to No. 5), 48, 719, 1969.
60. **Gerber, R., Karcher-Djuricic, V., and Ruch, J. V.,** Materiel presomptif odontogène et de topographie de l'épithelium dentaire dans la mâchoire inférieure de l'embryon de souris, *J. Biol. Buccale* 2, 249, 1974.
61. **Ooë, T.,** On the early development of human dental lamina, *Okajimas Folia Anat. Jpn.,* 30, 197, 1957.
62. **Pearson, A. A.,** The early innervation of the developing decidious teeth, *J. Anat.,* 123, 563, 1977.
63. **Kollar, E. J. and Lumsden, A. G. S.,** Tooth morphogenesis: the role of the innervation during induction and pattern formation, *J. Biol. Buccale,* 7, 49, 1979.
64. **Ruch, J. V., Karcher-Djuricic, V., and Gerber, R.,** Les déterminismes de la morphogenèse et des cytodifférenciations des ébauches dentaires de souris, *J. Biol. Buccale,* 1, 45, 1973.
65. **Dryburgh, L. C.,** Epigenetics of early tooth development in the mouse, *J. Dent. Res.,* 46, 1264, 1967.
66. **Heritier, M. and Deminatti, M.,** Rôle du mésenchyme odontogène dans l'orientation de la morphogenèse coronaire des dents chez la souris, *C. R. Acad. Sci. (Paris),* 271, 851, 1970.
67. **Kollar, E. and Baird, G.,** The influence of the dental papilla in the development of tooth shape in embryonic mouse tooth germs, *J. Embryol. Exp. Morphol.,* 21, 131, 1969.

68. **Kollar, E. and Baird, G.,** Tissue interactions in embryonic mouse tooth germs. I. Reorganization of the dental epithelium during tooth germ reconstruction, *J. Embryol. Exp. Morphol.*, 24, 159, 1970.
69. **Kollar, E. and Baird, G.,** Tissue interactions in embryonic mouse tooth germs. II. The inductive role of the dental papilla, *J. Embryol. Exp. Morphol.*, 24, 173, 1970.
70. **Osman, M., Karcher-Djuricic, V., Ruch, J. V.,** Interactions morphogènes entre constituants dentaires, *Arch. Anat. Microsc. Morphol. Exp.*, 66, 109, 1977.
71. **Grobstein, C. and Cohen, J.,** Collagenase: effect on the morphogenesis of embryonic salivary epithelium in vitro, *Science,* 150, 626, 1965.
72. **Slavkin, H. C. and Greulich, R. G., Eds.,** *Extracellular Matrix Influences on Gene Expression,* Academic Press, New York, 1975.
73. **Kollar, E. J.,** Effects of α,α'-dipyridyl on organ cultures of embryonic mouse tooth germs, *J. Dent. Res.*, 52, 145, 1973.
74. **Kollar, E. J.,** The role of collagen during tooth morphogenesis: some genetic implications, in *Development Formation and Evolution of Teeth,* Butler, P. M. and Joysey, K. A., Eds., Academic Press, New York, 1978.
75. **Ruch, J. V., Fabre, M., Karcher-Djuricic, V., and Stäubli, A.,** The effect of L-azetidine-2-carboxylic acid on dental cytodifferentiation in vitro, *Differentiation,* 2, 211, 1974.
76. **Dye, F. J. and Kollar, E. J.,** Inhibition of mouse molar morphogenesis in vitro by Hadacidin, *Exp. Cell. Biol.*, 46, 152, 1978.
77. **Hurmerinta, K., Thesleff, I., and Saxen, L.,** Inhibition of tooth germ differentiation in vitro by diazo-oxo-norleucine, *J. Embryol. Exp. Morphol.*, 50, 99, 1979.
78. **Thesleff, I. and Pratt, R. M.,** Tunicamycin inhibits mouse tooth morphogenesis and odontoblast differentiation in vitro, *J. Embryol. Exp. Morphol.*, 58, 195, 1980.
79. **Kollar, E. J.,** Tooth development and dental patterning, in *Morphogenesis and Pattern Formation,* Connelly, T. G., Brinkley, L. L., and Carlson, B. M., Eds., Raven Press, New York, 1980.
80. **Slavkin, H. C.,** The nature and structure of epithelial-mesenchymal interactions during tooth morphogenesis, *J. Biol. Buccale,* 6, 189, 1978.
81. **Hurmerinta, K., Thesleff, I., and Saxen, L.,** In vitro inhibition of odontoblast differentiation by vitamin A, *Arch. Oral Biol.*, 25, 385, 1980.
82. **Schiltz, J. R., Rosenbloom, J., and Levenson, G. E.,** The effects of ascorbic acid deficiency on collagen synthesis by mouse molar tooth germs in organ culture, *J. Embryol. Exp. Morphol.*, 37, 49, 1977.
83. **Domm, L. V. and Wellband, W. A.,** Effects of adrenalectomy, thyroidectomy, thyro-adrenalectomy and cortisone on eruption rate of incisors in adult female rats, *Proc. Soc. Exp. Biol. Med.*, 107, 268, 1961.
84. **Chibon, P.,** Vitesse de croissance et renouvellement des dents chez les amphibiens, *J. Embryol. Exp. Morphol.*, 42, 43, 1977.
85. **Hansson, L. E., Stenström, A., and Thorngren, K. G.,** Effect of thyroxine and growth hormone on dentin production in maxillary incisors in the rat, *Scand. J. Dent. Res.*, 86, 169, 1978.
86. **Moss, M. L.,** Analysis of developmental processes possibly related to human dental sexual dismorphism, in *Development Function and Evolution of Teeth,* Butler, P. M. and Joysey, K. A., Eds., Academic Press, New York, 1978.
87. **Ruch, J. V. and Karcher-Djuricic, V.,** Action de la 5-fluoro-deoxyuridine sur la différenciation in vitro de molaires d'embryons de souris, *Arch. Biol.*, 82, 115, 1971.
88. **Nogueira, T. O., Stene, T., and Koppang, H. S.,** Long-term effects of colchicine on dentinogenesis in rat incisors, *Scand. J. Dent. Res.*, 88, 15, 1980.
89. **Osborn, J. W.,** The control of tooth shape, *J. Dent. Res.*, IADR Abstr. 50, 57, 1975.
90. **Osman, M., Karcher-Djuricic, V., and Ruch, J. V.,** Rôle de la pulpe dentaire dans l'histogenèse de l'organe adamantin, *C. R. Soc. Biol.*, 173, 730, 1979.
91. **Olive, M. and Ruch, J. V.,** Does the basement membrane control the mitotic activity of the inner dental epithelium of the embryonic mouse first lower molar? *Dev. Biol.*, 93, 301, 1982.
92. **Slavkin, H. C., Beierle, J., and Bavetta, L. A.,** Odontogenesis: cell-cell interactions in vitro, *Nature (London),* 217, 269, 1968.
93. **Orams, H. J., Sim, F. R. P., and Reade, P. C.,** An in vivo and in vitro study of dissociated tooth germs of rats, *Arch. Oral Biol.*, 19, 288, 1974.
94. **Kollar, E. J.,** The development of the integuement: spatial, temporal and phylogenetic events, *Am. Zoologist,* 12, 125, 1972.
95. **Frank, R. M..** Etude autoradiographique de la dentinogenèse en microscopie électronique à l'aide de la proline tritiée chez le chat, *Arch. Oral Biol.*, 15, 583, 1970.
96. **Garant, P. R., Szabo, G., and Nalbandian, J.,** The fine structure of mouse odontoblast, *Arch. Oral Biol.*, 13, 857, 1968.
97. **Weinstock, M. and Leblond, C. P.,** Synthesis, migration and release of precursor collagen by odontoblasts as visualized by radioautography after 3H-proline administration, *J. Cell. Biol.*, 60, 92, 1974.

98. **Karim, A., Cournil, I., and Leblond, C. P.,** Immunohistochemical localization of procollagen. II. Electron microscopic distribution of procollagen. I. Antigenicity in the odontoblast and predentin of rat incisor teeth by a indirect method using peroxydase linked antibodies, *J. Histochem. Cytochem.*, 27, 1070, 1979.
99. **Lesot, H.,** Collagen type I trimer synthesis by cultured embryonic mouse molars, *Eur. J. Biochem.*, 116, 541, 1981.
100. **Lesot, H. and Ruch, J. V.,** Analyse des types de collagène synthétisés par l'ébauche dentaire et ses constituants dissociés chez l'embryon de souris, *Biol. Cell*, 34, 23, 1979.
101. **Munksgaard, E. C., Rhodes, M., Mayne, R., and Butler, W. F.,** Collagen synthesis and secretion by rat incisors odontoblasts in organ culture, *Eur. J. Biochem.*, 82, 609, 1976.
102. **Lesot, H., Osman, M., and Ruch, J. V.,** Immunofluorescent localization of collagens, fibronectin and laminin during terminal differentiation of odontoblasts, *Dev. Biol.*, 82, 371, 1981.
103. **Thesleff, I., Stenman, S., Vaheri, I., and Timpl, R.,** Changes in the matrix proteins, fibronectin and collagen during differentiation of mouse tooth germs, *Dev. Biol.*, 70, 116, 1979.
104. **Baume, L. I.,** The biology of pulp and dentine, *Monographs in Oral Science*, Myers, H. M., Ed., S. Karger, Basel, 1980.
105. **Linde, A.,** Glycosaminoglycans of the odontoblast-predentin layer in dentinogenically active porcine teeth, *Calcif. Tissue Res.*, 12, 281, 1973.
106. **Butler, W. T., Finch, J. E., and Desteno, C. V.,** Chemical characters of proteins in rat incisors, *Biochim. Biophys. Acta*, 257, 167, 1972.
107. **Veis, A. and Schlueter, R. J.,** The macromolecular organization of dentin matrix collagen. I. Characterization of dentin collagen, *Biochemistry*, 3, 1650, 1964.
108. **Hjerpe, S. and Engfeldt, B.,** Proteoglycans of dentin and predentin, *Calcif. Tissue Res.*, 2, 173, 1976.
109. **Jones, L. and Leaver, A. G.,** Glycosaminoglycans of human dentin, *Calcif. Tissue Res.*, 16, 37, 1974.
110. **Lazarides, E. and Weber, K.,** Actin antibody: the specific visualization of actin filaments in non muscle cells, *Proc. Natl. Acad. Sci. U.S.A.*, 71, 226, 1974.
111. **Brinkley, B. R., Fistel, S. H., Marcum, J. M., and Pardue, R. L.,** Microtubules in cultured cells: indirect immunofluorescence microscopy with cultured cells, *Int. Rev. Cytol.*, 63, 59, 1970.
112. **Franke, W. W., Schmid, E., Osborn, M., and Weber, K.,** Different intermediate size filaments distinguished by immunofluorescence microscopy, *Proc. Natl. Acad. Sci. U.S.A.*, 75, 5034, 1978.
113. **Weber, K. and Osborn, M.,** Microtubules and intermediate filament networks in cells viewed by immunofluorescence microscopy, in *Cell Surface Reviews*, Vol. 7, Post, G. and Nicolson, G. I., Eds., Biomedical Press, Amsterdam, 1983.
114. **Lazarides, E.,** Intermediate filaments as mechanical integrators of cellular space, *Nature (London)*, 283, 249, 1980.
115. **Bennet, G. S., Fellini, S. A., Croop, J. M., Otto, J. J., Bryan, J., and Holtzer, H.,** Differences among 100 A filament subunits from different cell types, *Proc. Natl. Acad. Sci. U.S.A.*, 75, 4364 1978.
116. **Lesot, H., Meyer, J. M., Ruch, J. V., Weber, K., and Osborn, M.,** Immunofluorescent localization of vimentin, prekeratin and actin during odontoblast and ameloblast differentiation, *Differentiation*, 21, 133, 1982.
117. **Garant, P. R.,** The organization of microtubules within rat odontoblast processes revealed by perfusion fixation with glutaraldehyde, *Arch. Oral Biol.*, 17, 1047, 1972.
118. **Ruch, J. V., Karcher-Djuricic, V., Staubli, A., and Fabre, M.,** Effets de la cytochalasine B et de la colchicine sur les cytodifferenciations dentaires in vitro, *Arch. Anat. Microscop. Morphol. Exp.*, 64, 113, 1975.
119. **Ruch, J. V., Karcher-Djuricic, V., and Thiebold, J.,** Cell division and cytodifferentiation of odontoblasts, *Differentiation*, 5, 165, 1976.
120. **Ruch, J. V. and Karcher-Djuricic, V.,** Mise en évidence d'un rôle spécifique de l'épithelium adamantin dans la différenciation et le maintien des odontoblastes, *Ann. Embryol. Morphol.*, 4, 359, 1971.
121. **Ruch, J. V., Karcher-Djuricic, V., and Gerber, R.,** Quelsques aspects du rôle de la prédentine dans la différenciation des adamantoblastes, *Arch. Anat. Microscop. Morphol. Exp.*, 61, 127, 1972
122. **Schwartz, S. A. and Kirsten, W. H.,** Tissue specific suppression of differentiation by 5-bromodeoxyuridine in vitro, *J. Dent. Res.*, 53, 509, 1973.
123. **Ruch, J. V., Karcher-Djuricic, V., Osman, M., Meyer, J. M. and Lesot, H.,** Action of 5-bromodeoxyuridine on tooth germs in vitro. I. Effects on cytodifferentiation, *J. Biol. Buccale*, 6, 267, 1978.
124. **Lesot, H., Karcher-Djuricic, V., Osman, M., and Ruch, J. V.,** Action of 5-bromodeoxyuridine on tooth germs in vitro. II. Effects on collagen synthesis, *J. Biol. Buccale*, 6, 281, 1978.
125. **Thesleff, I., Lehtonen, E., and Saxen, L.,** Basement membrane formation in transfilter tooth culture and its relation to odontoblast differentiation, *Differentiation*, 10, 71, 1978.
126. **Karcher-Djuricic, V., Osman, M., Meyer, J. M., Staubli, A., and Ruch, J. V.,** Basement membrane reconstitution and cytodifferentiation of odontoblasts in isochronal and heterochronal reassociation of enamel organs and pulps, *J. Biol. Buccale*, 6, 257, 1978.

127. **Osman, M. and Ruch, J. V.,** Secretion of basal lamina by trypsin isolated embryonic mouse molar epithelia cultured in vitro, *Dev. Biol.,* 75, 467, 1980.
128. **Slavkin, H. C., Matosian, O., Wilson, O. P., Bringas, P., Mino, W., Croissant, R. D. and Guenther, H.,** Epithelial specific extracellular matrix influences on mesenchyme collagen biosynthesis in vitro, in *Extracellular Matrix Influences on Gene Expression,* Slavkin, H. C. and Greulich, R. C., Eds., Academic Press, New York, 1975.
129. **Frank, R. M., Osman, M., Meyer, J. M., and Ruch, J. V.,** 3H-glucosamine electron microscope autoradiography after isolated labelling of the enamel organ or the dental papilla followed by reassociated tooth germ culture, *J. Biol. Buccale,* 7, 225, 1979.
130. **Osman, M. and Ruch, J. V.,** 3H-glucosamine and 3H-proline radioautography of embryonic mouse dental basement membrane, *J. Craniofacial Genet., Dev. Biol.,* 1, 95, 1981.
131. **Osman, M. and Ruch, J. V.,** Behavior of odontoblasts and basal lamina of trypsin or EDTA isolated mouse dental papilla in short term culture, *J. Dent. Res.,* 60, 1015, 1981.
132. **Manasek, J. F.,** The extracellular matrix: a dynamic component of the developing embryo, *Curr. Top. Dev. Biol.,* 10, 35, 1975.
133. **Thesleff, I., Barrach, M. J., Foidart, J. M., Vaheri, A., Pratt, R. M., and Martin, G. R.,** Changes in the distribution of type IV collagen, laminin, proteoglycan and fibronectin during mouse tooth development, *Dev. Biol.,* 81, 182, 1981.
134. **Meyer, J. M., Staubli, A., and Ruch, J. V.,** Ruthenium red staining and tannic acid fixation of dental basement membrane, *Cell Tissue Res.,* 220, 589, 1981.
135. **Cohn, R. L., Banerjee, S. D., and Bernfield, M. R.,** Basal lamina of embryonic salivary epithelia, nature of glycosaminoglycan and organization of extracellular materials, *J. Cell. Biol.,* 73, 464, 1977.
136. **Howell, S. L. and Whitfield, M.,** Cytochemical localization of adenyl cyclase activity in rat islets of Langerhans, *J. Histochem. Cytochem.,* 20, 873, 1972.
137. **Kempen, H. J. M., de Pont, J. J. H. H. M., Bonting, S. L., and Stadhouders, A. M.,** The cytochemical localization of adenylate cyclase: fact or artefact, *J. Histochem. Cytochem.,* 26, 298, 1978.
138. **Osman, M., Meyer, J. M., Staubli, A., and Ruch, J. V.,** Cytochemical localization of adenylate cyclase in embryonic mouse molars, *Acta Histochem.,* 68, 91, 1981.
139. **Kelly, R. O., Palmer, G. C., Crissman, H., and Nilson, J. H.,** Interactions of glycosaminoglycan and adenylate cyclase at the surface of cultured human diploid fibroblast, *J. Cell. Sci.,* 28, 237, 1977.
140. **Olive, M. and Ruch, J. V.,** Effects of diazo-oxo-norleucine on cell kinetics and odontoblast differentiation in cultured embryonic mouse molars, *Arch. Oral. Biol.,* 27, 505, 1982.
141. **Thesleff, I. and Pratt, R. M.,** Tunicamycin-induced alterations in basement membrane formation during odontoblast differentiation, *Dev. Biol.,* 80, 175, 1980.
142. **Karcher-Djuricic, V. and Ruch, J. V.,** Culture d'associations interspécifiques de constituants mandibulaires d'embryons de souris et de poulet, *C. R. Soc. Biol.,* 167, 915, 1973.
143. **Kollar, E. J. and Fischer, C.,** Tooth induction in chick epithelium, expression of quiescent genes for enamel synthesis, *Science,* 207, 993, 1980.
144. **Slavkin, H. C., Cummings, E., Bringas, P., and Honig, L. S.,** Epithelial derived basal lamina regulation of mesenchymal cell differentiation in *Proc. Int. Soc. Dev. Biologists IX Congr.,* Weber, R. and Burger, M., Eds., Alan R. Liss, New York, 1982.
145. **Cummings, E. G., Bringas, P., Grodin, M. S., and Slavkin, H. C.,** Epithelial-directed mesenchyme differentiation in vitro, model of murine odontoblast differentiation mediated by quail epithelia, *Differentiation,* 20, 1, 1981.
146. **Banerjee, S. D., Cohn, R. H., and Bernfield, M. R.,** Basal lamina of embryonic salivary epithelia. Production by the epithelium and role in maintaining lobular morphology, *J. Cell. Biol.,* 78, 445, 1977.
147. **Brownell, A. G., Bessem, C. C., and Slavkin, H. C.,** Possible functions of mesenchyme cell-derived fibronectin during formation of basal lamina, *Proc. Natl. Acad. Sci. U.S.A.,* 78, 3711, 1981.
148. **Ruch, J. V., Lesot, H., Karcher-Djuricic, V., Meyer, J. M., and Olive, M.,** Facts and hypothesis concerning the control of odontoblast differentiation, *Differentiation,* 21, 7, 1982.
149. **Ruch, J. V. and Karcher-Djuricic, V.,** On odontogenic tissue interactions, in *Extracellular Matrix Influences on Gene Expression,* Slavkin, H. C. and Greulich, R. C., Eds., Academic Press, New York, 1975.
150. **Meyer, J. M., Staubli, A., and Ruch, J. V.,** Ultrastructural localization of concanavalin A binding sites on the surface of differentiating odontoblasts, *Biol. Cell,* 42, 193, 1981.
151. **Bornstein, P., Duskin, D., Balian, C., Davidson, J. M., and Crouch, E.,** Organization of extracellular proteins on the connectine tissue cell surface: relevance to cell-matrix interactions in vitro and in vivo, *Ann. N.Y. Acad. Sci.,* 312, 99, 1978.
152. **Heggeness, M. H., Ash, J. F., and Singer, S. J.,** Transmembrane linkage of fibronectin to intracellular actin-containing filaments in cultured human fibroblasts, *Ann. N.Y. Acad. Sci.,* 312, 414, 1978.
153. **Yamada, K. M., Olden, K., and Hahn, L. H. E.,** Cell surface protein and cell interactions, in *The Cell Surface: Mediator of Developmental Processes,* Subtenly, S. and Wessells, N. K., Eds., Academic Press, New York, 1980.

154. **Steiner, M.,** 3′-5′ cyclic AMP binds to and promotes polyassociation of platlet tubulin, *Nature (London),* 272, 834, 1978.
155. **Nath, K., Shay, J. W., and Bollon, A. P.,** Relationship between dibutyryl cyclic AMP and microtubules organization in contracting heart muscle cells, *Proc. Natl. Acad. Sci. U.S.A.,* 75, 319, 1978.
156. **Moe, H. and Mikkelsen, H.,** Light microscopical and ultrastructural observations on the effect of vinblastine on ameloblasts of rat incisors in vivo, *Acta Pathol. Microbiol. Scand. (Sect. A),* 85, 73, 1977.
157. **Wolters, J. M. L.,** The transfilter transmission of 3H-proline labeled material in cultured rat tooth germs, *Arch. Oral Biol.,* 23, 51, 1978.
158. **Slavkin, H. C., Bringas, P., Croissant, R., and Bavetta, L. A.,** Epithelial-mesenchymal interactions during odontogenesis. II. Intercellular matrix vesicles, *Mech. Ageing Dev.,* 1, 139, 1972.
159. **Wolters, J. M. L. and Van Mullem, P. J.,** Electron microscopy of epithelio-mesenchyme intercellular communication in transfilter cultures of rat tooth germ, *Arch. Oral. Biol.,* 22, 705, 1978.
160. **Slavkin, H. C. and Bringas, P.,** Epithelial-mesenchyme interactions during odontogenesis. IV. Morphological evidence for direct heterotypic cell-cell contact, *Dev. Biol.,* 50, 428, 1976.
161. **Kallenbach, E. and Piesco, N. P.,** The changing morphology of the epithelium-mesenchyme interface in the differentiation zone of growing teeth of selected vertebrate and its relationship to possible mechanisms of differentiation, *J. Biol. Buccale,* 6, 229, 1978.
162. **Slavkin, H. C., Trump, G. N., Brownell, A. G., and Sorgente, N.,** Epithelial-mesenchymal interactions: mesenchymal specificity, in *Cell and Tissue Interactions,* Lash, J. W., Ed., Raven Press, New York, 1977.
163. **Meyer, J. M., Fabre, M., Staubli, A., and Ruch, J. V.,** Relations cellulaires au cours de l'odontogenèse, *J. Biol. Buccale,* 5, 107, 1977.
164. **Thesleff, I. and Hurmerinta, K.,** Tissue interactions in tooth development, *Differentiation,* 18, 75, 1981.
165. **Kefalides, N. A., Ed.,** Biology and chemistry of basement membranes, in *Proc. 1st Int. Symp. Biol. Chem. of Basement Membrane,* Academic Press, New York, 1978.
166. **Brunner, G.,** Membrane impression and gene expression, *Differentiation,* 8, 123, 1977.
167. **Mider, N. A.,** The dentitions of tabby and crinkled mice (an upset in mesodermal:ectodermal interaction), in *Development, Function and Evolution of Teeth,* Butler, P. M. and Joysey, K. A., Eds., Academic Press, New York, 1978.

Chapter 4

ULTRASTRUCTURE OF DENTIN AND DENTINOGENESIS

Sheila J. Jones and Alan Boyde

TABLE OF CONTENTS

I. INTRODUCTION

Ultrastructural studies of dentinogenesis rely on two main methods of microscopy: transmission electron microscopy (TEM) and scanning electron microscopy (SEM). Each method may be amplified by different ancillary techniques that extend its range of investigative power. TEM enables one to sample very small slices of the tissue at high magnification but its usefulness is limited by its sampling rate. However, it is preeminent in the investigation of ultrastructural details of cells such as odontoblasts. SEM cannot provide the high resolution of TEM but scores on its excellent sampling rate, its greater depth of focus, and its versatility. It is the tool of choice to unravel the complex three-dimensional organization of the matrix of calcified tissues such as dentin. Our task with both methods is to interpret the artifacts we have created in the terms of living biology. It is an uncompleted task as the following exposition shows.

II. ODONTOBLASTS

A. Differentiation of Odontoblasts

Odontoblasts (Figures 1 to 6) differentiate from ectomesenchymal cells adjacent to the inner enamel epithelial cells.[1] A *basal lamina*, adherent microfibrils, dense aggregates, and amorphous electron dense material separate the two cell layers.[2] Slavkin and colleagues[3,4] have proposed that these extracellular matrix macromolecules, produced by the two sets of cells, participate in the morphogenetic processes during their differentiation. In particular, they have stressed the importance of the mesenchymal side of the basal lamina, with its associated microfibrils, in the epithelial-mesenchymal interactions that accompany differentiation of odontoblasts and dentinogenesis.[5] Several substances may contribute to the morphogenetic influence of this layer. Kollar[6] found that normal collagen synthesis was necessary for odontoblast differentiation although collagenase does not always seem to disrupt the process,[7] and others cite evidence for an important role for glycoproteins and glycosaminoglycans.[8] The nonbanded fine fibrils attached to the basal lamina are probably proteoglycans.[9] Contact between the susceptible differentiating cells and the extracellular layer is essential,[10] and Slavkin and colleagues[3,5,11-13] have suggested a role for extracellular RNA and matrix vesicles as morphogens.

Once the basal lamina is breached by the preameloblasts,[14] direct contact is made between the finger-like projections of the preameloblast and the processes of the odontoblast. These junctions are considered to provide morphological evidence for *epithelial-mesenchymal interaction*.[15]

The sequence of events may be summarized thus: the secretion of a basal lamina by inner enamel epithelial cells, differentiation of *preodontoblasts* (from mesectodermal cells) which send long cell processes toward the epithelial cells, followed by differentiation of odontoblasts from the preodontoblasts.[16] The last stage is characterized by cessation of cell division, elongation of the cell, polarization, and synthesis and secretion of *predentin* matrix components[17] (Figure 3). Additionally, it has been mooted that the preodontoblast is responsible for degradation of the basal lamina by enzyme secretion from cell processes or via matrix vesicles[18] because the basal lamina disintegrates before there is direct contact between the two layers of cells.[10]

As the odontoblasts retreat from the epithelial layer, their *processes* (Figures 4 to 8) become encased in the matrix of collagen, phosphoproteins, proteoglycans, glycoproteins,

FIGURE 1. (Above) Early dentinogenesis in rat molar, TEM. EO = enamel organ, OP = odontoblast process. Note peripheral fine fibers perpendicular to basement membrane and fine mineral particle clusters. (Magnification × 32,000.) (Below) Longitudinally sectioned odontoblasts. (Magnification × 5000.) (Courtesy of Professor Edward J. Reith.)

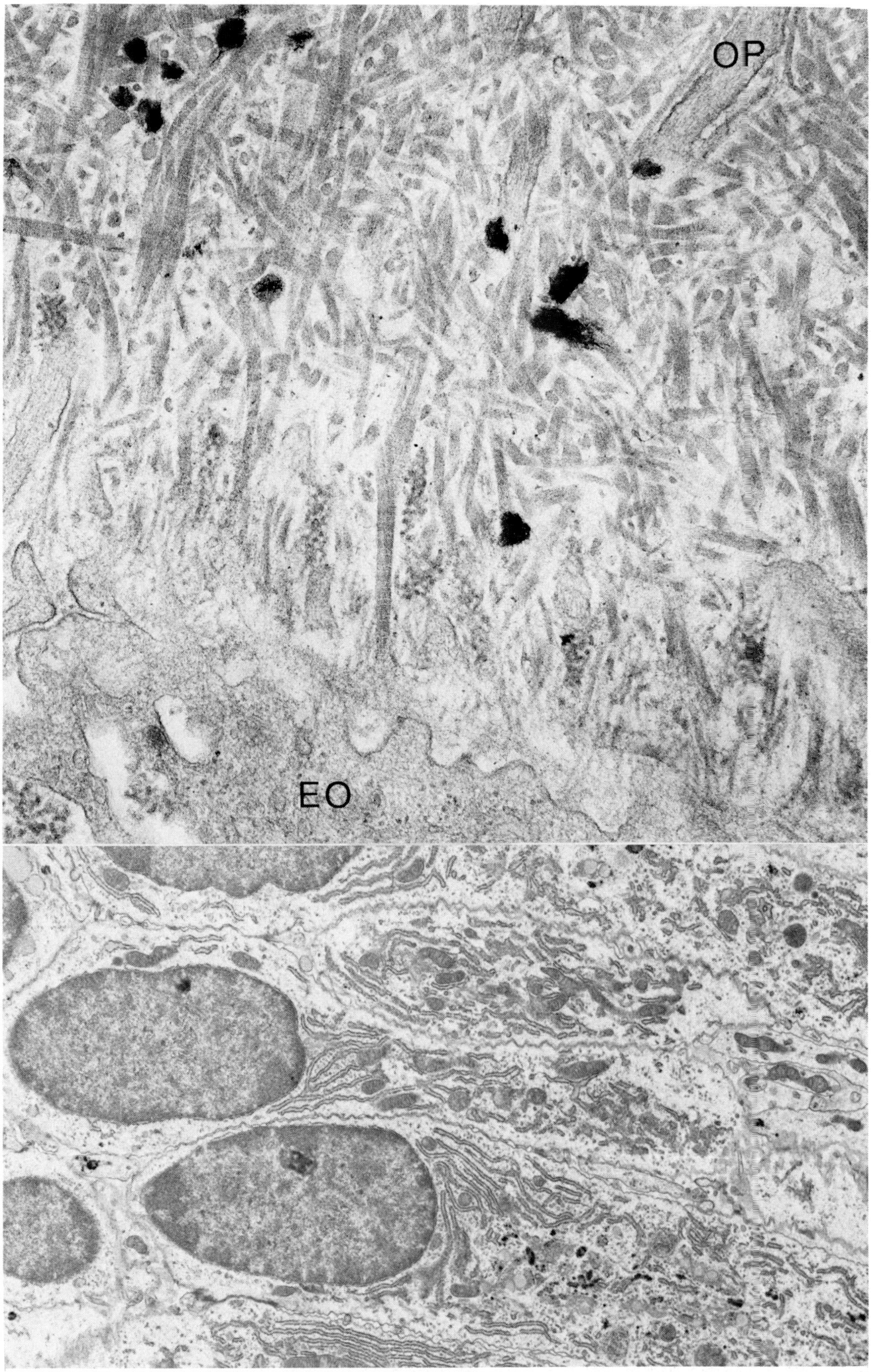

FIGURE 1.

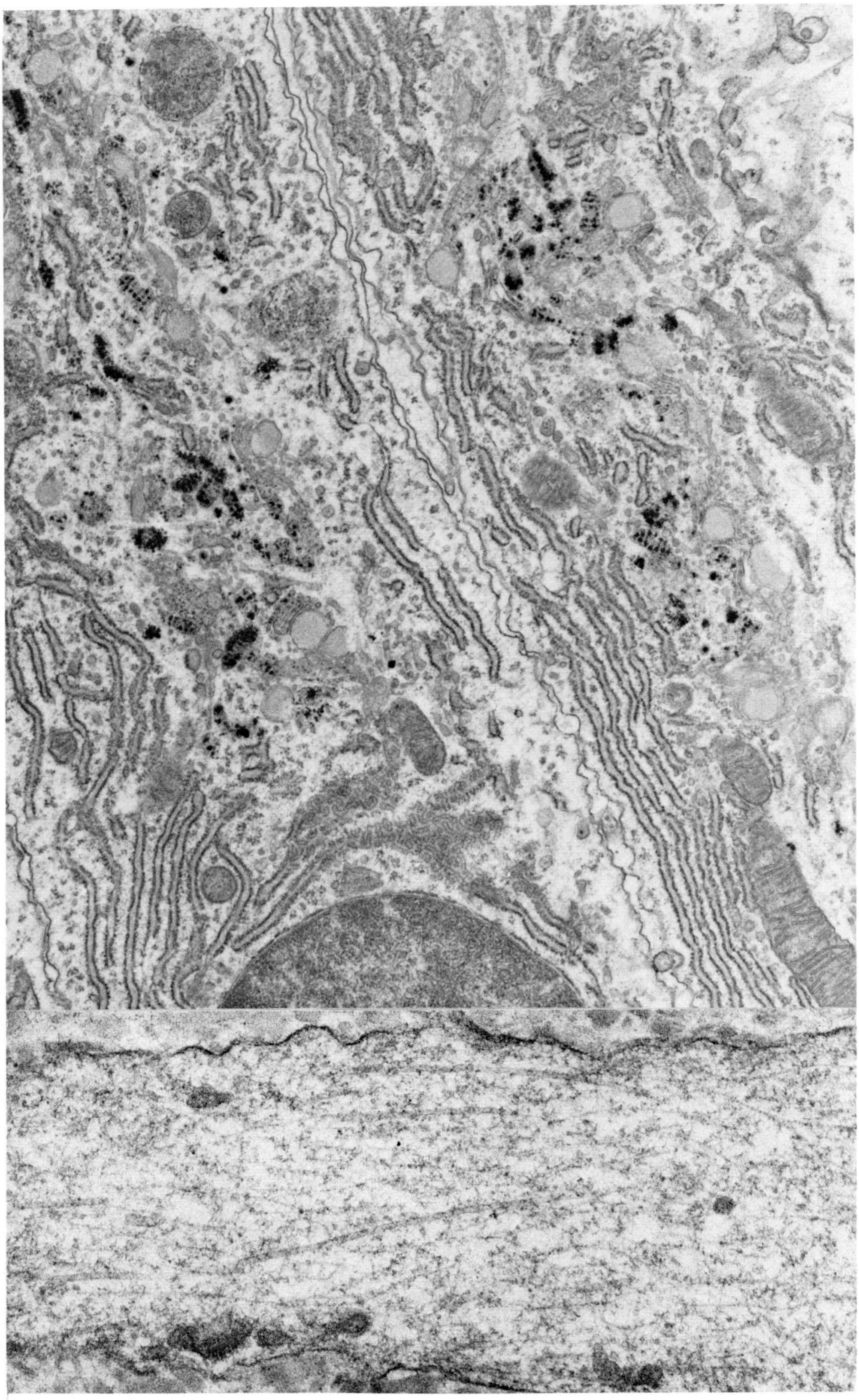

FIGURE 2.

and phospholipids that are being secreted. The odontoblasts gradually acquire the full complement of organelles of actively secreting, matrix-forming cells.[19] They become organized into a coherent layer, each cell fastened to its neighbors apically by a junctional complex. The formation of the structural features of the *terminal bar apparatus* marks the final phase of full differentiation and separates spatially the two main functions of the odontoblasts, synthesis occurring in the cell body and secretion via the cell processes. Although the major synthetic effort is the formation of the components of the intercellular matrix for export from the cell, a not inconsiderable tax on the biosynthetic apparatus is applied by the elongation of the cell process itself involving a significant increase in total cell volume. The differentiation of preodontoblasts, as assessed by mitotic rates in the cervical tissues of rat incisors, shows a circadian rhythm,[20] but the controlling factors have not been studied or analyzed.

B. The Functioning Fully Differentiated Odontoblast

1. The Cell Body

The structure of the typical odontoblast midway through dentinogenesis has been reviewed by Leblond and Weinstock[21] and Frank.[22] There appears to be little difference between the odontoblasts of rodents, cat and man,[22] and there is a good consensus of opinion on their cytological features. The odontoblast (Figures 1 and 2) is an elongated cell with its nucleus at the basal end. Parallel stacks of rough *endoplasmic reticulum,* aligned parallel with the length of the cell, are present at the apical side of the nucleus and at the apical end of the cell on either side of the *Golgi apparatus*. This latter structure is prominent in odontoblasts and has several stacks of flattened sacculi. These connect at the forming face of the cisternae with the rough endoplasmic reticulum. Distended saccules occur at the mature surface of the apparatus and free vesicles or secretory granules are seen nearby in the cytoplasm. These are like the ones found in the apical regions of the cell and in the odontoblast process. Exocytosis of *secretory granules* is believed to take place at these latter sites. An extensive morphological classification of the types of vesicles seen in odontoblasts was proposed by Nagai.[23]

Apical junctions between cells isolate the intercellular space from that of the predentin and dentin which house the odontoblast process[24] (Figures 4 and 6 to 9). The latter elongates synchronously with the pulpward retreat of the odontoblasts. Transverse microfibrils at the level of the *terminal web* mark morphologically the separation of cell body and cell process.

Electron microscope radioautographs using labeled proline have been used to demonstrate the pathway of collagen secretion.[22,25] The label first appeared solely in the rough endoplasmic reticulum, then in the Golgi apparatus, and finally in presecretory and secretory granules before appearing in the predentin, presumably after exocytosis. This entire process was completed in 4 hr in the rat. Labeled proline did not appear in the dentin for approximately a day.

Other organic components of dentin show a similar pathway but are incorporated in dentin more rapidly. Phosphoproteins, glycoproteins, and proteoglycans accumulate in dentin within minutes rather than days, passing rapidly through the predentin to the dentin border where they are incorporated as mineralization proceeds. Since these substances rapidly accumulate at the border zone for calcification, it has been suggested that they may play a regulatory role in that process.[21,26,27] Hypophosphatemia is associated with interglobular dentin and it is possible that this is due to an impairment of phosphoprotein production.[28] We still await ultrastructural studies showing the pathway of phosphoprotein production and delivery under normal and hypophosphatemic conditions.

FIGURE 2. (Above) Higher magnification of middle portion of odontoblast cell body. (Magnification × 16,150.) (Below) Portion of odontoblast process in predentin of rat molar. (Magnification × 48,000.) (Courtesy of Professor Edward J. Reith.)

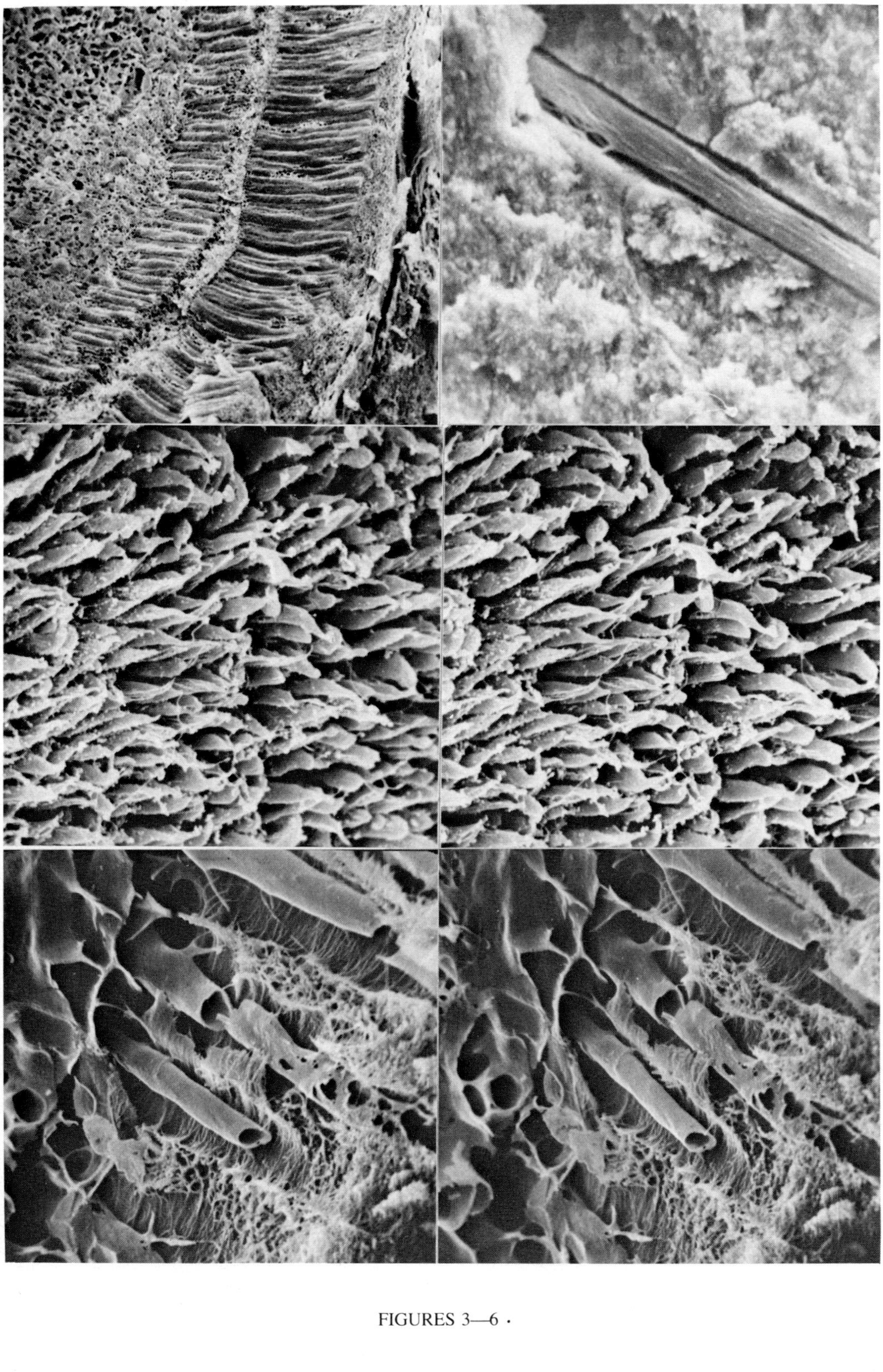

FIGURES 3—6 ·

Odontoblasts do not divide, even in conditions that would be expected to provide the maximum stimulation.[29] This is curious, for it is possible to induce osteoblasts, perhaps the cells most akin to odontoblasts, to "dedifferentiate" and divide although they too are generally considered to be in a postmitotic state.[30] Recruitment of new odontoblasts does occur, but the identity of the precursor cell and the processes controlling recruitment remain obscure and intriguing.

The ultrastructural details of the terminal bar apparatus have been described by Garant et al.,[31] Frank,[32] and Goldberg et al.[24] Scattered intercellular contacts comprising *desmosomes, gap,* and *tight junctions* also occur between odontoblasts.[33] SEM evidence suggests that the *junctional complex* forms a continuous and effective mechanical seal.[34]

Tetracycline entry into dentin is as slow as its entry into enamel beneath striated border maturation zone ameloblasts. The latter each have a complete distal terminal bar apparatus. In contrast, the transitional nonstriated border ameloblasts at the border regions between the striated border and smooth-ended type of cell do not have a complete apparatus and allow immediate access for tetracycline.[35]

Goldberg and colleagues[24] considered that the arrangement of the desmosomal and gap junctions between rat odontoblasts would still allow a passage between the cells for the diffusion of calcium and serum-derived matrix components.

Capillaries from the subodontoblastic region may extend between the odontoblasts, but do not cross the barrier of the terminal bar apparatus during most mammalian dentinogenesis.[34] Jessen[36] found capillaries to weave between rat odontoblasts at a level of about 10 μm from the predentin surface. This considerably reduces the blood-predentin distances for the transport of ions and other substances.

2. *The Odontoblast Process*

The odontoblast process has fewer cytological features than the cell body. Its structure reflects its secretory role[37] and it is therefore devoid of the synthetic organelles that are a feature of the cell body of the odontoblast.[38] The features present show an arrangement that reflects its own elongated form.[39] Reith[38] reported that the base of the odontoblast process contains fine filaments and microtubules. Fine filaments and microtubules were also found throughout the length of the process, but only microfilaments were constant features of the side branches (Figure 4).

Reith[38] also observed dense bodies, smooth and coated vesicles, and occasionally small granules. His findings were paralleled by Katchburian and Holt,[40] who reported acid phosphatase activity in the dense bodies and vesicles and an extensive lysosomal system, and by Frank.[32] Costacurta and colleagues[41] also found polyribosomes in the process in addition to vesicles containing electron dense material. Proteoglycans have been identified in elongated secretory vesicles by histochemistry, and these have been shown to be associated with microtubules.[42] Mitochondria are observed only as rarities in odontoblast processes in contrast with secretory granules, dense bodies, large bristle-coated vesicles, and smooth membrane structures which are common.[25,36]

Two types of vesicles that fuse with the cell membrane of the odontoblast process have been described by Frank.[22] One type was an elongated, rod-shaped vesicle containing dense

FIGURE 3 (Upper left). Pulp (left), odontoblasts, thin layer of dentin matrix, and preameloblasts in freeze-fractured, freeze-dried (FD), fresh unfixed rat incisor, dry-dissected. (Magnification × 420.) FIGURE 4 (Upper right). Freeze-fractured, critical point dried (CPD), prolonged glutaraldehyde-fixation, human premolar dentin. Slight shrinkage of odontoblast process has emphasized cytoskeleton. (Magnification × 4200.) FIGURE 5 (Center). Stereopair. Rat incisor odontoblasts, fixed 2% OsO_4 in boric acid borate buffer, CPD, and dry-dissected. Distal ends of odontoblasts, which were previously in contact with predentin, and first part of process still adherent to a few cells. (Magnification × 1550.) FIGURE 6 (Below). Stereopair. Freeze-fractured, freeze-dried, fresh, unfixed rat upper incisor odontoblasts and predentin. Ice crystal growth in center of odontoblast processes pushes cytoplasmic components to periphery creating a hollow center. (Magnification × 7700.)

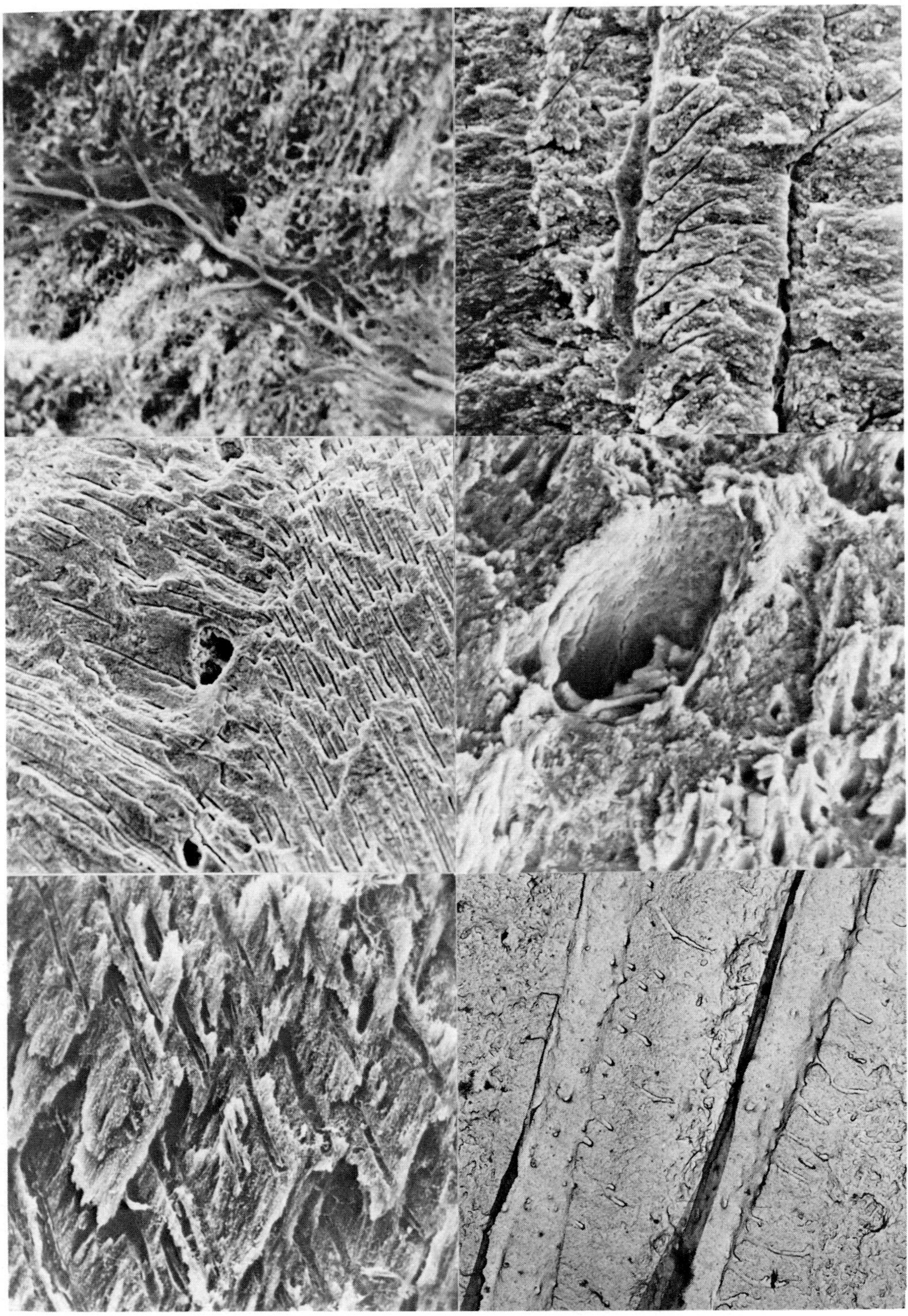

FIGURES 7—12.

filamentous and granular material. The others were coated vesicles, thought to be involved in pinocytosis. Frank[22] observed that one could not tell whether or not one secretory granule might carry both collagen precursors and noncollagenous proteins.

The shape and size of the neck region (Figure 13) of the odontoblast process varies between species and at different stages of dentinogenesis.[43] This will affect the orientation of the fibrous elements in the predentin. The junction between the process and the cell body may be long and smoothly tapered (Figure 5) or short and abrupt. The former shape is often found in fast dentin formation while the latter is associated with slower formation. The diameter of tubules, and presumably of the processes that they formed around, is narrower in the root than the crown in the cat[43] and in man,[44] and this may also be ascribed in part to a slower secretory rate.

There is a terminal arborization of the odontoblast processes below the enamel-dentin and cement-dentin junctions (Figure 7). The end branches may be very fine or rather distended, and may also arch through the peripheral dentin. Backscattered electron images of a plane in the dentin readily display their rich variety of form.

The odontoblast processes have numerous side branches (Figures 7 and 8) leaving the main stem either at right angles or making an acute angle with the distal extension. These offshoots themselves frequently branch, and may connect with the lateral branches of other odontoblasts. Their diameter is best judged by the lumen of the tubuli that house them. Because most are below the level of the resolution of the light microscope, the frequency of the branching can be determined most reliably from examining the internal surface of tubules that are lined with peritubular dentin by scanning electron microscopy. The homogeneous sheet of peritubular dentin is seen to be perforated by minute holes leading into the intertubular regions, and the number of side branches of the first order may therefore be assayed at high magnification with accuracy.

In conjunction with other histological markers, such as the amount and distribution of peritubular dentin and mantle dentin, the numbers of side branches, the angle they form with the main stem, and the numbers of anastomoses could be used to identify different mammalian orders.

The structural elements of the odontoblast process are essential for its secretory function[42] and may also be the elements responsible for alignment of the maturing extracellular matrix.[45] Vinblastine has been found to not only prevent secretion but also to change the rate of maturation of the predentin matrix, causing a premature matrix aggregation and a disorganization of collagen structure. From these experimental results, Goldberg et al.[45] have argued that a flow occurs in the predentin zone with secretion occurring from the proximal part of the odontoblast process, material flowing back toward the apical cell surface then being reflected through the central bulk of the predentin toward the mineralizing front. They suggested that parts of the process close to the dentin might have an absorptive rather than a secretory role. Phosphatases are located at the predentin-dentin interface,[9] and it is known that the constitution of the matrix changes at the dentin-predentin border where enzymatic degradation of proteoglycans and glycosaminoglycans probably occurs.[46] This may necessitate the removal of degradation products by endocytosis. It will not be easy to obtain unequivocal results when testing this hypothesis.

FIGURE 7 (Upper left). Side branches of odontoblast process in peripheral region of human premolar dentin. (Magnification × 4200.) FIGURE 8 (Upper right). Freeze-fractured, freeze-dried rat incisor labial dentin showing numerous lateral branches from a main dentin tubule. (Magnification × 4400.) FIGURE 9 (Center left). Blood vessel canals at junction of primary and secondary dentin. Anorganic, fractured viscacha molar. (Magnification × 425.) FIGURE 10 (Center right). Primary osteonal canal lined by bone in anorganic, fractured dentin of sheep molar. (Magnification × 610.) FIGURE 11 (Lower left). Tubules, many with odontoblast processes retained, crossing incremental layers at about 45°. Fixed demineralized, freeze-fractured CPD human premolar. (Magnification × 850.) FIGURE 12 (Lower right). TEM carbon replica of fractured anorganic deciduous calf dentin showing numerous fine side branch canals in peritubular dentin. (Magnification × 5000.)

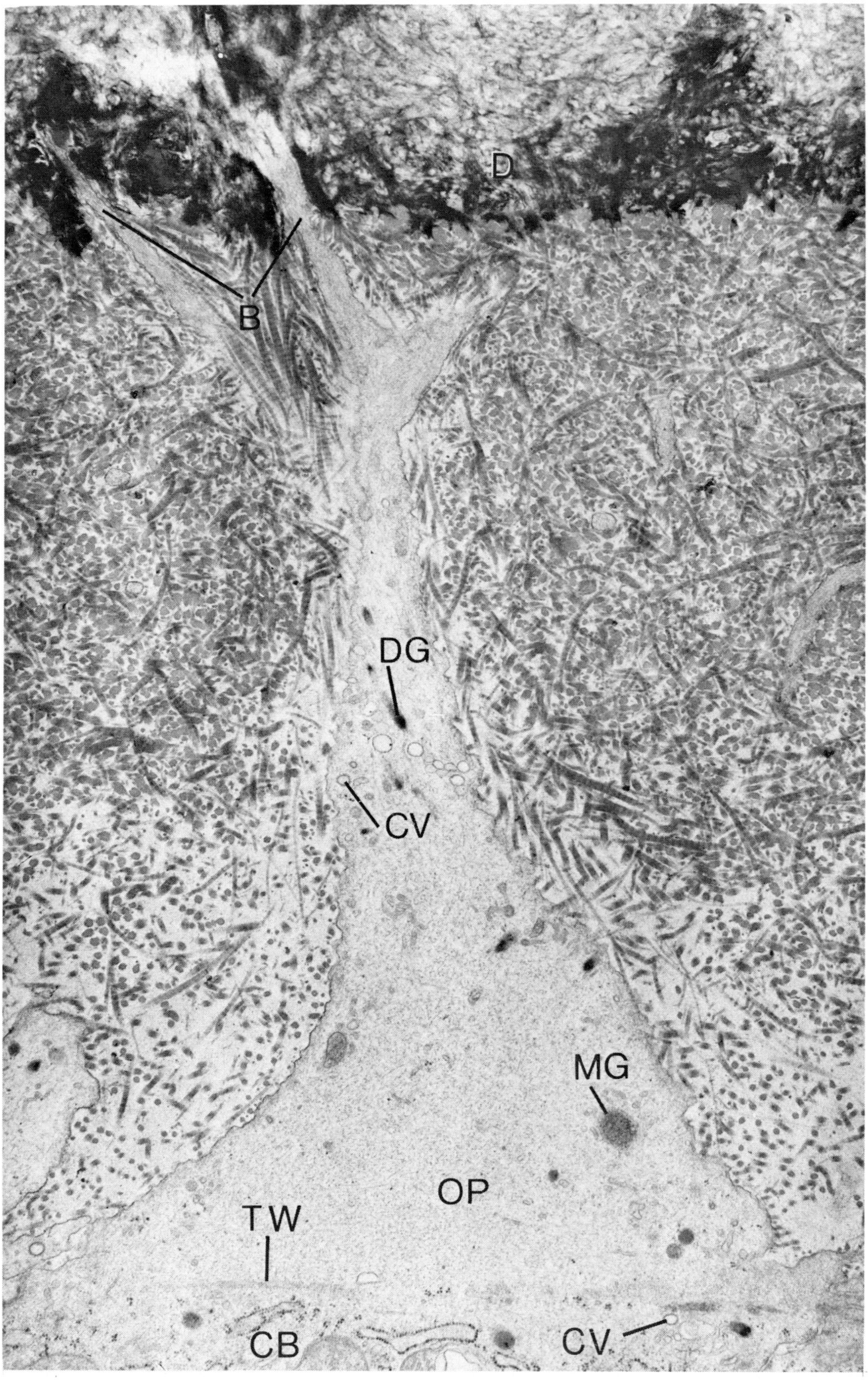

FIGURE 13.

There is a significant decrease in the available space for the noncollagenous components of the matrix from the surface of the predentin matrix adjacent to the cell and the deeper layers of the predentin just prior to mineralization. The collagen fibrils increase in diameter and are much more closely packed (Figure 13). Either there is a withdrawal of water and an increase in density of all the components or some noncollagenous material is withdrawn or expressed. This would require a reverse flow of material through the odontoblast process, as Goldberg and co-workers[45] have suggested, or through the predentin matrix itself back to the cell layer. The odontoblast layer forms an uninterrupted sheet (Figures 3 and 5) with circumferential junctional complexes binding the apical ends of the cells mechanically and isolating the predentin compartment.[34] It is likely that any material outflow from the deep layers of the dentin would either contribute to the last formed predentin or be absorbed by the cells, rather than traversing the intercellular spaces.

The preodontoblast is thought to be responsible for the degradation of the basal lamina, perhaps by collagenase production,[16] but it is not known whether the odontoblast and its process also function to control by enzymatic means the maturation of the matrix once secreted.

C. Resting or Aging Odontoblasts: Limitation on Function

Resting or aging odontoblasts have not been the subject of many ultrastructural studies; they are encased within the pulp and are difficult to fix adequately *in situ*. It is not known how the amount of primary dentin to be formed is controlled. However, there is the obvious circumstantial evidence from comparative odontology that continuous eruption is associated with continuous dentin apposition so that there is occlusion of the pulp chamber in advance of attrition. This is an extreme example of the secondary dentin formation which is also found in teeth which do not erupt continuously. The dentin fulfilling this function generally varies in structure from the bulk of the circumpulpal dentin and sometimes involves the recruitment of new odontoblasts. It is the subject of another chapter in this volume.

Primary dentin formation may be governed by the same type of control that limits the production of enamel by ameloblasts or bone by osteoblasts. Given that there might be a maximum volume of matrix that any one postmitotic cell could produce or a maximum number of days on which it might secrete, it remains a mystery as to what genetic, systemic, or local factors normally limit the expression of its full productive potential at any one site in the tooth. Evidence for limiting genetic factors can be deduced from the aberrant dentin formation in some human taurodontism, for example.[47] The formation of secondary dentin itself, which occurs after the external form of the tooth is completed as a slow, regular, but distinctive continuation of primary dentin formation, attests to local control mechanisms. This is an area in which much interpretative and experimental work is required for elucidation.

There is a considerable variation in the shape of odontoblasts within a functioning tooth, from columnar to round or low cuboidal.[48] They appear more columnar in coronal regions and are pseudostratified. This could be related to two factors: crowding and secretory activity. Fox and Heeley[48] have also suggested that the coronal cells of the human deciduous canines that they studied retain a columnar shape because of their readiness to respond to attrition, while the odontoblasts of the root do not have that requirement.

The shape and size of the cells certainly vary during the functional life cycle of the odontoblast as the synthetic apparatus is developed, attains its maximum potential, and finally is reduced as dentinogenesis slows or even stops.[17] Older odontoblasts in the rat incisor reach a length of 60 μm before shortening to 20 μm or less. The organization in

FIGURE 13. Rat molar odontoblast process (OP) showing wide base, separated by terminal web (TW) material from cell body (CB) of odontoblast. At top of figure branches (B) have become surrounded by mineral and are now within dentin (D). CV, coated vesicles; MG, multivesiculated granules; DG, dense granules. (Magnification × 20,000.) (From Reith, E. J., *J. Ultrastructure Res.*, 21, 383, 1968. With permission.)

the older cell becomes less rigid, with the Golgi apparatus becoming less polarized, and the number of ribosomes attached to the endoplasmic reticulum being reduced. Intercellular spaces widen and intercellular connections are reduced.[17] Holland[33] also reported wide intercellular spaces between odontoblasts of canines from young adult cats and a lack of complete junctional complexes. The cat odontoblasts Holland studied had sporadic desmosomal attachments and specialized junctions, which were identified tentatively as gap junctions, between the odontoblasts and between odontoblasts and putative nerve fibers.

D. Dentin Tubule Contents: Odontoblast Processes, Nerves, and the Periodontoblastic Space

Dentin tubules contain odontoblast processes; that is why they form in the first place. Initially, within the latest predentin, their border is the newly secreted intertubular matrix in which collagen fibrils are forming and increasing in size within a noncollagenous ground substance (Figure 13). These fibrils reach their ultimate size before the dentin-predentin border where mineralization begins. At this level, the peritubular matrix may already be forming and mineralizing, providing a new housing for the cell process. This much is generally agreed, and not difficult to demonstrate since this part of the tissue is readily available for good fixation. The structure of the contents of the tubules deeper within the dentin is more controversial, because the penetration of fixatives by diffusion is inadequate to preserve cellular detail[49,50] even when the dentin is fractured into small fragments immediately upon extraction of the tooth. This has resulted in the apparently simple problem as to whether odontoblast processes reach to the dentino-enamel junction, or are withdrawn as dentinogenesis proceeds, being the subject of much controversy.[44] Many scientists have recorded their failure to demonstrate odontoblast processes in the peripheral regions of dentin by ultramicroscopy[36,51-59] and most of these have been well aware of the difficulties of preparation of the tissue.

We have always been able to exhibit the peripheral retention of odontoblast processes in small teeth by either freeze-fracturing and freeze-drying, or by dry-fracturing critical point dried material (Figures 4, 7, and 11). There are now published reports that odontoblast processes persist in the outer dentin of monkey and man. These studies have taken advantage of the greater sampling rate to be gained from studying fractured surfaces of dentin using SEM.[60,61] Two main difficulties attend such preparations: the processes tend to be lost from the fracture surface, particularly in the middle third of the dentin according to Kelley and colleagues,[60] and shrinkage of the process during drying distorts it[62] and causes problems in distinguishing it from longitudinal intratubular collagen. Additionally, the cytoplasm within the process may not be preserved even close to the pulp, and the cell membrane itself may be incomplete.[57] A common artifact of freeze-drying, freeze-fractured unfixed dentin is the translocation of cytoplasmic components to a subplasmalemmal location during the freezing out process so that the odontoblast process subsequently appears hollow (Figure 6). A similar effect can be noted in some TEM preparations.[50]

Since it has been so difficult to demonstrate the major structure contained in dentin tubules, the interpretation of other contents, particularly deep within the dentin, must be viewed critically. Brännström and Garberoglio[57] believed that an amorphous lining to the tubule coated the odontoblast process but said its presence altered along the length of the tubule; other workers have shown annular hyaline material,[52] a tubular membranous structure with fibrous components that represent unmineralized peritubular centers,[63] unmineralized collagen fibers free of an embedding cement,[58,64,65] or rods of unidentified material.[66] Scanning electron micrographs may be especially difficult to interpret[67,68] with regard to the composition of fibrous strands and the appearance of granular extracellular material coating odontoblast processes. It is usually necessary to coat specimens for SEM and the thickness of the coating can obscure real structure or confer its own texture. Fracture of the dentin tears and dislodges its components (Figure 11) and shrinkage of the unmineralized features further distorts the original form and relationships. Narrow strands of material within tubules then defy attempts to classify them from this evidence alone.[69]

The peritubular matrix may be retained in demineralized dentin and itself be mistaken for the odontoblast process. Precipitation artifacts, particularly prevalent at structural boundaries, are probably the cause of the so-called limiting membrane on the inner surface of the peritubular matrix.[59]

It is accepted that sensory nerve fibers are present in the tubules, in inner parts of dentin, and in predentin.[51,70] They have not been traced throughout the depth of the dentin and it has been assumed that they extend relatively further into the dentin with time merely because they are overtaken by dentinogenesis.[71] Fearnhead,[72] on the other hand, indicates that the density of innervation of dentin increases with the age of the newly completed tooth as a consequence of the continuous, peripheral growth activity of fine terminal branches of nerve fibers. Frank[73] reported a complex infolding of nerve endings with the odontoblastic process and tight junctions between them which were later identified as gap junctions by Holland.[33] The nerves are frequently seen lying adjacent to the odontoblast process in a groove, have an irregular course, and may branch within the tubule.

The certain identification of nerve fibers in dentin tubules is not without difficulty by TEM;[32,73,74] it is unlikely by SEM.[67] Auxiliary methods of identification, such as labeling axon-transported protein,[75] are required for positive identification. Dentin innervation is discussed in detail in a separate chapter.

E. The Role of the Odontoblast in the Mineralization of Dentin

Mineralization of dentin matrix occurs extracellularly. Apatite crystals have never been satisfactorily demonstrated in odontoblasts, and it is reasonable to assume that they are not there. Early TEM work purporting to show calcium phosphate crystals intracellularly is currently discredited as artifactual by most, but not all, investigators.[76] However, that is not to say that the odontoblasts do not, in some way, regulate the ingress of calcium salts into dentin; the processing of calcium need not cause an accumulation adequate to be detected by radioautography.[77] It is possible that calcium is briefly accumulated in mitochondria,[78] rather as occurs just prior to the calcification zone in cartilage.[79] The barrier between the calcification front and the serum varies in each of the calcified tissues, but in all there are strong morphological indications that the cells do play a controlling role in the rate of access.[34,35] Nagai and Frank[78] found evidence for two routes of calcium transit to the front using electron microscopic autoradiography. In the first, calcium passed through the inter-odontoblastic space; in the second, calcium was traced through the odontoblast, accumulating in the Golgi apparatus and mitochondria, but not in secretory vacuoles.

Pyroantimonate has been used for the ultramicroscopical identification of sites of accumulations of calcium ions in odontoblasts.[80] Parts of the Golgi apparatus, particularly *abacus bodies*[38,81] stain heavily with pyroantimonate, as do secretory granules at the apical end of the cell. Reith[80] concluded from these preparations that calcium is bound by Golgi elements in which collagen precursors were also present. However, according to later work, the pyroantimonate method is discredited because it is not specific for calcium and involves fixation which causes both redistribution of electrolytes, and an ingress of calcium to the cell. Quantitative electron probe analysis demonstrates a high concentration of calcium in the distal secretory pole of odontoblasts.[82]

F. Matrix Vesicles

The other way in which odontoblasts may control mineralization is by the production of matrix vesicles which are budded from the cells, accumulate calcium, and act as initiation sites for mineralization. They have three ultrastructural components: the extravesicular layer of bound proteoglycans, the trilaminar membrane, and an intravesicular domain.[83]

Matrix vesicles are easy to demonstrate in the initial stages of dentinogenesis of peripheral dentin,[19,21,84-89] but not in circumpulpal dentin.[88,90] This could mean that they are not produced in the formation in the latter tissue or, on the other hand, the poor sampling rate of TEM and the infrequency of new initial loci of mineralization in the bulk of the tissue could result in their occurrence being missed. The incidence of a band of interglobular dentin sited at the junction of the outer region of dentin containing many small spherical calcospherites, with a middle region of large arcade-shaped calcospherites is, perhaps indicative of a fairly abrupt change in the rate of budding off of matrix vesicles, perhaps combined with a change in the predominant nucleation method.[91] We speculate that matrix vesicles become fewer and widely separated. The spread of mineralization is therefore mainly by accretion at existing surfaces rather than through new nucleation sites. The gap in time and therefore space at the changeover in the rate of vesicle production means that a band of dentin becomes sealed off by a continuous mineral front before the peripheral spread of the large parabolic calcospherites can extend to entirely fuse with the spherical calcospherites.

Matrix vesicles are rich in alkaline phosphatase which is thought to be bound to the cell membrane.[89] However, Linde and Granström[92] have pointed out that the association with the odontoblast cell membrane is an artifact of glutaraldehyde fixation for electron microscopical histochemistry and the true location of alkaline phosphatase in dentinogenically active odontoblasts is on the membranes of intracellular vesicles in the odontoblast process and the Golgi region. In an ultrastructural study aimed at localizing alkaline phosphatase in rat odontogenesis, Orams and Snibson[9] concluded that the enzyme activity was present throughout the vesicles but confined to the plasmalemma of the odontoblasts. Further studies are required to define the location of enzymes in the living state.

Theories on the functioning of matrix vesicles are addressed in a separate chapter of this volume.

G. Rhythmic Variations in Functioning of Odontoblasts

It is believed that odontoblasts, like most secretory cells, show rhythmic variations in their secretory functions because the matrix that they produce shows rhythmic compositional changes.[93] However, rhythmic alterations in the cytological features of these cells have not yet been demonstrated. Beside the circadian rhythm associated with von Ebner's incremental growth lines that may be demonstrated with tetracycline labeling,[94] Rosenberg and Simmons[95] have identified circadian, ultradian, and infradian rhythms of dentinogenesis. They found that the Ca (mineralization) and S (proteoglycan deposition) rhythms were independent and had complex phase relationships in rabbit incisors, and discussed some aspects of the physiological basis for dentin rhythms at the structural and chemical levels. The Ca and S levels on the labial and lingual aspects of the rabbit incisors differed, the Ca difference being much more pronounced,[96] and this reflected differences in growth rates. The concentrations were inversely proportional. The authors made the interesting comment that the odontoblasts might each have a limited daily budget of Ca to transport into whatever volume of matrix was produced, and this would result in the faster growing labial dentin being less well mineralized. Rosenberg and Simmons[96] extended their argument to propose that the presence of a relatively high degree of mineralization in the layer of mantle dentin on the labial side compared with the circumpulpal dentin and its absence on the lingual side could simply be a consequence of the increased growth rate on the labial side. Their studies emphasize the importance of the cellular control of mineralization and raise the question as to whether the timing of the formation of junctional complexes between the odontoblasts may vary in the two sides of the tooth and contribute to the difference in the degree of mineralization in the most peripheral layers.[34] Even in profound disturbances in the mineralization of circumpulpal dentin due to hypophosphatemia, the mantle dentin beneath the enamel is well mineralized,[28] perhaps due to the abundance of initial calcification foci in that region,[88] as well as the lack of intercellular seals at the time of its formation.

H. The Subodontoblastic Cells

The knowledge of the structural organization of the subodontoblastic region has been excellently reviewed by Baume.[44] He considered that the cells closest to the odontoblasts were sufficiently different from cells of the remainder of the pulp to retain their proper noun designation as *Höhl's subodontoblastic cells*. The degree of organization in this peripheral region of the pulp varies,[48,97,98] but at its most extreme is divided into a cell-free zone containing processes both from the basal ends of the odontoblasts and from the parallel bipolar or sometimes multipolar cells of the subjacent cell-rich layer.[99]

The subodontoblastic cells have the same complement of organelles as other synthetic, matrix-producing connective tissue cells and presumably contribute to the substance of the pulp. On the basis of histochemical studies it has been speculated that they produce von Korff fibers and assist in their maturation. However, since the subodontoblastic cell layer is not well defined during either peripheral or later primary dentin formation, this is a dubious claim. Additionally, autoradiographic studies indicate sparse labeling of pulpal cells and lateral cell spaces and do not support a pulpal origin for predentin collagen.[22]

Gotjamanos[97] postulated a special role for the cells in assisting the odontoblasts metabolically. Indeed, the plasmalemma of the cells in the subodontoblastic layer is rich in alkaline phosphatase during odontogenesis, although why is not known.[9] Many other investigators have suggested that subodontoblastic cells form a pool for the provision of odontoblasts in secondary dentin formation.[44] At present, it seems that we have to acknowledge a hiatus in our information on any specialized secretory or regulatory function, if any, that these cells possess.

Subodontoblastic cells may sport a single cilium associated with a centriole.[99] This is a feature shared with, amongst other cells, odontoblasts, chondroblasts, and osteoblasts. It has been suggested that the cilia may be an indication of the migratory history of ectomesenchymal cells. The arrangement of these structures shows a (9 + 0) configuration of microtubules; this is atypical for motile cilia in which (9 + 2) is standard. As they are always connected with centrioles, their presence could be a reflection of a postmitotic, differentiated status, or have no special significance.

Specialized cell junctions occur between the subodontoblastic cells, and between these cells and the overlying odontoblasts. Desmosomes and gap junctions have been reported.[44] The significance of gap junctions between odontoblasts and subodontoblasts is unknown.

III. TISSUE JUNCTIONS

A. Dentin-Enamel Junction

The junction between dentin and enamel is the first hard tissue interface to develop during tooth formation. Although dentin formation precedes the deposition of enamel matrix, it is simplistic to state that the enamel is laid down on a preformed template of dentin. The topography of the junction changes as each tissue continues to mature and intermingle with the other at their common origin.[100]

Most studies of the dentin-enamel junction have examined its sectional appearance viewed by light microscopy. There have been relatively few ultrastructural studies illustrating topography finer than the escalloping of the border. It is accepted that the plane of the junction may be, but is rarely, flat, but that the degree of relief varies from one region of a tooth to another, from one tooth to another, and in different species.[101-103] Staley[102] also described circumferential ridging on the outer dentin surface of incisors which he related to incremental lines, and clusters of horizontal ridges of limited extent. It is not easy to tell from his data whether these are partly due to a shrinkage artifact produced on drying the demineralized crowns.

The shape of the junction in human teeth is usually said to confer strength and prevent

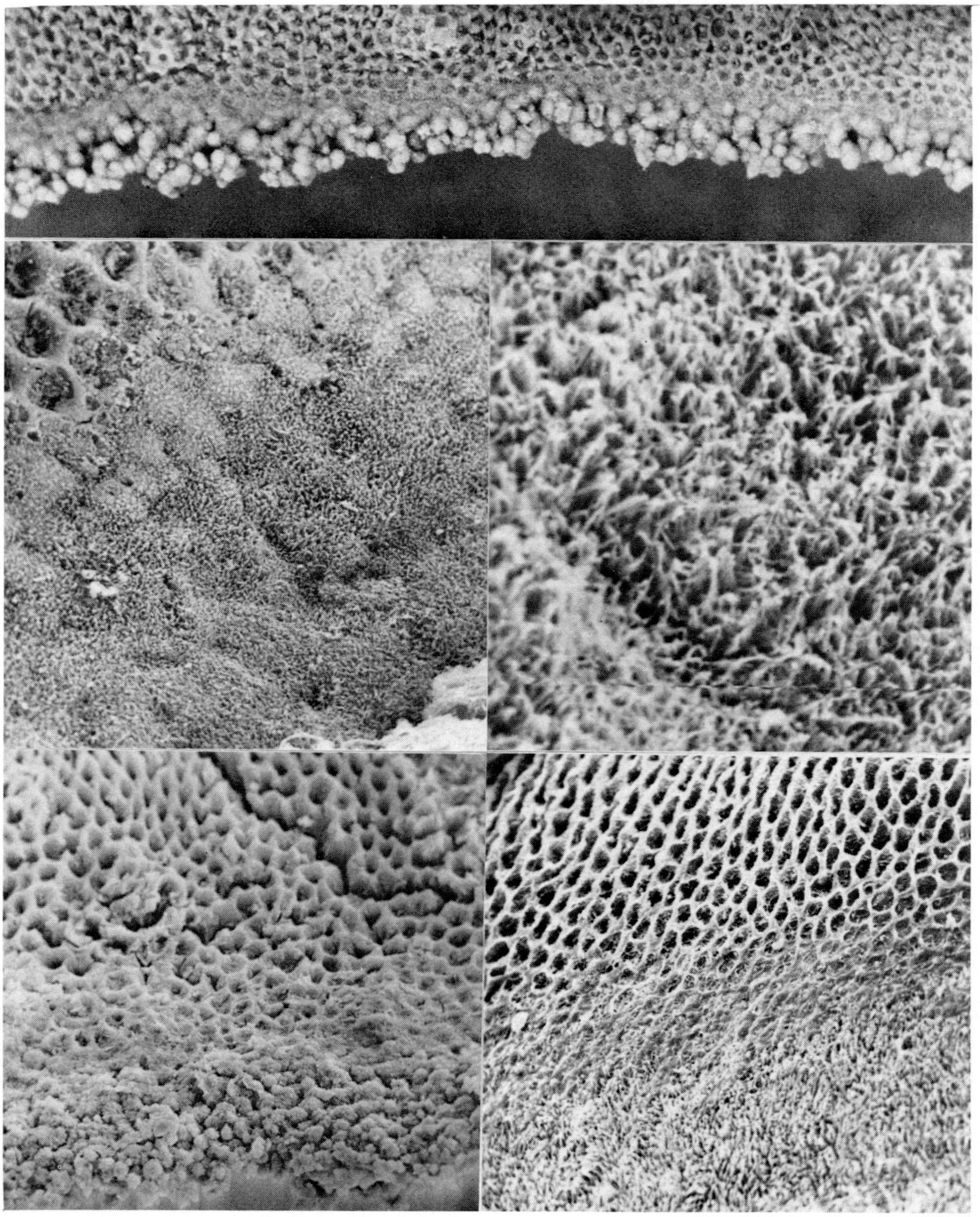

FIGURE 14 (Above). Plasma-ashed, growing edge of crown of human female 12 year lower third permanent molar, viewed from enamel aspect, showing fusion of dentin calcospherites to form a relatively smooth surface before deposition of first enamel matrix. (Magnification × 325.) FIGURE 15 (Center left). External surface of growing edge of same crown as Figure 14, critical point dried only. Enamel (top left) forming on dentin surface. (Magnification × 950.) FIGURE 16 (Center right). Higher magnification of Figure 15 of dentin surface on which enamel was about to be deposited. (Magnification × 4700.) FIGURE 17 (Lower left). Anorganic preparation of growing end of crown of orangutan lower second deciduous molar, showing fusion of dentin calcospherites to create relatively smooth mineral surface before deposition of enamel matrix. (Magnification × 450.) FIGURE 18 (Lower right). External surface of freeze-dried, developing crown of *Metachirus nudicaudatus* cheek tooth showing dentin fibrils perpendicular to surface over which enamel formation is spreading. (Magnification × 870.)

the two tissues parting during function. However, there is no evidence that such an increase in the surface area of the junction by scalloping is functionally significant — certainly it is not a feature of other primate teeth. The intermingling of the tissues at a finer scale (Figures 15 and 16) would appear to provide more than adequate mechanical adhesion.[100] Indeed, investigators have always found that it is necessary to desiccate the tooth tissues, or to chemically remove one phase, in order to see the junction face on. When dried, teeth crack just within the enamel, not precisely at the junction or within the dentin. Additionally, there is a brief report that teeth affected by dentinogenesis imperfecta show similar junctional topography to that of normal teeth, yet the enamel of these may separate close to the dentin-enamel junction.[104]

Where escalloping of the dentin-enamel junction (Figures 19 and 20) is present, its size is such that it mimics the appearance of a reversal line. This has led to speculation that resorption of the dentin may precede amelogenesis. There is a precedent for such a sequence of events in the resorption of superficial enamel prior to coronal cementogenesis in, for example, the horse.[30] However, these are two centrifugally produced tissues, the production of one having to cease, and its formative cells to be displaced, prior to the deposition by the other. During this process, there can be a ready access for odontoclasts. Amelogenesis and dentinogenesis are not sequential processes and there is no call for the epithelial layer to be breached, nor any evidence that it is.

The tissue surfaces purporting to be at a dentin-enamel junction of an internally resorbed tooth in the paper by Sela et al.[105] cannot be that. The enamel surface shows typical resorption bays. The dislodged "dentin" surface which appears to fit into the enamel, and contains fragments of enamel on it, must be reparative bone that has fractured away in specimen preparation. Such bone would also show openings of canaliculi and could be misinterpreted as dentin.

Svejda and Bures[106] attempted to relate enamel prism organization to the depressions in the dentin surface using SEM. They illustrated their concept diagrammatically, showing groups of parallel prisms located in each escallop, the orientation of each group of prisms differing slightly from that of its neighbors. This clear organization is not easy to envisage from the micrographs published. A finer imprinting of the ends of individual prisms (Figure 19) was demonstrated by Whittaker[103] at the dentin frontier of decalcified monkey teeth. He concluded that the newly formed dentin must have retained sufficient plasticity to distort during the initial formation of prisms which reached right to the junction. Matching enamel surfaces of human teeth (retrieved after treating specimens with hypochlorite, drying, and dissecting away the dentin) showed projecting prism ends. Where escalloping was lacking, Whittaker[103] reported that concave prism ends reached the junction with dentin although no comparable reverse image of this was illustrated on the opposing dentin surface.

In our view, the appearance of enamel prism outlines indentations on an enamel-dentin junction surface, whether prepared by demineralization, or by fracturing an anorganic specimen, is due to the retention of enamel on the dentin surface. In demineralized preparations, enamel matrix protein, from tuft and prism boundary locations in particular, may help to emphasize the borders of the real escallops at the junction and show the sites of the prisms (Figure 19). The retention of organic matrix debris from enamel will be greater in immature and fixed teeth. In anorganic preparations, the fracture plane passes through the enamel very close to the junction; thus enamel prisms may be seen on the dentin.

The timing of the development of the escallopment is controversial. The junction between odontoblasts and inner enamel epithelial cells is usually described as flat or forming a straight or slightly wavy line in section. After early dentin and enamel formation in human teeth, Whittaker[103] reported the junction to show little scalloping. However, because of the great variation in the degree of scalloping in completed teeth, his sample may not have been adequate to examine this point properly. We have not noted escalloping of the future enamel-

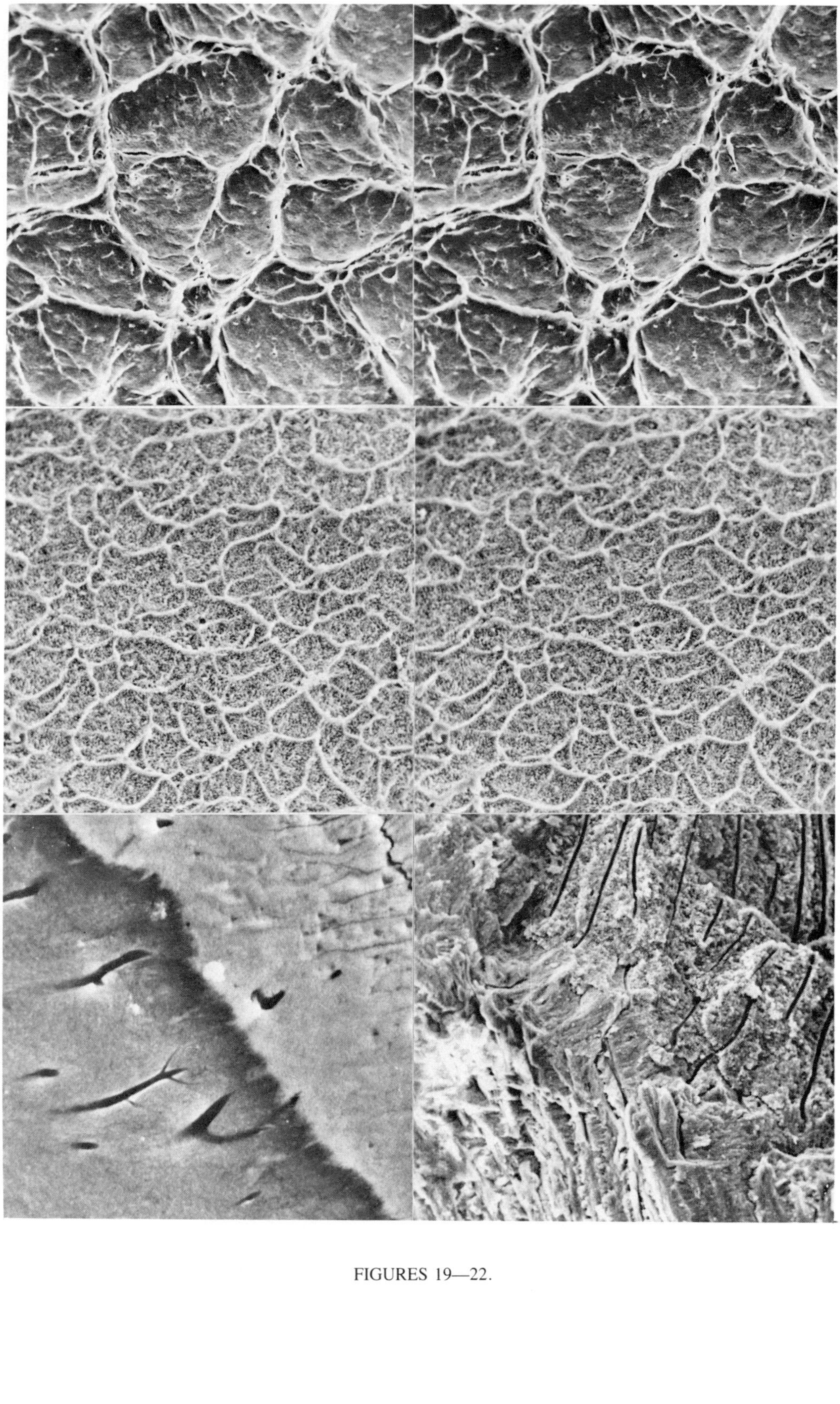

FIGURES 19—22.

dentin junction in a survey of late stages of crown development in human third permanent molars (Figures 14 to 16).

We have compared the appearances of the developing junction with the recovered one in several species. The outer limit of the dentin shows fine fibrils lying vertical to the junction[107] and it is upon this that the first evidence for enamel is seen (Figures 15, 16, and 18). Deep to the surface fibrils, and within the thickening tissue, the outlines of calcospherites can be visualized. In anorganic preparations, the calcospherites have fused and the surface dentin appears to be completely mineralized before enamel (mineral) is recognized (Figures 14 and 17). Demineralization of the fully formed crowns of unfixed teeth allows the vertical fibrillar pattern to be recovered in freeze-dried and critical point dried material (Figure 20). However, Svejda and Bures[106] and Whittaker[103] figure a fine network of fibrils parallel with the surface of the dentin at the junction — a situation at odds with developmental evidence on the orientation of the first-formed fibrils.[107] Whittaker[103] has tentatively suggested that the edges of the scallops, where present, may be the location of von Korff fibers which lie approximately at right angles to the frontier. There is no evidence, however, that they are confined to such regions.

Dentin tubules may cross the dentin-enamel junction and pass into the enamel where they become enamel tubules (Figures 21 and 22). At their simplest, they are thought to have contained the terminal part of the odontoblast process. Enamel tubules are especially well developed in all marsupials[108,109] but the wombat (Figure 22). We believe it to be significant that wombats are also unique amongst marsupials in having an abundance of large von Korff fibers parallel to the junction in the peripheral dentin which may preclude odontoblast processes reaching the junction. For contrast, an ultrastructural study of kangaroo dentin, prepared by ion-beam thinning, indicated that tubules branching in the dentin rejoin in the enamel[110] but the authors were unable to explain their formation or give their contents.

It has never been shown how enamel spindles are formed though their continuity with dentin is usually taken for granted. They may represent aggregations of dentin matrix and odontoblast processes protruding beyond the position of the basement membrane prior to or in the initial steps of amelogenesis; they are, perhaps, von Korff fibers. Further studies should examine the development of these structures.

B. Dentin-Cement Junction

It is not the form, but the exact location, of the dentin-cement junction that has provided the most controversy. The junction should be located at the original site of the basal lamina formed by the epithelial root sheath.[111] Odontoblasts differentiate and begin to lay down dentin prior to the disintegration of the basal lamina. Subsequent to the interruption of the latter and precementum deposition, the junction becomes obscured as the dentin and cement mineralize.[112] The hyaline layer of Hopewell-Smith is a light microscopical feature which lies in the region of the junction of the two tissues and peripheral to the granular layers of Tomes. The hyaline layer has been thought to be part of the cementum[113] or alternatively the dentin.[114-117] Others have also implied that the hyaline layer is cementum, in assuming that the granular layer of Tomes is adjacent to the cementum, whether caused by the inclusion of epithelial cells[118] or by the failure of continued extension of mineralization of the initial spherical calcospherites.[119] Shellis[120] identified the hyaline layer as a 10-μm thick layer of

FIGURE 19 (Above). Stereopair: dentin surface of enamel-dentin junction. Enamel matrix residue obscures fine detail of dentin. (Magnification × 410.) FIGURE 20 (Center). Stereopair of enamel-dentin junction. Demineralized human deciduous canine, showing fine dentin fibrils end-on to the junction. (Magnification × 410.) FIGURE 21 (Lower left). Backscattered electron (BSE) image of micro-milled surface of enamel-dentin junction in human third molar, showing dentin tubules with terminal branches and hypomineralized dentin zone subjacent to enamel. (Magnification × 1000.) FIGURE 22 (Lower right). *Macropus* fractured enamel-dentin junction showing dentin tubules (top right) continuous with enamel tubules (bottom left). (Magnification × 960.)

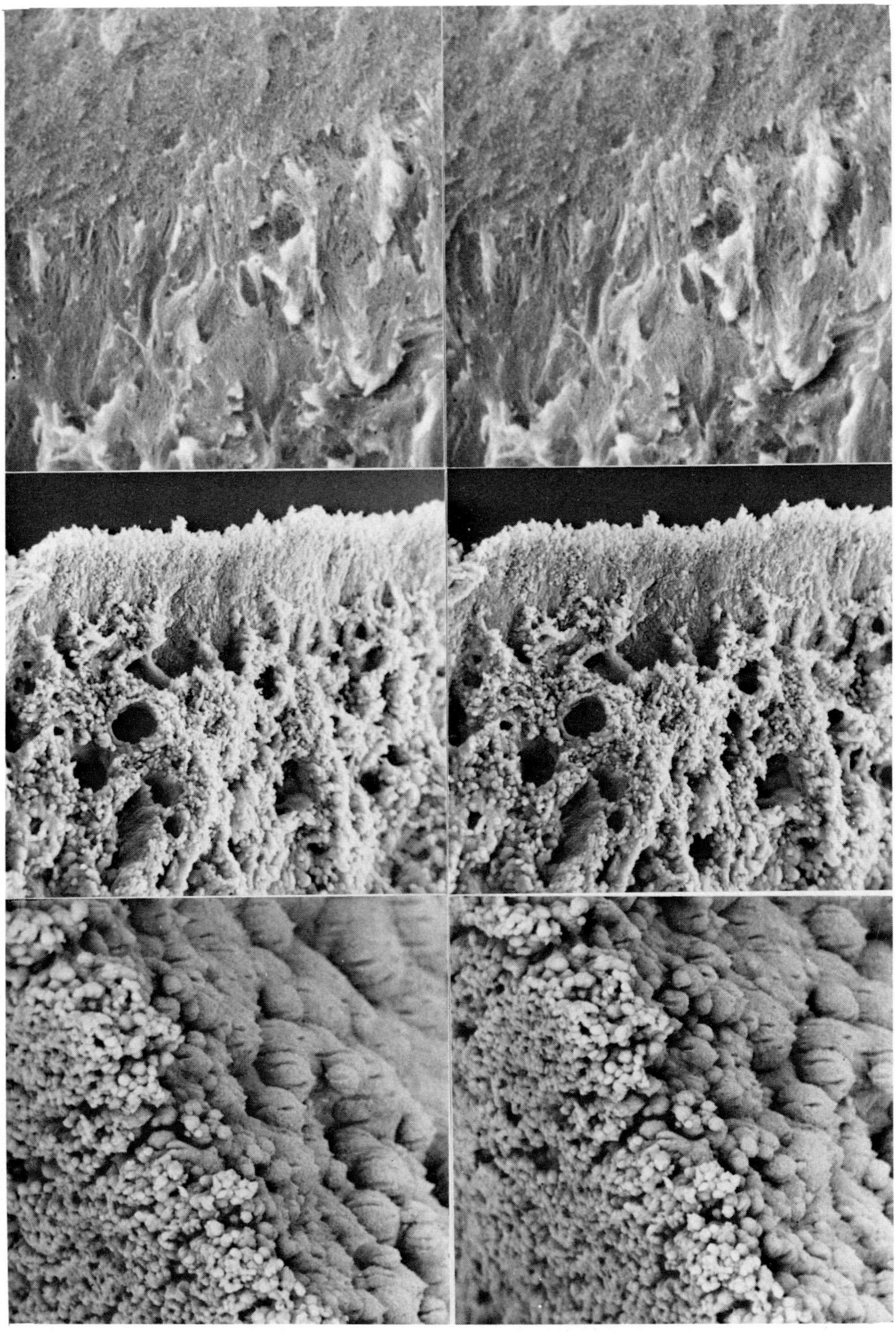

FIGURES 23—25.

dentin, and said it corresponded to the coronal mantle dentin, contained radially oriented collagen fibers, and small, tightly packed calcospherites.

The identification of this layer as dentin rather than cement would appear to depend on the occurrence within it of dentin tubules — although if one compares this situation with that pertaining at the dentin-enamel junction, the possession of tubules is not an adequate proof of the origin of the tissue. The dentin-enamel junction is readily identified by the transition from a collagenous matrix with small apatite crystals to a noncollagenous matrix with much larger crystals. Such a difference in structure is not available at the cement-dentin interface.

In microradiographs a radiodense line is usually seen peripheral to the radiolucency caused by the granular layer of Tomes,[121,122] but whether this radioopaque zone lies in dentin[123] or cement, or bridges both tissues[124] is disputed. If one considers the TEM of demineralized root dentin from mouse molars published by Ten Cate,[125] it would seem likely that there the hypermineralized band lies in a narrow layer with sparse, fine collagen fibrils, and presumably more proteoglycans, that forms immediately below the basal lamina of the epithelial root sheath during the very first stages of dentinogenesis. This may later merge with the product of cementoblasts, for Selvig[126] reported that the first indication of cementum formation was the deposition of ground substance and occurrence of crystals at the border. One may compare this with the development of resting lines and reversal lines in bony tissues generally, and with the development of peritubular dentin and perilacunar bone, where a dearth of collagen fibrils but richness of ground substance is allied to a higher degree of mineralization. Ten Cate[125] found in the mouse that this layer, about 1-μm thick, persisted deep to the next region of dentin which contained coarse fibrils, the mantle dentin, and thought that it was possibly the murine equivalent of the layer that Hopewell-Smith[113] described in human teeth. However, he also considered that both the epithelial cells and the newly differentiated odontoblasts contributed to this layer. Thus, there still seems to be confusion in the correlation of the light and electron microscopical views on the identification of the layers in this region.

We believe that this perplexity results from the considerable variation that occurs in the structural organization and degree of mineralization of the dentin and cementum in the region of their junction (Figures 23 to 40). We have found that the granular layer of Tomes may extend right to the junction or be separated from it by a more homogeneously mineralized layer of varying depth which we would identify as the so-called hyaline layer. The most peripheral part of the dentin appears to enhance its mineralization from the cemental side (Figure 32) and, just inside the junction, may become more highly mineralized than the bordering dentin or cementum. There is an intermingling or continuity of all components of the two tissues (Figures 23 and 30 to 40). We base this interpretation on backscattered electron (BSE) images of the junction which show an increase in mineral content in the dentin just opposite the ends of Sharpey's fibers (Figures 32 and 35). This would place the hypermineralized layer, which is an inconstant feature, in dentin just below and at the junction. It explains our previous finding[126] that one could trace Sharpey's fibers extending into the hypermineralized layer in anorganic preparations; the mineral phase does project from Sharpey's fibers across the border in some regions and fades in intensity with depth into dentin.

Besides the fine intermingling of the tissues at the junction, the plane of the junction is

FIGURE 23 (Above). Stereopair: cement-dentin junction of demineralized, freeze-fractured, and freeze-dried human premolar with Sharpey's fibers at right. Fibrils from dentin and cement mingle at the junction. (Magnification × 1700.) FIGURE 24 (Center). Stereopair of outer surface of anorganic developing root of rat molar showing cellular cement forming on mineralized and mineralizing dentin. (Magnification × 715.) FIGURE 25 (Below). Stereopair: anorganic preparation of edge of growing root of human lower third molar. Large deficiencies in mineralization on root surface (left) represent nonmineralized spaces of granular layer of Tomes. (Magnification × 420.)

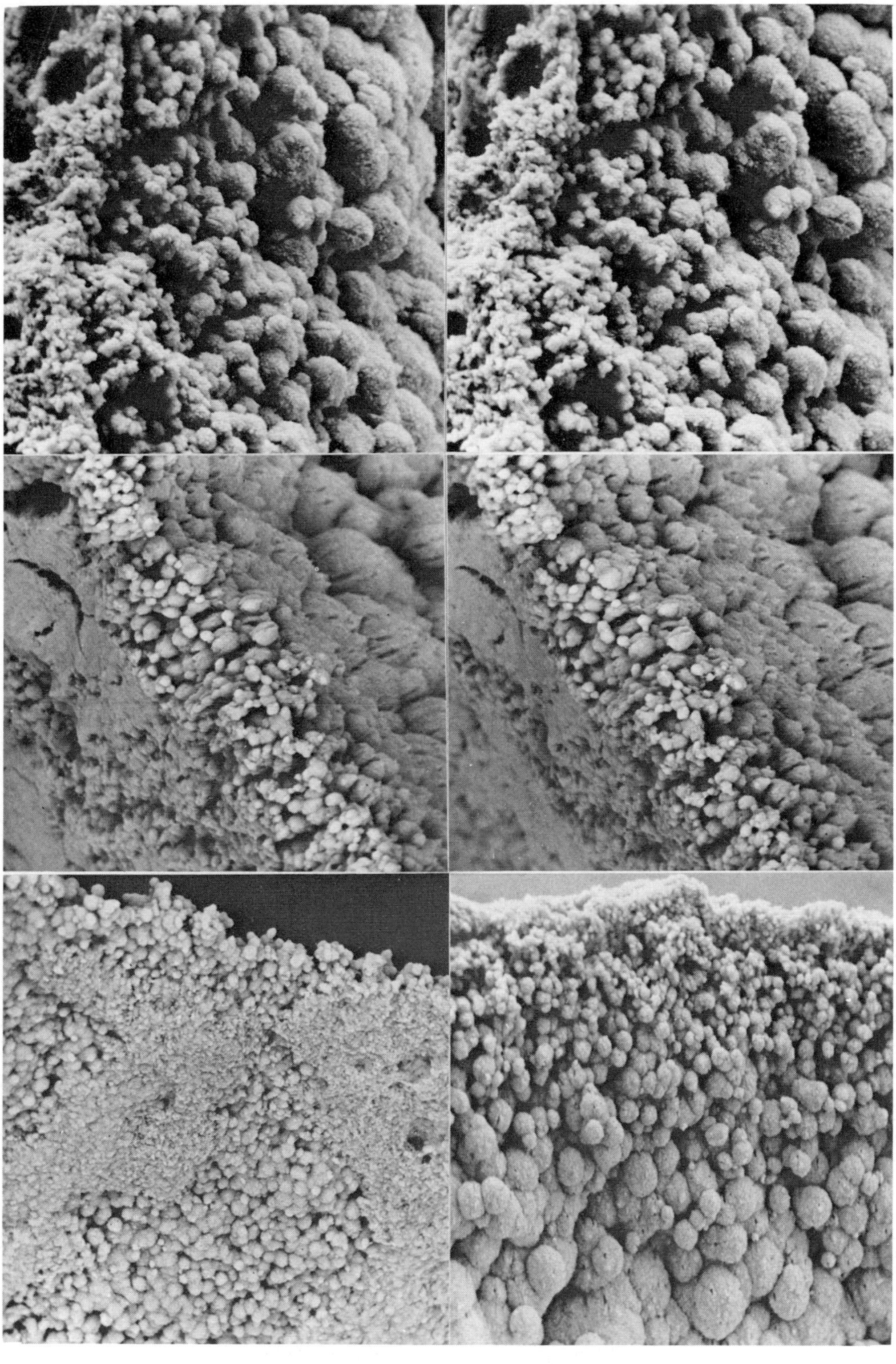

FIGURES 26—29.

often irregular on a grosser scale. Longitudinal pleating and horizontal ridges or waves record the accommodation of the epithelial root sheath to varying rates of growth and eruption and change in shape of the root.

IV. FORMATION OF DENTIN

A. Mantle Dentin

1. Coronal Mantle Dentin Matrix

Coronal mantle dentin is the first-formed, peripheral dentin which eventually lies adjacent to enamel in the crown of a tooth. It is a layer of variable thickness, extending from virtually nothing to tens of micrometers. It is characterized by the presence of collagen fibers that are arrayed differently from those in the circumpulpal dentin that forms the bulk of the dentin (see reviews by Lester and Boyde[108] and Moss[127]). Circumpulpal dentin usually forms so that the fine collagen fibrils lie within the plane of the developing surface[64] and therefore, parallel to the incremental lines of the organic matrix. By contrast, the mantle dentin contains coarser fibrils that may be grouped into fibers[108] (Figure 42). They lie with their long axes parallel to the odontoblast processes in cuspal and occlusal surface regions, but deviate rootward on lateral aspects of the crown and there may be parallel to the dentin-enamel junction. The existence of this layer and the orientation of its fibers was described by polarized light microscopy.[127,129]

Confusion has reigned over whether the radial fibers, usually called *von Korff fibers,* originate in the pulp and are thus extrinsic fibers in the dentin, or whether they are formed by the odontoblast, the collagen precursor being liberated from the odontoblast process or apical end of the cell.[41] The problem arises because of the difficulty of identification in light microscopical preparations of argyrophilic material deep to, between, and peripheral to, the odontoblast cell bodies during initial dentinogenesis[125,130] and the problem of differentiating artifact from structure in some dried specimens.[131] Electron microscopical observations on the odontoblast layer during initial dentinogenesis provide conflicting evidence for the incorporation into dentin of fibers produced from the subodontoblastic layer. These would have to be passed by the odontoblasts in their centripetal migration and would be seen in the intercellular spaces. Collagen fibrils have been illustrated between odontoblasts in human tooth germs,[132] in cat teeth,[133] and in rat molars,[81] but Ten Cate[125] found these to be peripheral to a junctional complex system in murine teeth. Ten Cate's work supported that of Sisca and Provenza[84] who failed to find collagen between the odontoblasts of human teeth, and Costacurta and co-workers[41] in their study of dentinogenesis in rat incisors. Whether all such fibers lie peripheral to the terminal bar apparatus in all species is a point requiring further investigation. It would be surprising if collagen fibers could pass through the close intercellular junctions once the terminal bar apparatus is fully established.[34]

The question of the origin of the collagen fibrils in mantle dentin is thus not entirely clear.[22] On balance, it would seem that we should drop the term ''von Korff fibers'', which has been applied to two different classes of feature and thus has led to unnecessary confusion in the literature. The first class is that of the large fibers which do exist in mantle (peripheral)

FIGURE 26 (Above). Stereopair: anorganic preparation of growing root end of human lower premolar, converted BSE image. Presumed location of cement-dentin junction indicated by cleft in this surface. Mineral particle clusters in cement side (left) of this line are slightly finer than those in the peripheral dentin. (Magnification × 780.) FIGURE 27 (Center). Stereopair: anorganic preparation of growing root of human lower third permanent molar. Patchy cement formation (left) on surface of dentin. (Magnification × 410.) FIGURE 28 (Lower left). Anorganic preparation of growing root edge of human lower third molar, viewed from root aspect. Fine mineral particle clusters are presumed to be cement matrix mineralization which is seen here to be patchy. Larger calcospherites are those of the peripheral dentin. (Magnification × 365.) FIGURE 29 (Lower right). Anorganic preparation of growing root end of human lower premolar, viewed from dentin side showing increase in size of forming calcospherites from close to cement-dentin junction to deeper within dentin. (Magnification × 390.)

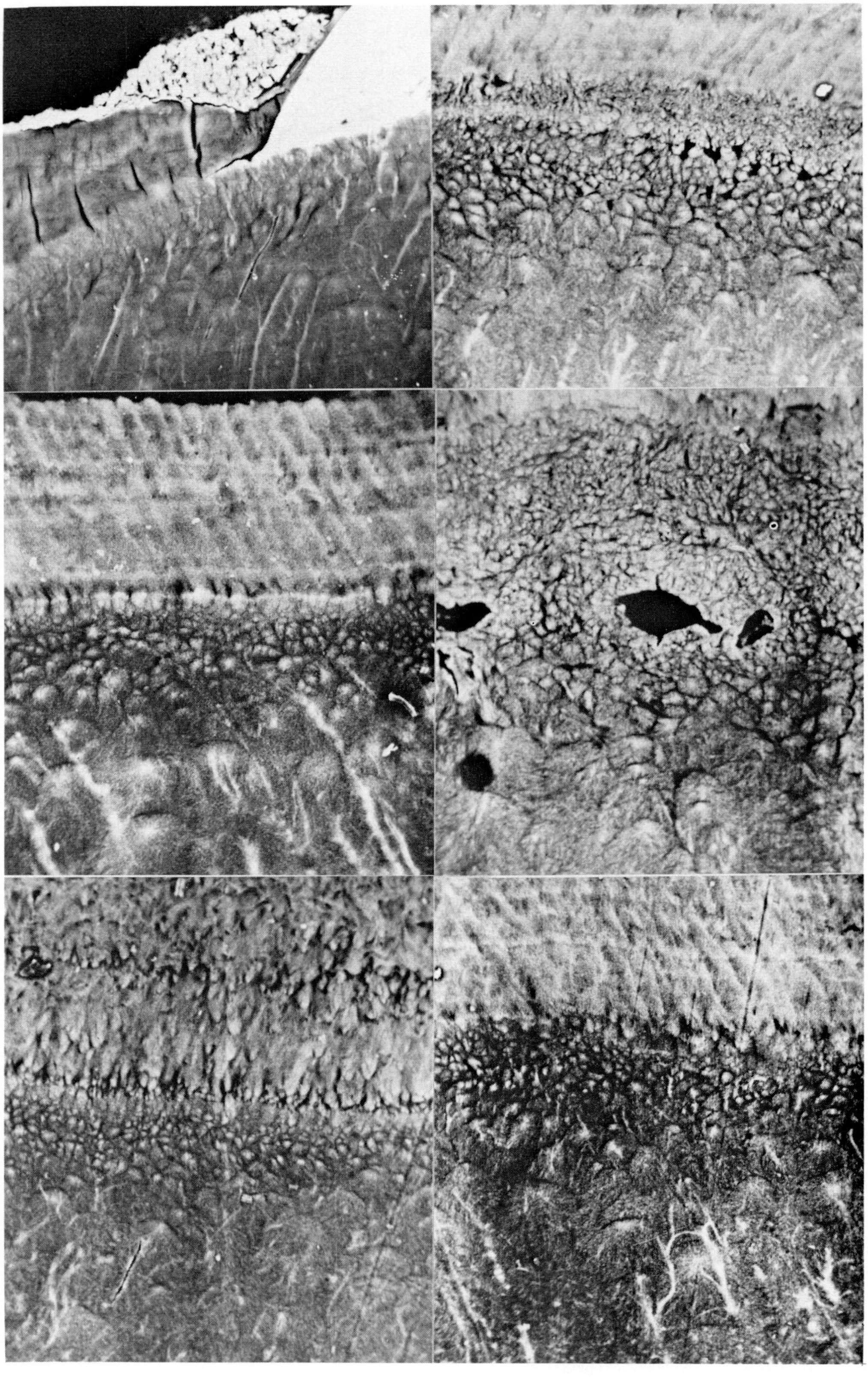

FIGURES 30—35.

dentin, and are particularly easily demonstrated by SEM because of its rapid surveying possibilities (Figures 41 and 42). The second is that of the "corkscrew" variety which was thought by Han,[134] and has been shown by Ten Cate[125] to be an artifact of the Ag staining technique; they may be demonstrated in late circumpulpal dentinogenesis where the SEM shows no fiber bundles perpendicular to the formative surface. They lie between the odontoblasts but they do not contact the predentin.

The coarse collagen fibrils in the peripheral mantle dentin are most likely, though this is not proven, the earliest collagen produced solely by the immature odontoblasts[127] and aggregate and align in directions characteristic for their site in the tooth, presumably related to cell movement and differentiation occurring during the early stages of dentinogenesis. Moss[127] made the interesting suggestion that if odontoblastic cytodifferentiation determined the type of dentin laid down, as indeed Herold's data[135] on dentinogenesis imperfecta indicate, a more extensive investigation of other conditions where dentin formation is abnormal might be instructive.

Once the organization of the odontoblast layer is completed, the terminal bar apparatus established at the apical pole, and a steady, rhythmic production of dentin underway, the coarse fibers are no longer formed and the more regular, circumpulpal dentin with finer, randomly arranged fibrils lying in the plane of the developing surface, that is, parallel to the available cell surface, is produced (Figures 43 to 46). There will be a transition between these two patterns.[108] Interestingly, the opposite interpretation is made by Portilla[136] concerning the relationship between the collagen fibrils and the odontoblasts. This author states that von Korff fibers originate in the pulp, can be traced into circumpulpal dentin, and that they, rather than the basement membrane,[107] play a major role in the orientation of the odontoblasts during their dentin forming process.

In this respect it is difficult to separate the discussion from that of the situation in the teeth of certain odontocete species where coarse fibers may be found throughout the thickness of the dentin,[137] where collagen parallel to the dentin tubules and forming its wall comprises a large component of the matrix. The relationship of the fibrillar orientation to the cell surface is a recurring theme in ultrastructural studies of dentinogenesis[31] to which we shall return (Section IV.B.1).

The first appearance of the coarse fibrils is close to, and intermingling with, the aperiodic, very fine, fibrils linked to the basal lamina.[85] This association would be expected to be closest where the orientation of both is the same — perpendicular to the lamina.[125] Lester and Boyde[108] reported a very narrow region between the enamel and the mantle dentin devoid of coarse fibrils — a situation which is also seen peripheral to radicular mantle dentin, and this is confirmed in our recent data from SEM studies of the development of the enamel-dentin junction in several species. The transmission electron micrographs of Whittaker and

FIGURE 30 (Upper left). Surface of diamond-polished longitudinal ground section of human canine, showing enamel, dentin, cement, and adherent calculus. BSE image. (Magnification × 380.) FIGURE 31 (Upper right). LS of human premolar, micro-milled surface. A hypermineralized layer in the superficial dentin lies deep to the junction above large unmineralized spaces in granular layer of Tomes. Note dense centers of calcospherites and tubules occluded by peritubular dentin. BSE, 20 kV. (Magnification × 520.) FIGURE 32 (Center left). LS human premolar, micro-milled surface, BSE image. Cement-dentin junction marked by most hypermineralized line. Mineralization appears to have increase in dentin opposite ends of Sharpey's fibers. No large interglobular spaces present in peripheral layer with small calcospherites. BSE, 20 kV. (Magnification × 490.) FIGURE 33 (Center right). LS human premolar, micro-milled surface. Carbon-coated BSE image. Large spaces at junction of cement with dentin have dimensions equivalent to those of cell lacunae in bone and cement. (Magnification × 550.) FIGURE 34 (Lower left). LS human premolar, micro-milled surface, BSE image. Diffuse hypermineralized layer in dentin below cement-dentin junction is presumed to correspond to hyaline layer of Hopewell-Smith. Note abrupt change from small to large calcospherites. BSE, 20 kV. (Magnification × 525.) FIGURE 35 (Lower right). BSE image of human premolar root, micro-milled surface. There is no hypermineralized layer at the cement-dentin junction. Looping anastomotic branches of dentin tubules at center bottom. Radial orientation of dense streaks from dense initiation point in larger calcospherites. BSE, 20 kV. (Magnification × 490.)

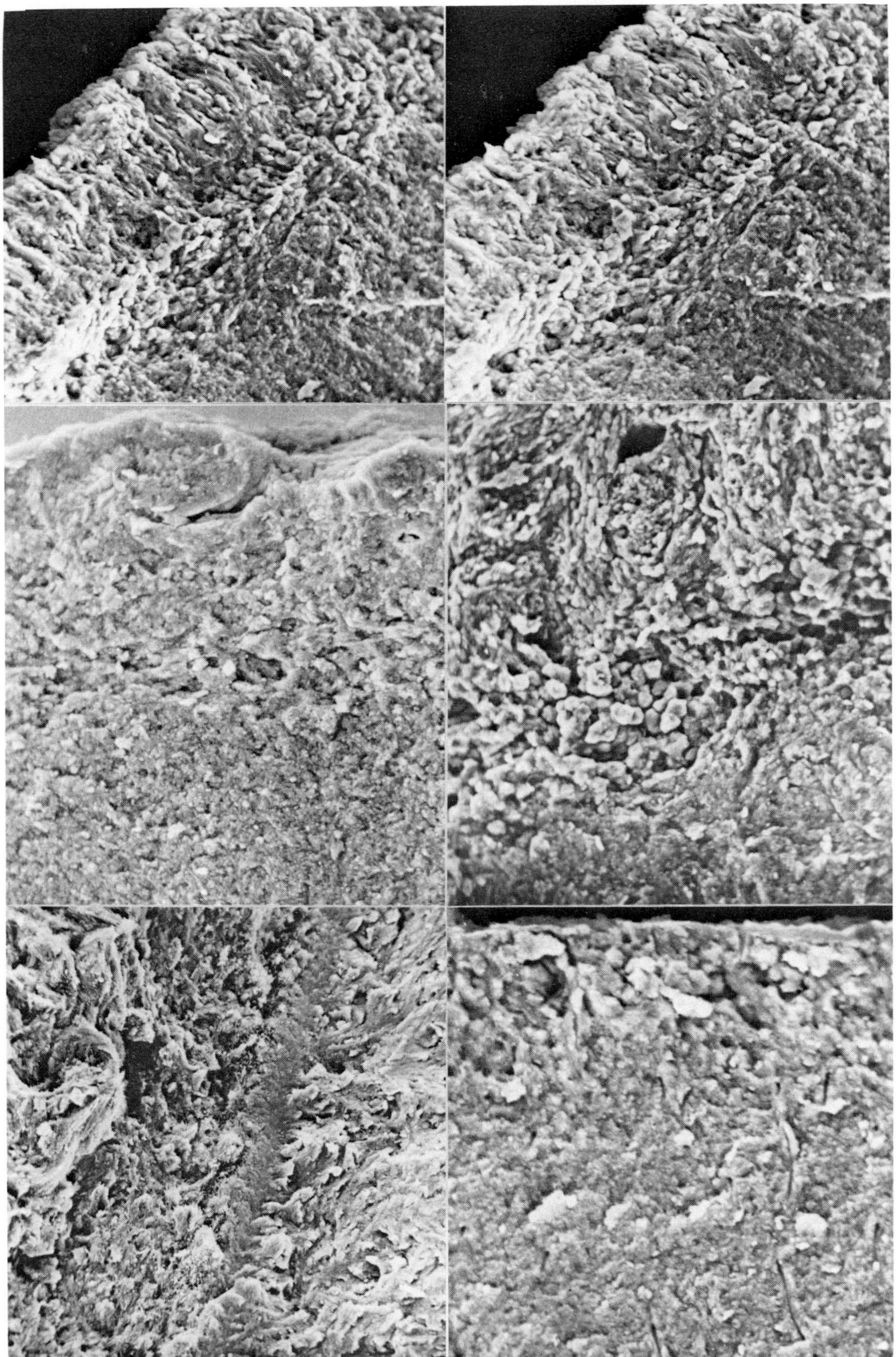

FIGURES 36—40.

Adams[132] also show a narrow gap between the basal lamina and the banded collagen fibrils, filled by very fine aperiodic fibrils perpendicular to and attached to the basal lamina. These fine aperiodic fibrils are a constant finding in association with the basal lamina, but may become obscured if the collagen fibrils of the mantle dentin extend amongst them.[138]

The distribution of the coarse mantle dentin fibers has been implicated in the shaping of the dentino-enamel junction during maturation of both tissues.[103] However whether the density and grouping of the fibers, which alter from one region of the interface to another, control or contribute to the escalloping of the margin is not known.

There is some evidence from autoradiographic studies that the dentin closest to the enamel acquires some enamel protein when amelogenesis begins, but this is probably a negligible contribution.[22]

2. Radicular Mantle Dentin Matrix

Mantle dentin is found in the root as well as the crown and is peripheral to the granular layer of Tomes[127] (Figure 23). It is said to be not as constant a layer as the coronal but, where present, contains similar, coarse collagen fibrils.[125] Radicular mantle dentin has not attracted as much attention as its coronal counterpart and its position relative to other proper-named layers is unclear. Many equate the hyaline layer of the root with the coronal mantle dentin.[140] It has been reported to be absent below cementum in rat, rabbit, and guinea pig incisors,[127] but present as a thick (8 to 15 μm) radioopaque layer below cementum in the dog,[139] and to be 15- to 30- μm thick in primates.[140]

The formation of this layer has been well described in the ultrastructural study of Ten Cate.[125] However, he was unable to clarify the confusion over the terminology of the differently composed layers in the region of the dentin-cement junction. It would appear that, in the mouse at least, the development of the mantle dentin layer follows that of a narrow band containing few fibrils close to the basal lamina. The organization of the coarse fibrils is usually parallel to the basal lamina, not perpendicular to it as is often the case in the crown. It would seem that the apical, secretory ends of odontoblasts develop junctional complexes early in root dentinogenesis. That may explain why the orientation of the coarse fibers in the root is similar to that of the finer circumpulpal fibers; they also form tangential to the available cell surface which is the apical one, and cannot be influenced by the lateral cell surfaces. A slower rate of differentiation and dentinogenesis in the root may favor a more advanced stage of cellular organization prior to collagen precursor production.

Accepting that the fibril orientation is a factor related to the secretory cell surface, and this changes with differentiation of the cells, the question remains as to why the fibrils of mantle dentin are wider in diameter and may be grouped into larger bundles with a parallel array. We have noted that the collagen component in mantle dentin is much greater than that in circumpulpal dentin at an equivalent distance from the secretory surface. This could be because the ratio of the fibrous component produced compared to the nonfibrous proteoglycans is higher, or the rate of dentinogenesis is so slow that there is time for a greater aggregation of collagen molecules onto fibrils. Towards the end of dentinogenesis, greater

FIGURE 36 (Above). Stereopair: granular layer of Tomes in peripheral dentin reaches junction with cement (left). LS fractured anorganic root of tapir tooth. (Magnification × 820.) FIGURE 37 (Center left). Coarse granular texture of peripheral layer of dentin contrasts with more homogeneously mineralized dentin (below) and cellular cement with vascular channel (above). Anorganic fractured molar root, Finlayson Siamese squirrel. (Magnification × 1030.) FIGURE 38 (Center right). Fusiform mineral clusters in Sharpey's fibers of cellular cement (above) can be followed to cement-dentin junction and hypomineralized peripheral dentin with small discrete calcospherites. More homogeneously mineralized deeper dentin lies below. Anorganic preparation, fractured walrus root. (Magnification × 860.) FIGURE 39 (Lower left). More homogeneous layer of fine fibrils in peripheral dentin next to cement-dentin junction is equivalent to hyaline layer. LS fractured human molar. (Magnification × 830.) FIGURE 40 (Lower right). Peripheral layer of dentin with small, incompletely fused calcospherites reaches almost to root surface as cement is very thin in this developing dog deciduous molar root. Anorganic LS fracture. (Magnification × 880.)

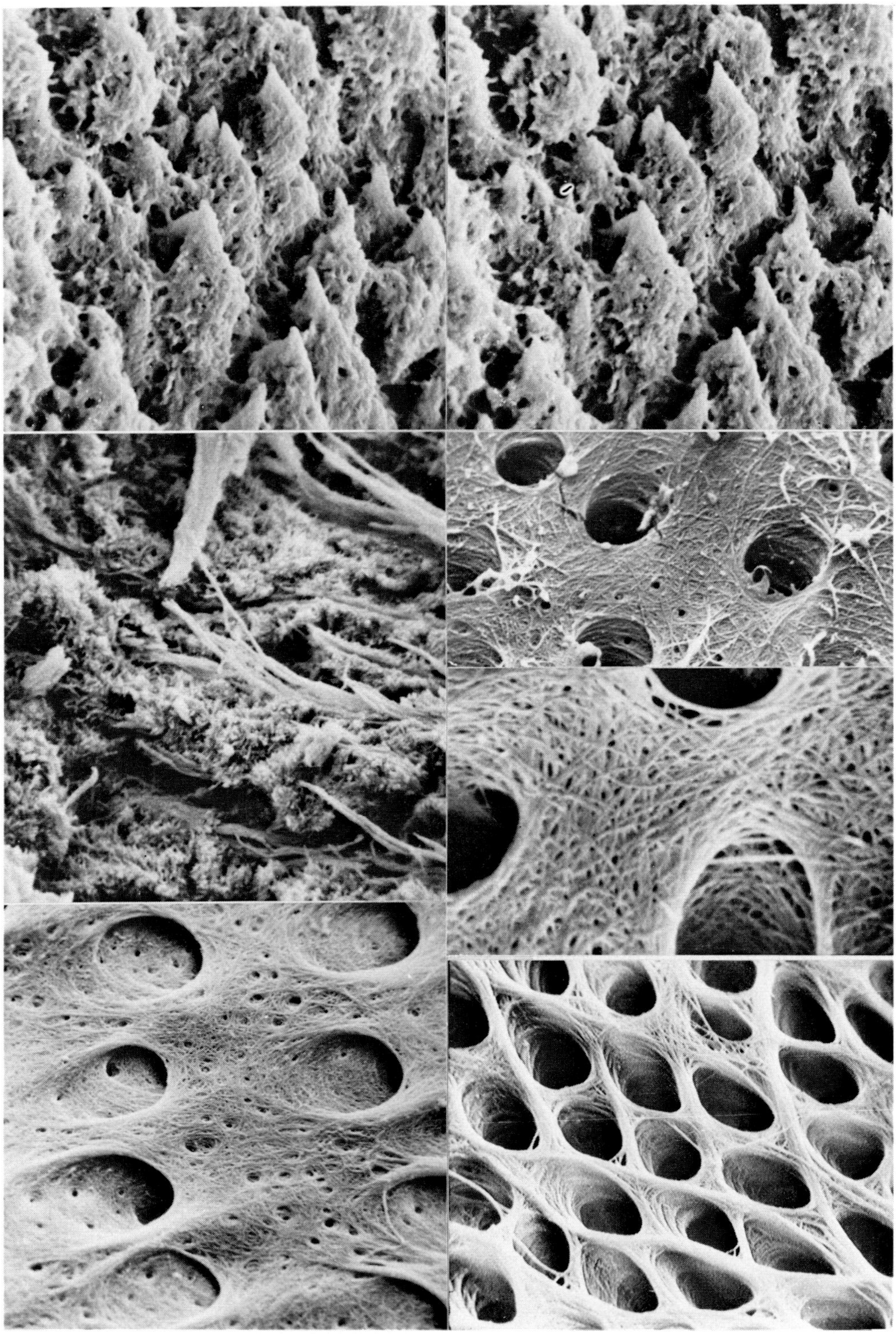

FIGURES 41—46.

grouping of fibrils also occurs, but whether each fibril is also coarser we do not know. Individual chondrocytes secrete different types of Type II collagen at different stages in chondrogenesis. By analogy, it is possible that the coarse fibrils in dentin also differ chemically from the fine ones, being, perhaps, Type I trimer[141] or Type III[22] which are reported to be present in small amounts, but have not been located.

a. Granular Layer of Tomes

The granular layer of Tomes forms one of the most prominent features in the dentin of the root in a ground section. It is peripherally located below the cementum, and thought either to extend to the cement-dentin junction[112] or to be separated from it by mantle dentin[127,139] or the hyaline layer.[140] The neat distinction between these layers suggested linguistically is not structurally correct[126,137] and this has caused some of the confusion in the literature as we have discussed previously.

The one feature of the granular layer that is not disputed is that the region with a granular light-microscopical appearance is hypomineralized. The cause, or even location, of this hypomineralization is ascribed to different features. Ten Cate[112] proposed that it was due to an increase in the spaces occupied by the odontoblast process because the development of the process was out of phase with the rate of matrix production and retreat of the cell body from the dentin-cement junction. This led to looping or buckling of the processes, an increase in the proportion of tubular to matrix volume, and hence to an overall decrease in mineral density of the layer. Ten Cate reported that he found no looping of dentin tubules below the enamel and that this supported his interpretation since the granular layer is absent in the crown. Ten Cate supposed that as dentinogenesis in the crown was more rapid than the root, process and matrix formation would proceed at the same rate, and buckling not arise. Equally, to support his argument, he could have called upon the relief that the extension of odontoblast processes into enamel would give to any buildup of pressure caused by their growth.[109] However, dentinogenesis close to the dentin-cement junction is more rapid than in the rest of the root dentin.[142] One would therefore expect, if Ten Cate's proposal is correct, that the granular layer of Tomes extends throughout the dentin of the root and would become more marked with increasing distance from the peripheral border, unless his argument also supposes a greater proportional diminution in the rate of process formation with time.

The other main reason postulated for the hypomineralization of this layer is a deficient mineralization of the matrix in this layer. Shackleford[139] found that the layer was hyperorganic compared with the adjacent dentin, and proposed that the "granules" were due to the presence of an unmineralized organic reticulum in which most of the components were oriented longitudinally. He considered that the reticulum could be largely amorphous although one component was fibrous. However, Furseth[143] demonstrated that the unmineralized areas contained collagen fibers.

A different explanation of the deficiency in the mineralization of the matrix is that it contains small calcospherites which fail to fuse, leaving small interglobular spaces (Figures 25 to 40). This is an explanation favored by many textbooks[124,144,145] and strongly supported

FIGURE 41 (Above). Stereopair: mineralizing front in peripheral dentin of rat incisor on the enamel-covered side of the tooth. Spike protuberances in anorganic preparation of mineralizing front relate to centers of large diameter (von Korff) fiber bundles. (Magnification × 2650.) FIGURE 42 (Center left). *Tursiops truncatus* (dolphin) fractured dentin showing large diameter (von Korff) fiber bundles parallel with dentin tubules in peripheral dentin. (Magnification × 2650.) FIGURE 43 (Center right above). Surface of dentin matrix of tapir molar with main tubules and side branch openings. Fibrils encircle the tubules. (Magnification × 3300.) FIGURE 44 (Center right below). Calf molar predentin, cleaned by enzyme treatment showing collagen fibril network. (Magnification × 7400.) FIGURE 45 (Lower left). Horse deciduous molar predentin surface showing extreme obliquity of entry of dentin tubules and large number of side branch tubule openings. (Magnification × 1840.) FIGURE 46 (Lower right). Human permanent canine, pulp chamber dentin showing close packing of wide dentin tubule openings and constraint of fibrils to run as bundles between these openings. (Magnification × 2900.)

by scanning electron microscopical evidence and transmission electron microscopy.[119,143] The numbers of initial loci of mineralization must be very high compared with those of later dentin production, and the surface area available for the accretion of mineral consequently greater. It is possible that before these calcospherites have time to extend to encompass all the matrix, a layer now superficial to them is already mineralizing and taking up most of the available mineral ions, effectively sealing off the region. A further influx of mineral could occur peripherally upon the disruption and replacement of the epithelial root sheath cells leading, at times, to a narrow region of increased mineralization at the cement-dentin junction. This concept is also supported by the work of Heritier and Fernandez[146] who found that a fine layer of collagen fibrils remained unmineralized below the epithelial cells until they moved away and cementogenesis began, leading to the merging of both tissues. However, this secondary mineralization does not reach back into the granular layer.

The delay in the completion of mineralization in the matrix in the granular layer of Tomes, contributed to by the longer blocking of access of ions from the outside by the epithelial root sheath cells, may also mean that the matrix loses some of its capacity to mineralize or the calcospherites lose the ability to grow. The mineralizable zone with its special environment[147] will have moved on. It is in any case clear from the natural history of both bone and dentin mineralization that failure to mineralize at roughly the right time leads to a permanent failure to mineralize.

As with other puzzles in the structure of dentin, it is difficult to relate the artifacts of the light microscopical view to the ultrastructure of the tissue. Incompletely fused small calcospherites (Figures 30 to 40) and looping (Figure 35) or expanded odontoblast branches both occur in the peripheral region of dentin in the root; both might contribute, albeit unequally, to the familiar appearance of the granular layer of Tomes. The problem would be best resolved by the examination of undecalcified tissue by TEM, or by the sequential study of a plane through the dentin-cement junction using light microscopy then BSE images for density, followed by SEM images of the same plane in an anorganic preparation.

The inclusion of epithelial cells from the disintegration of the epithelial root sheath is occasionally responsible for unmineralized areas in the root at the cement-dentin junction (Figure 33). This inclusion can occur sporadically in any tooth, but is reported to be a common feature in the apical half of rat molar.[128]

3. *Mineralization of Mantle Dentin*

The first dentin to mineralize is the mantle dentin below the tips of the cusps. Here there is a wealth of fibers approximately perpendicular to the dentino-enamel junction, centers of mineralization occurring in matrix vesicles[85-87] amongst these fibers. Mineralization spreads along their lengths to the full thickness of the layer.[148] Some workers[149] held that matrix vesicles do not occur in mantle dentin, but TEM of the first stages of dentinogenesis confirms their presence, if not their necessity.[150] The contrasting opinion was that matrix vesicles occur in mantle dentin, but not in circumpulpal dentin.[88,90] The inward spread of mineral along the bundles of coarse fibrils of the mantle layer has also been effectively demonstrated in some species by SEM,[151-154] and is the predominant pattern in that narrow coronal layer (Figure 41). Mineralization also spreads back along the fibers to the dentin-enamel junction, reaching it in the cat developing tooth when the predentin is 100-μm thick, and then into the newly developing enamel.[14]

Although granular regions do not occur in the same manner in the crown, the initial dentin formed below the enamel does seem, on microradiographic evidence, to be less well mineralized than the circumpulpal dentin.[124,155] BSE images of section surfaces show a very thin layer of lower density at the dentin-enamel junction (Figure 21), peripheral to the layer in which fine branching of the tubules occurs, but no granular layer of unfused calcospherites, as is easily recognized in the root with the same technique (Figures 31 to 35). The layer of greater radiolucency below the enamel appears thicker than the width of mantle dentin in microradiographs, but this is likely a result of using relatively thick sections. It has been supposed that this may be due to the coarser fibrils and the fibril groupings present in the coronal mantle dentin, a situation also present in the root. Alternatively, such a diffuse appearance could be due to an abundance of side branches of odontoblast processes or a relatively lower quantity of peritubular dentin.

However, it is significant that coarse fibrillar dentin of lower vertebrates is less well mineralized than the finer fibrillar dentin[135] and of course, the nonfibrillar peritubular dentin is best mineralized of all. Totally uncalcified bundles or cores of bundles do not seem to exist and therefore cannot be the cause of increased radiolucency, in contrast to the other bony tissues. It could be just that intrafibrillar mineralizaton does not occur and thus not only is a higher volume proportion excluded from the mineralization process, but the surface area available as a template for mineralization, perhaps through the linkage offices of one of the other matrix components, is reduced by the greater fibrillar diameter.

Mantle dentin in the root, as in the crown, shows two directions of spread of mineralization from the initiation sites within the dentin. The mineral spreads back toward the outer limit of the dentin (Figures 25 and 28) to what will become the dentin-cement junction, and also pulpward. Additionally, a second input of mineral may come from the root aspect once the cement begins to form, as we have discussed previously. Tetracycline labeling of developing roots confirms that the leading edge of mineralization is just within the dentin, not at the dentin-cement junction.[156] This centrifugal spread has caused some confusion especially in work based solely on low resolution light microscopy,[116,157] and in species where the cementum is extremely thin.

Owens[158,159] has suggested that this peripheral dentin layer, in the rat and the dog at least, may be contributed to by some secretion of the epithelial cells before their disruption as a limiting layer. His reasoning for this is, first, that the cells look like secretory ones; second, that this layer stains differently from the remainder of the dentin; third, that the lingual side of the incisal tip of rabbit incisors is covered by a thin layer of enamel matrix.[160] His opinion is contested by Heritier and Fernandez[146] who consider the epithelial cells not to be secretory.

Katz and Li[161] have postulated that the ability of the dentinal collagen to mineralize depends on the molecular packing; the intermolecular gaps of about 6 Å permit the large phosphate ions to enter intrafibrillar regions. It is not known whether there is a molecular packing difference between the coarse and fine fibrils of dentin. Small quantities (<3%) of Type I trimer collagen have been recovered from normal bovine dentin,[141] but whether this mineralizes differently or is confined to mantle dentin fibrils is unknown.

B. Circumpulpal Dentin

Circumpulpal dentin forms the bulk of the calcified connective tissue in mammalian teeth and is laid down rhythmically as the odontoblasts move centripetally. It is penetrated throughout with a wealth of tubules housing the main processes of the odontoblasts and their side branches. It comprises two main regions, designated *intertubular* and *peritubular dentin.*

1. Intertubular Matrix

Collagen forms from procollagen extracellularly. Occasionally, centrosymmetrical cross-banded structures are seen in the matrix which look like SLS collagen, that is procollagen.[162,163] These may possibly be an artifact of preparation but are reported to be a constant finding.

The intertubular matrix of circumpulpal dentin has a collagen fibril and fiber organization of varying complexity. At its simplest, fine fibrils form a feltwork within the plane of the developing surface[64,154,164] that is entirely random (Figures 43 to 45). The fibrils of circumpulpal dentin usually also show a circular orientation immediately next to the tubule,[64,165]

(Figure 47) an organization that reminds one of encircling intrinsic fibers that sometimes occur adjacent to Sharpey's (extrinsic) fibers in cement and bone.

Some degree of linear orientation of the circumpulpal dentin collagen may also occur due to one or more of the following three factors:

1. The collagen is grouped into bundles by the constraint offered by the narrowness of the interval between adjacent odontoblast processes at the most superficial level of the predentin (Figure 46). Thus, this can occur in any tooth in later stages of dentinogenesis when the odontoblasts become crowded. It can be seen by examining the predentin surface.
2. Many dentin also have collagen fibers with their long axes lying parallel to the dentin tubules (Figure 48).[129] These fibers are parallel to an extensive formative surface related to a long taper on the (first) proximal portion of the odontoblast process. There are many published electron micrographs which illustrate the presence of these collagen fibrils lying parallel and adjacent to the odontoblast process.[38,81,137,164,166] In some cases these fibers form a sizeable proportion of the matrix, are clearly at right angles to the intervening, interweaving fibrils, but may not be present equally on all aspects of the tubule wall.[137] Tubule parallel collagen can also be seen by SEM of fractured predentin and suitably oriented specimens of intact predentin.
3. In teeth with extensive formative surfaces where the incremental planes lie nearly parallel with the tooth long axes and the enamel- or cement-dentin junction and in which dentin formation is rapid, the obliquity of entry of the dentin tubules is considerable (Figure 66). In plain view of the predentin surfaces the openings of the tubule appear as elongated, pointed ellipses and the collagen is mostly oriented roughly parallel to the long axis of these ellipses, the tooth, the junction, and the tubules. It is, of course, also parallel to the element of translation of the odontoblast across the predentin. Both cell movement and constraint of space, then, may help to provide the linear orientation seen here.

It has been suggested that the orientation of the collagen fibrils changes in successive layers of circumpulpal dentin rather like the change that occurs from one lamella to the next in bone, and that this is the basis of von Ebner's incremental lines.[129,140] This regular lamination is not easy to demonstrate in ultrastructural studies and we know of no published electron micrographs that illustrate it. The likeliest way to exhibit such a structure would be an oblique step-wise fracture or tear through mineralized dentin so that parts of several successive developmental planes could be seen face-on using scanning electron microscopy. This should be more fruitful than such rupture through predentin because here the fibrils have not yet aggregated to their full thickness in the most superficial part, yet our preparations of this nature fail to show any such orientation-dependent layering, at least in human permanent dentin (Figure 11).

If the orientation of the fibrils did change in layers, it would be necessary to assume that

FIGURE 47 (Upper left). Fractured human 12 year third mandibular molar showing fibrillar organization in coronal intertubular predentin. Fibrils lining the tubules are circularly or randomly arranged. (Magnification × 2000.) FIGURE 48 (Upper right). Fractured predentin of developing crown of lower third molar of 12 year human showing some longitudinal collagen fibrils in walls of the tubules. (Magnification × 4900.) FIGURE 49 (Center left). Ethanol freeze-fracture of glutaraldehyde-fixed developing rat molar at predentin (right)-dentin junction, showing packing of collagen fibrils in predentin. (Magnification × 17,000.) FIGURE 50 (Center right). Human 12 year mandibular third molar, fracture passing through predentin (below) and dentin showing peritubular matrix formation at level of mineralizing front. (Magnification × 5000.) FIGURE 51 (Below). Stereopair: *Metachirus nudicaudatus* (rat-tailed opposum). Anorganic preparation of pulpal surface of tooth, showing nearly complete mineralization of collagen fibrils at arrested mineralizing front. (Magnification × 9350.)

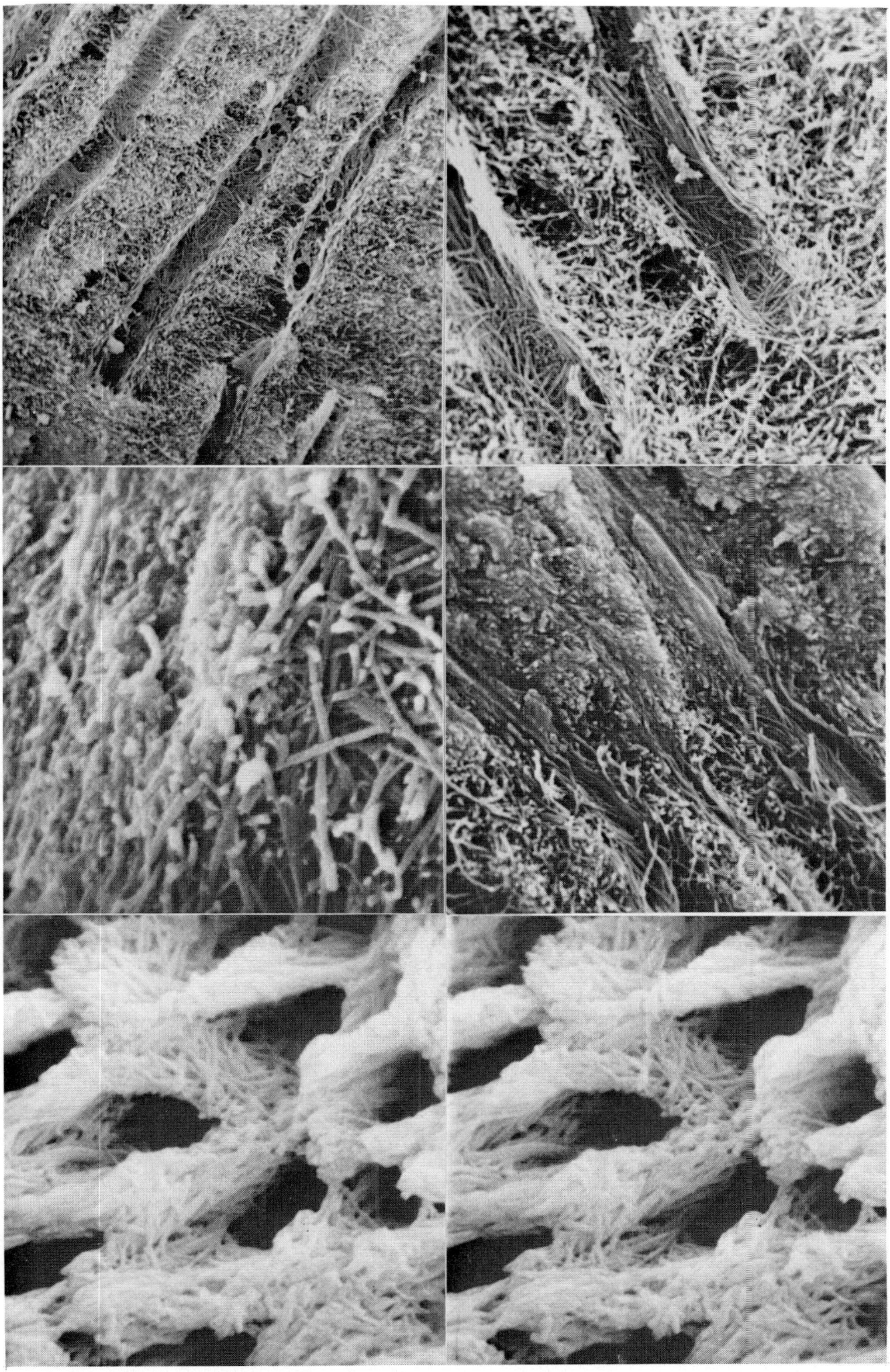

FIGURES 47—51.

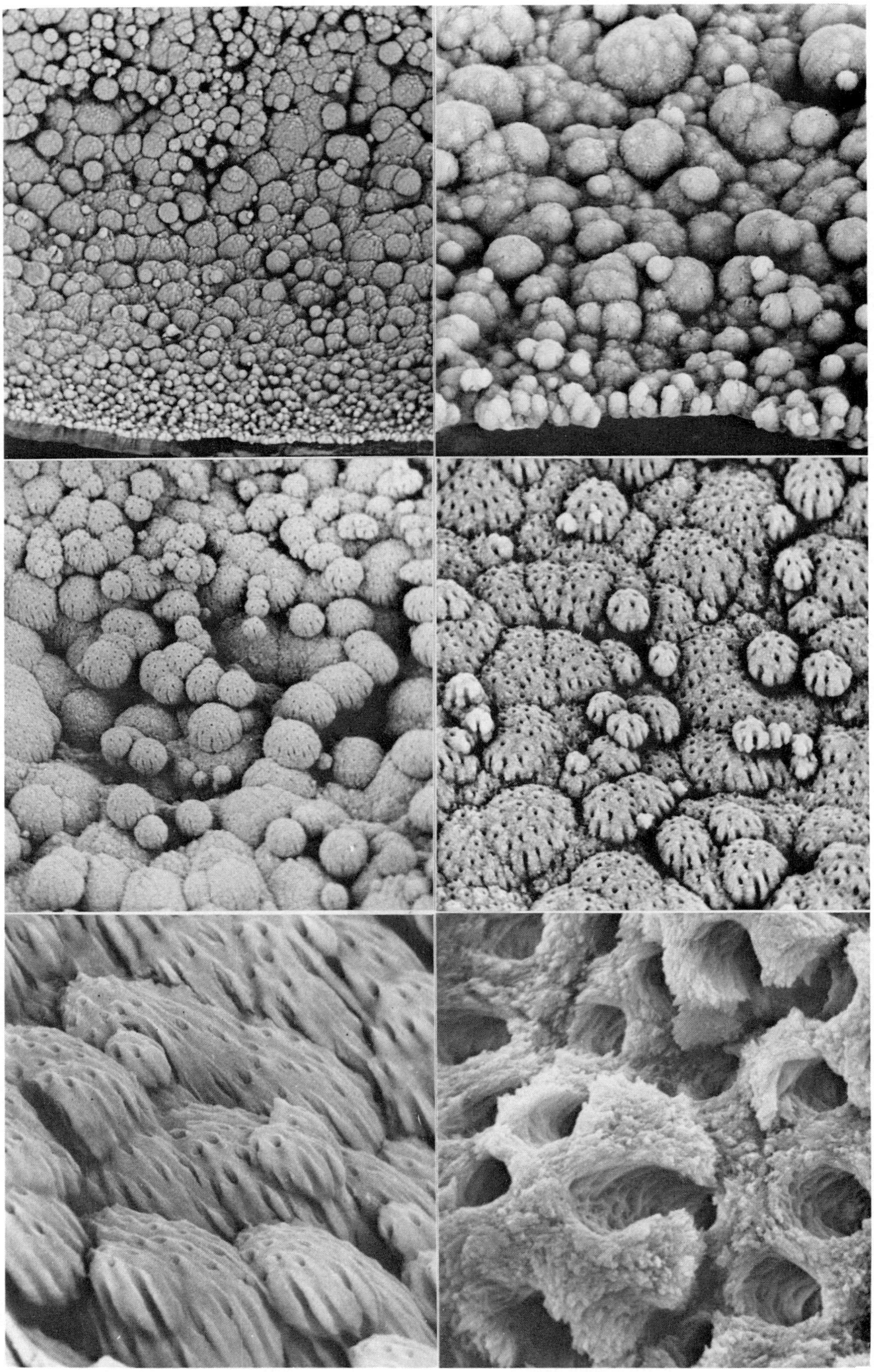

FIGURES 52—57.

some circadian change in the rate of production was associated with an alteration in the movement of the cell in relation to the formative surface. Von Ebner's lines have been shown to have a diurnal periodicity in the pig.[94] Cell movement across the forming dentin surface is difficult to conceive for the odontoblasts because they are anchored by their processes and have a small secretory territory. They are therefore not free to change their shape and to translocate across the matrix surface in the same way as osteoblasts. However, the secondary curvatures of dentin tubules, emphasized in the larger lines of Owen, indicate that the processes at least do not follow a straight line. The deviation of dentin tubules in a way that must express the relative movement of groups of cells is most clearly seen in elephant ivory.[167]

Kaye and Herold[168] put forward an interesting idea concerning the possible role of odontoblast side processes in the ordering of collagen fibrils. Because of the abundance of lateral branches, they speculated that these might direct the formation and orientation of their investing matrix. If this were so, an angular change in the main direction of the processes at any one level to the next could result in a lamination in the fibrous structure. A compositional change must also be occurring in such rhythmic deposition and this will later be reflected in alterations in the level of mineralization as the predentin subsequently becomes dentin.

The ultrastructural localization of the nonfibrous elements of the dentin matrix is especially difficult because they are masked in the untreated tissue and methods to recover them after removal of the mineral, or mineral and collagen, result in their total or partial loss. Staining techniques may be quite informative for predentin,[42] but much less so for dentin.[169] A limited study of predentin matrix in rat incisors sampled in pairs of sibling rats at 4 hr intervals over a 24-hr period[170] has shown that the rate of noncollagen ground substance components to collagen next to the odontoblast varies dramatically. If this indication that the composition of the matrix changes according to a circadian rhythm could be confirmed, it would explain the clear demonstration of the daily (von Ebner) incremental lines following the use of, for example, 24-hr hematoxylin staining. The demonstration of these lines by polarized light microscopy might then be explained by the presence of varying proportions of the ground substance component in which crystallites might be oriented perpendicular to the plane of a relatively flat mineralizing front.

2. *Mineralization of Intertubular Matrix*

Predentin transforms into dentin when mineral salts are deposited in the organic matrix (Figures 49 to 51). The calcification border may be broad with many discrete loci of mineralization (Figures 52 to 67), or it may be a continuous plane if the mineralization is proceeding very slowly. The patterns of mineralization may be described at several levels of magnification.

The most characteristic form is calcospheritic (Figures 52 to 62). Accumulations of crystals form, and growth of the mineral phase occurs in all directions, more or less evenly until

FIGURE 52 (Upper left). Anorganic preparation of growing edge of crown of human 12 year lower third molar, viewed from dentinal aspect. Note very fine calcospherites in peripheral dentin and rapid increase in size of calcospherites further coronally. (Magnification × 80.) FIGURE 53 (Upper right). Same preparation as Figure 52, higher magnification. Mineralization has spread furthest around each tubule adding a second relief to the surface of the calcospherites. (Magnification × 395.) FIGURE 54 (Center left). Anorganic preparation, converted BSE image of mineralizing front in coronal dentin, roof of pulp chamber in human lower third molar. Unmineralized regions extend deep into the dentin. (Magnification × 450.) FIGURE 55 (Center right). Oxygen plasma-ashed human lower third permanent molar developing coronal dentin. Peritubular dentin is mineralizing at same level as intertubular dentin. (Magnification × 360.) FIGURE 56 (Lower left). Anorganic 12 year human lower third molar; shows oblique entry of dentin tubules and relative advance of mineralizing front surrounding each tubule. (Magnification × 830.) FIGURE 57 (Lower right). Human lower second permanent molar coronal dentin mineralizing front. Complete collagen fibril mineralization can be seen in wall of tubule which has no peritubular dentin. (Magnification × 2815.)

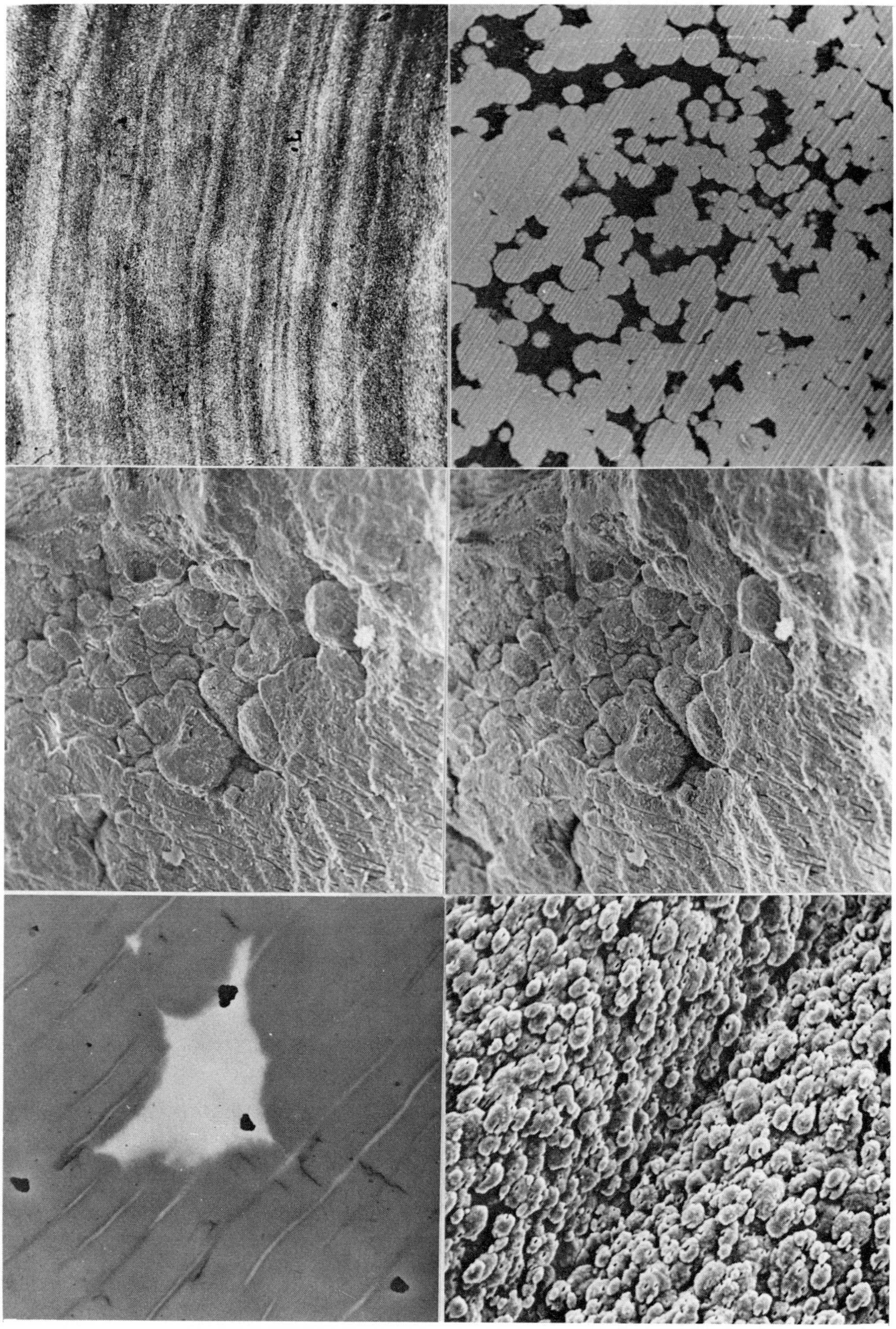

FIGURES 58—62.

the *calcospherite* impinges on the surrounding ones. Growth will then proceed on the remaining available surface for so long as a plentiful supply of ions reaches the mineral-accreting surface. The initiation of spheritic mineralization is generally considered to be associated with matrix vesicles, which are small, membrane-bound structures, budded off from the odontoblasts and lying free within the intertubular matrix. Matrix vesicles have rarely been demonstrated in circumpulpal dentin.

The number of calcospherites formed may exceed the numbers of matrix vesicles and their density is thought to be an expression of the cell surface activity of the odontoblast at any one time. Additionally, Slavkin[12] reported that not all matrix vesicles accumulate calcium and phosphate ions and initiate calcospherites. As we have already discussed, matrix vesicles are a feature of the earliest phase of dentinogenesis,[85-87] but they are also reported to occur in reparative dentin.

The size of calcospherites, and their ultimate shape varies in different regions of the dentin[151,152,165] (Figures 24 to 35 and 52 to 57). They can be excellently displayed in anorganic specimens prepared for scanning electron microscopical study, but it is necessary to recall that the separate calcospherites will not be retained.[171] In human teeth they are smallest, most numerous, and spherical close to the peripheral limits of dentin but rapidly increase in size and decrease in incidence (Figures 52 to 57). In this middle layer, which lies in the outer third of the primary dentin, the shape of the completed calcospherites is a parabolic cone extending pulpward. The calcospherites in the inner half of the dentin are again smaller, yet not so small as those of the initial layer, and with their centers more widely spaced (Figure 52). The abundance of the two main forms of calcospherites, spheres and paraboloids, varies in different species[129] and was thought to be related to the depth of predentin or the rate of dentinogenesis.

The evidence of polarized light microscopy suggests that a proportion of the crystals in a calcospherite spread radially from the growth center.[172] The highly mineralized center of the calcospherite and the ''spokes'' in the radial spread may be demonstrated by BSE images (Figures 31 to 35). Scanning electron microscopy of anorganic preparations shows that mineralization will track along collagen fibrils encountered in the growth of the calcospherites, but this does not alter the general radial pattern of spreading (Figures 67 and 68). By presumption, therefore, the crystals which are demonstrated by polarized light microscopy are located in the interfibrillar ground substance.

Interglobular spaces of unmineralized dentin result from incomplete fusion of calcospherites (Figures 59 to 61). This is especially prevalent in human teeth where there has been a deficiency in vitamin D during dentin formation, or conditions such as vitamin D-resistant rickets (Figure 59) or severe fluorosis.[28] Because of the limitation of their growth, calcospherites tend to remain spherical in these cases. However, interglobular spaces may be found in most human teeth, and are the norm in poorly mineralized teeth of, for example, some odontocetes[137] (Figures 58 and 62). Longitudinal grooves in the formative front of narwhal dentin relate to radial mineralization deficiencies within the dentin The grooves have smaller calcospherites that fail to fuse properly (Figure 62).

In calcospherites proper, the main advancing edge of the dentin initially appears mounded without regard for the siting of the tubules and several openings of the tubule may pass

FIGURE 58 (Upper left). Polished surface of TS of sperm whale mandibular tooth, showing incremental lines due to variation in degree of mineralization BSE, 30 kV. (Magnification × 25.) FIGURE 59 (Upper right). Longitudinal diamond saw cut surface of molar tooth from case of familial hypophosphatemia, showing prominent calcospherites in interglobular dentin. BSE, 30 kV. (Magnification × 83.) FIGURE 60 (Center). Stereopair: anorganic, fractured root of tapir tooth showing large region of interglobular dentin. (Magnification × 300.) FIGURE 61 (Lower left). Micro-milled LS human molar, negative BSE image of interglobular dentin space (white = low degree or zero degree of mineralization). (Magnification × 590.) FIGURE 62 (Lower right). Narwhal (*Monodon monoceros*) anorganic preparation showing mineralizing front of tusk. Oblique valley from lower left to upper right is longitudinal spiral groove. (Magnification × 280.)

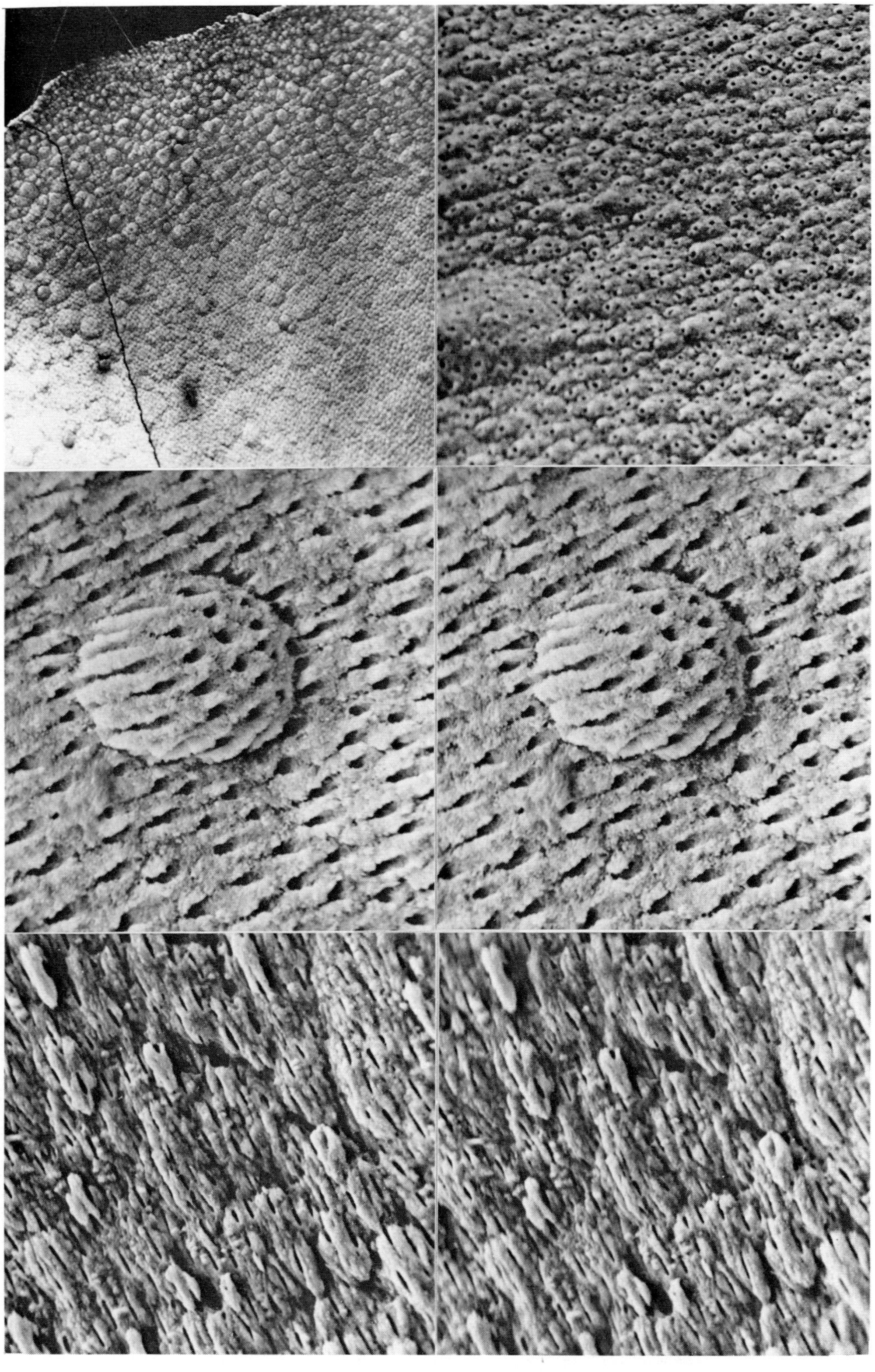

FIGURES 63—66.

through one mound (Figures 52 to 57 and 65 to 67). Anorganic preparations of such calcospherites may emphasize the cogwheel perimeter caused by partly incorporated processes.[151,152,165,173] The calcospherites ahead of the main mineral front first appear to be perched on the surface, their deep surfaces undercut. Later, they merge more with the surface, with no undercut. At this stage one can detect a small rampart around each tubule, as tubule-centered mineralization of the intertubular matrix adds a finer relief to the calcospheritic pattern.

Some regions of the dentin-predentin border in some animals, such as the rhesus monkey, rat, and dog have more prominent projections of the mineralizing front which are centered around dentin tubule openings.[151,152,154] These mineralization fronts are always seen as continuous layers and it is likely that a basically linear spread of mineralization has extended most rapidly next to the odontoblast process (Figures 53, 56, 63, and 64), presumably a source of ions. Mineralization of peritubular dentin below, level with or in advance of mineralization of the intertubular dentin, is a further element in the topography of the predentin-dentin border.

In most cases, tetracycline delineates both the mineralization border around isolated calcospherites in predentin and the advancing ends of the fused parabolic cones. It probably binds to both the mineral and organic phases of the dentin, because fluorescence is still apparent after demineralization.[174] Thin sections of dentin affected by sequential doses of tetracycline show concentric accretion in the calcospherites.

Locally, the border between dentin and predentin may not be parallel with the predentin surface, and calcification disorders will therefore not necessarily be aligned with the incremental lines. However, changes in the relative quantities of collagenous and noncollagenous components in matrix at the formative predentin surface may show later as changes in the degree of mineralization.

Besides regions of hypomineralization in the intertubular dentin, regions of hypermineralization also occur. Eda and Takuma[175] found batches of dentin in which the level of mineralizaton in the intertubular matrix almost equalled that of peritubular dentin. It is important to consider the origin of such dentin though, for exposure to oral fluids could cause an increase in the level of mineralization.[176]

The crystals which form the mineral phase of intertubular dentin are thought to be a calcium hydroxyapatite[177,178] and are usually described as plates or needles. Daculsi and coworkers[179] gave width and thickness values of 30 and 3 nm similar to Johansen's figures[180] and said that during carious attack they could grow to twice that thickness. The values from laser diffraction studies obtained by Höhling et al.[181] for both bone and dentin were not too dissimilar. However, dentin undergoes plastic deformation during cutting and it is therefore likely that long crystals, should they be present, would break in preparing TEM sections. Ion beam thinning excludes this possibility and dentin prepared in this way (Figure 69) exhibited circular and, compared with ultramicrotomed sections, *very long* tramline profiles of the mineral phase.[182] It is possible that the mineral phase ensheaths the microfibril of collagen, forming a tube with an inner diameter of from 3.8 nm upwards, and a length that equals that of the microfibril.[149,182] Boyde and Pawley[183] have pointed out that the widely accepted view that the crystallites in dentin are ~64 nm or less in length would mean that

FIGURE 63 (Upper left). *Macaca mulatta* anorganic preparation of permanent molar. Growing edge showing increase in size of calcospherites from peripheral dentin — top of micrograph — to very large calcospherites and then a smooth mineralizing front in which the small protuberances are each centered around a dentin tubule. (Magnification × 88.) FIGURE 64 (Upper right). Tubule centered mineralization over most of field partly masked by calcospherite, bottom left. Anorganic molar, *Macaca mulatta*. (Magnification × 430.) FIGURE 65 (Center). Stereopair: oblique entry of tubules emphasized on calcospherite. Anorganic macaque monkey molar. (Magnification × 1520.) FIGURE 66 (Below). Stereopair: rat incisor dentin on labial side. Anorganic preparation. Location 8 mm from growing apex. (Magnification × 900.)

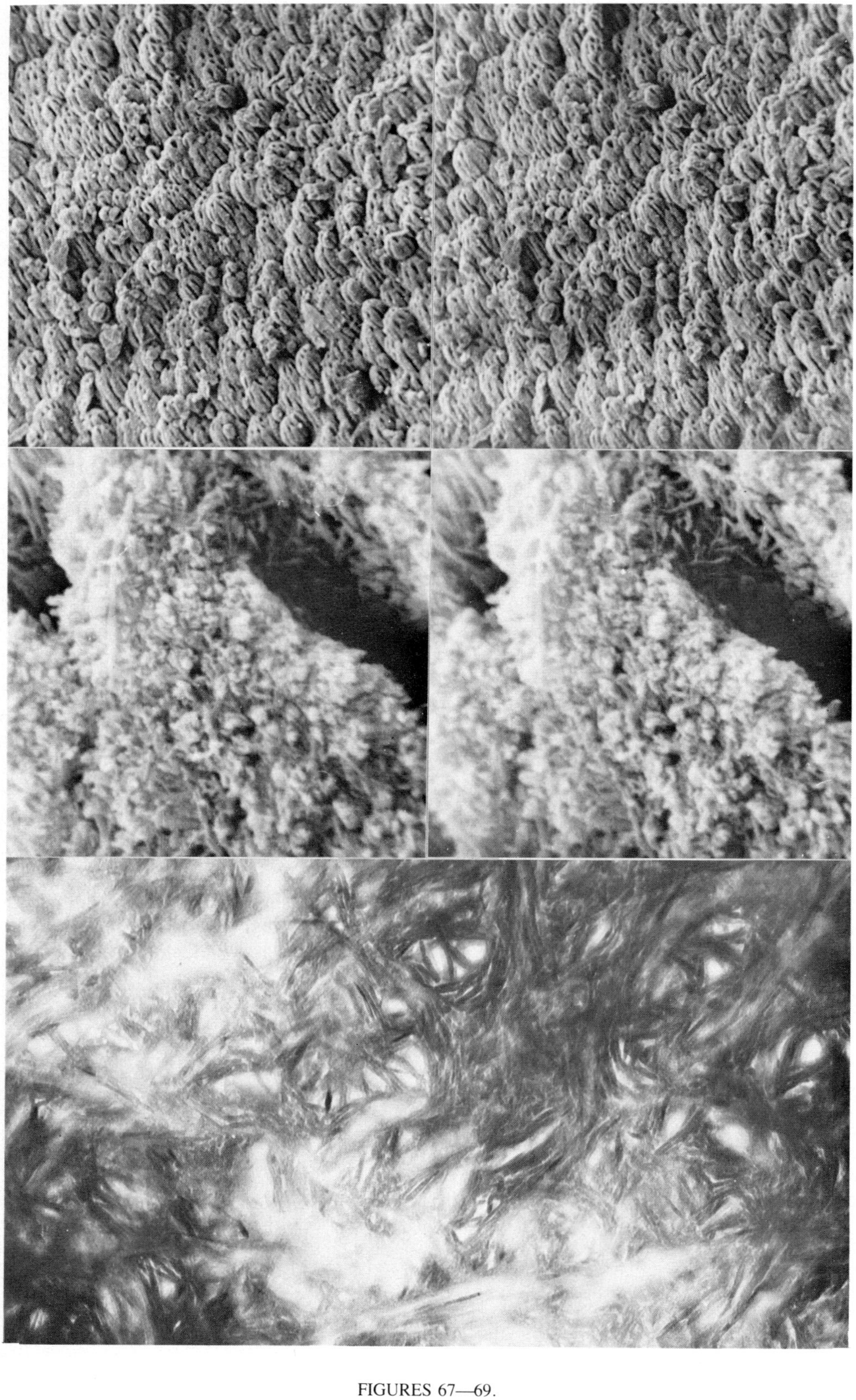

FIGURES 67—69.

anorganic dentin would be a suspension of fine crystals, whereas in fact, it retains its original size and shape, suggesting that the crystals are both longer and continuous. The details of early stages of crystal growth in dentin and other mineralizing connective tissues have been considered in detail by Höhling's group.[149,181,184-186] Höhling believes that dentin crystals grow from the coalescences of "dot-like nuclei", to form "chains" which eventually fuse to become "crystals". His chapter in Volume II should be consulted for further details.

3. Peritubular Matrix

The matrix of peritubular dentin is really *intra*tubular, forming between the intertubular matrix and the odontoblast process. Fortuitous fractures through dentin may reveal the abrupt junction between peritubular and intertubular dentin[64,128] (Figure 73). Peritubular dentin is not always present, but when it is, it may mineralize before, at the same time as, or later than, intertubular dentin.[151,152] The secretion of the matrix of peritubular dentin occurs after the deposition of the intertubular predentin, and may take place quite rapidly at the junction of dentin and predentin[175] (Figure 50).

The amount of peritubular matrix that develops varies greatly between species;[189-192] it is, for example, particularly plentiful in the cow (Figure 12), horse,[175] and elephant[154] (Figures 72 and 73), and scarce in the rabbit and coypu.[189] Toda and co-workers[56] have reported it to be present in mantle dentin in the dog, but not in circumpulpal dentin. It develops eccentrically around the tubule in some ungulates, especially where the tubule enters the dentin obliquely (Figures 74 and 75). Here the greatest thickness of peritubular dentin is found on the aspect of the tubule which faces more toward the dentin-enamel junction.[192]

The quantity of peritubular dentin also varies along the length of any one tubule and the variation in quantity may occur in a rhythmic fashion. Eda and Takuma[175] considered that this reflected an incremental pattern that gave rise to bands of radiolucency and opacity of the dentin.

In some odontocetes mineralization is lower in the intertubular dentin, with a failure of fusion of calcospherites, in alternate layers; in these layers of incomplete mineralization peritubular dentin may be entirely absent or very sparse.

The matrix of peritubular dentin contains either no collagen fibrils at all[192] or very few.[164,193] Observed in fractured surfaces, the smoother texture of the afibrillar, peritubular dentin differs greatly from that of the fibrous nature of the intervening richly collagenous intertubular dentin and this makes its identification easy[57,64,69,154,165,194,195] (Figure 73). It is commonly supposed that the matrix of peritubular dentin is the same as the noncollagenous component of the matrix of intertubular dentin, but this has not been adequately investigated and one report at least indicates it is not so.[196]

There are occasional reports of a limited number of fibrils embedded within the densely calcified peritubular dentin matrix but these are not always positively identified as collagen.[197] Large bundles of collagen fibers parallel to the tubules (Figure 48) should be more correctly assigned to intertubular dentin.[198] Because the collagenous component is lacking or very low, decalcification often causes the peritubular matrix to be entirely or partly lost from thin sections.[199] Careful demineralization after sectioning preserves a fine lacework in which Allred[200] and Johnson and co-workers[201] could see no substructure. Their findings were supported by Höhling and colleagues[186] and Goldberg and colleagues.[45] The dissenting report published by Plackova et al.,[202] in which replicas of etched dentin showed some patterning in the peritubular regions that they believed to be unmasked collagen, is probably unreliable

FIGURE 67 (Above). Stereopair: sheep molar. Anorganic preparation showing calcospherites in mineralizing front. (Magnification × 300.) FIGURE 68 (Center). Stereopair: sheep molar, higher magnification of Figure 67. Anorganic preparation showing collagen fibril centered mineralization within surface of a single calcospherite. (Magnification × 10,000.) FIGURE 69 (Below). TEM: ion beam thinned section of sperm whale dentin. (Magnification × 97,000.)

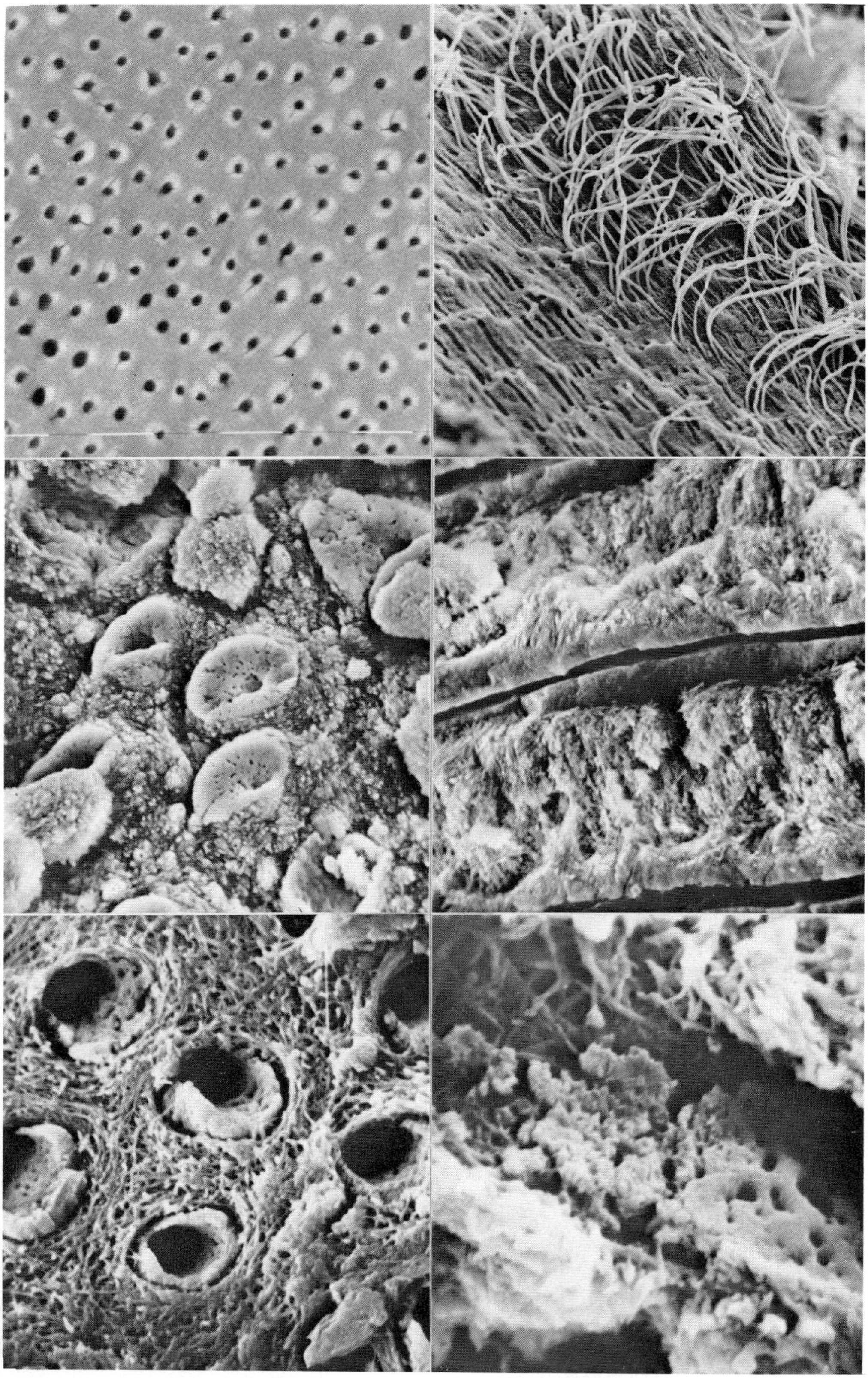

FIGURES 70—75.

because etching procedures can dissolve peritubular dentin and probably allow translocation of material. The peritubular matrix may be well preserved with some fixation and decalcification procedures and be seen as "Neuman's sheaths"[44] in fortuitous SEM preparations (Figure 71).

Peritubular dentin increases in thickness at the expense of the lumen of the tubule[52,203] and one factor in this may be occlusal attrition.[66,204] It was this gradual increase in man with time and function that led to the still widely held, but too limited, belief that the formation of peritubular dentin is basically an aging or protective response of the odontoblast. This phase is often mineralized at the same time as intertubular dentin in the crowns and first portion of the roots in human third permanent molars[229] (Figures 52 to 56).

Hypercalcified peritubular regions are not usually found in interglobular dentin of normal teeth.[67,205,206] A tubule which lies only partly in an interglobular region may have peritubular dentin adjacent to the calcified intertubular dentin and be lacking it next to the uncalcified matrix.[198] Whether the noncollagenous intratubular matrix forms in that region, but remains uncalcified, is not known; ultramicroscopy of undecalcified sections would be required to demonstrate it, if it were there, and care would be needed to ensure that the delicate and soluble matrix was not inadvertently lost in the preparation of the specimen.[45] The difficulty would be to compare the mineralized and demineralized views of the tissue. Unmineralized peritubular matrix is certainly evident in unmineralized regions at the predentin-dentin border,[164] but whether peritubular matrix forming deeper within dentin could remain unmineralized is another matter. Perusal of microradiographs showing interglobular regions published by Blake[205] leads one to question whether mineralization is entirely absent, rather than at a much lower level, in all parts of the interglobular dentin. A thin rim of mineralized peritubular matrix has been identified in the profuse interglobular dentin of dentinogenesis imperfecta[207] but whether its organic matrix was of normal constitution was not clear. Our own BSE images of such dentin tend to confirm this mineralization. The quantity of peritubular dentin formed in this condition is, anyway, far greater than usual, perhaps as a response to attrition.[208]

4. *Peritubular Mineral Phase*

The mineral phase of peritubular dentin differs from that of intertubular dentin in its distribution, density, structure, and crystal size. We have previously noted[175] its unequal distribution along the tubule length, often giving rise to an incremental pattern.

The extra density of peritubular dentin is its most remarkable feature[209] (Figure 70) — it is about 40% more highly mineralized than intertubular dentin.[186] It has a homogeneous structure[210] and the crystalline phase is evenly dispersed throughout the matrix which itself appears finely granular after the mineral (and some soluble products) has been removed.

Lester and Boyde[64,128,211] found closely packed, equidiametrical mineral clusters of about 25 nm in diameter in fracture planes of peritubular dentin extracted with ethylenediamine. Similar particles were observed, but less clearly, in untreated material. They described the mineral clusters as roughly spherical or polygonal, forming a regular mosaic pattern in all

FIGURE 70 (Upper left). BSE image of micro-milled human third molar dentin surface, showing extent of hypermineralized peritubular dentin zones in coronal dentin. (Magnification × 1000.) FIGURE 71 (Upper right). N HCl etched human deciduous tooth, showing Neuman's sheaths, i.e., peritubular dentin matrix remnants. (Magnification × 350.) FIGURE 72 (Center left). Elephant molar coronal dentin mineralizing front showing peritubular zones locally proud of mineralizing front of intertubular dentin. Peritubular dentin forms so rapidly that tubules are largely occluded a few microns deep to the surface. (Magnification × 900.) FIGURE 73 (Center right). Elephant molar coronal dentin, fractured perpendicular to surface. Anorganic preparation showing extent of peritubular dentin zones. (Magnification × 1025.) FIGURE 74 (Lower left). Calf molar dentin digested with papain producing a surface close to the mineralizing front, showing a predominantly one-sided location of peritubular dentin which forms close to the level of the mineralizing front in the intertubular dentin. (Magnification × 4600.) FIGURE 75 (Lower right). Calf molar. Fractured anorganic preparation, showing mineralization of peritubular dentin at the level of the mineralizing front in the intertubular dentin. Note the short distance of 2 to 3 μm over which the peritubular dentin mineralizes and fuses to become a compact homogeneous layer. (Magnification × 10,000.)

planes of fracture. A fine mineral particle size of 2.5 nm ± 30% has been reported by Vahl and Mierau,[212] while Höhling et al.[181,185] have described dot-like nuclei and short chains of nuclei.

Lefevre et al.[213] studied peritubular dentin using secondary ion mass spectrometry microscopy. They recorded that calcium, phosphate, and magnesium ion levels were higher than in intertubular dentin, magnesium reaching 1% in weight, and thought whitlockite was present. From TEM evidence, the whitlockite may have been in the intratubular region, as Frank et al.[214] have also found.

The level of mineralization in peritubular dentin is reported to be more variable than that of intertubular dentin,[215] but this variability might decrease with age. Certainly it has a patchy distribution initially. As long as the odontoblast process remains vital and extends along the tubule, peritubular dentin can increase at the expense of the tubular volume and the degree to which this occurs can differ greatly in adjacent tubules and with the general degree of sclerosis.[69,176,204,215-217]

Occlusion of the tubules may also be the result of the deposition of large crystals in their lumen. These may be remineralization crystals associated with dental caries, abrasion, or attrition.[64,192,197] They are usually easy to distinguish from the proper peritubular dentin which contains a finer mineral phase[64,192,201] although occasionally investigators have not agreed that this is so.[212] Such crystalline deposits are also reported to be more acid-resistant to etching procedures[218] than the surrounding peritubular dentin which might result, in the case of the so-called caries crystals, from their formation in a more acid environment. Attempts have been made to identify the intralumenal crystalline deposits from their morphology. The crystalline component of peritubular dentin is considered to be apatite,[216] but it has also been referred to as amorphous calcium phosphate. In contrast, the larger intratubular crystals have been tentatively identified as whitlockite, octacalcium phosphate, a carbonate apatite, or tricalcium phosphate.[64,192,201,214,219,220]

V. RESORPTION AND REPAIR OF DENTIN

There have been few ultramicroscopical studies of resorption of dentin, either occurring as the physiological process of exfoliation of deciduous teeth,[64,128,219,221] or during adaptation to functional stress. Unless protected by a layer of formative cells, either secretory or not, calcified tissues are liable to resorption.[223,224] Dentin may, therefore, be resorbed from any aspect; from the direction of the pulp if the odontoblasts are no longer providing a barrier, or from the outer aspect of the root following a breach in the cementum. Whatever the cause, the cell responsible for removal of the dentin is the *odontoclast,*[221] a cell identical in all respects to the osteoclast.[225] The cytological features of such cells are well documented and their putative origin from cells of the monocyte-macrophage series has been extensively investigated though not proven.[226] Whether any other cells assist in the removal of calcified tissues, including dentin, is a contentious point.[227]

The topography of the resorbed dentin surface is best examined by transmission electron microscopy of replicas or by scanning electron microscopy[222] (Figures 76 to 79). Demineralization precedes the removal of organic matrix, as in bone resorption, cyclical and reprecipitation crystals may occur on the resorbed surface. Scanning electron microscopy can also provide quantitative data on the size of resorption lacunae.[228] An extension of the

FIGURE 76 (Above). Stereopair: resorptive surface of human deciduous tooth. (Magnification × 360.) FIGURE 77 (Center left). Human deciduous molar, resorbing surface of dentin. (Magnification × 2500.) FIGURE 78 (Center right). Araldite replica of resorbing dentin surface in human deciduous tooth. (Magnification × 180.) FIGURE 79 (Below). Stereopair: enzyme preparation of pulpal aspect of resorbed dentin surface of human deciduous lower incisor, which has been repaired by cement (above). Ends of Sharpey's fibers are seen amongst intrinsic fibers. (Magnification × 415.)

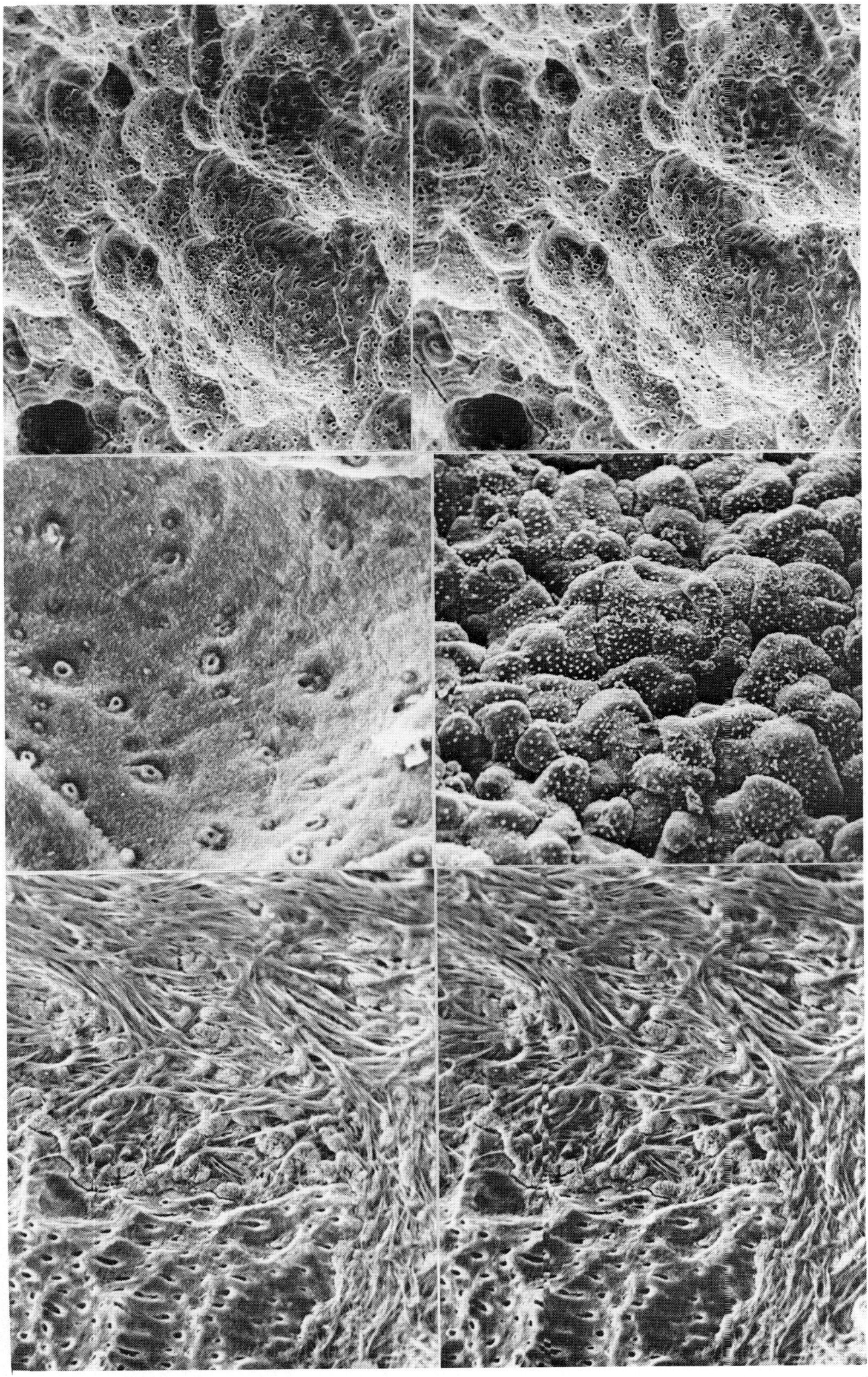

FIGURES 76—79.

protocol used in such studies could allow for the dimension of time and provide a rate for the dissolution of dentin by odontoclasts under controlled conditions. More information on hormonal control or modification of odontoclasia by the three main bone hormones, parathyroid hormone, calcitonin, and calcitriol (1,25 dihydroxy-vitamin D_3), is needed.

Because dentin is heterogeneous in structure, not all of it resorbs equally fast. Peritubular dentin is relatively resistant to resorption, and stands slightly proud in the resorbing dentin surface surrounded by a moat (Figure 77). One would also expect that regions of interglobular dentin would be immediately recognizable in a resorbing front, with a step at the outer limit of the borders of calcospherites. Equally, there should be a discernibly different texture in the region of the granular layer of Tomes, but we know of no published work describing such features. Resorption lacunae in dentin tend to be more limited in lateral extent but deeper than those found in lamellar bone.[228]

Baume[44] showed, close to the resorbed surface, argyrophilic fibers purporting to be recovered from mantle dentin of a deciduous root undergoing physiologic resorption, but there was no evidence for their origin or constitution. He suggested that these might be von Korff fibers that, unlike ordinary dentin collagen, were resistant to enzymatic lysis. With its superior sampling power, scanning electron microscopy should enable one to see such a recovering of fibers at the resorption surface with great ease; indeed as remnants they would obscure the Howship's lacunae as they projected from or lay upon the resorbed surface. We have never observed them ultrastructurally, and find it difficult to accept conceptually that a resorptive process that has the chemical mechanism to demineralize and degrade the matrix of five quite different tissues should balk at one group of collagen fibers.

Repair of dentin resorbed during physiological shedding of teeth or during functional readjustment of the root surface is by cementum (Figure 79). The two tissues are bordered by a scalloped reversal line with characteristics which mimic those between any other two similar or dissimilar calcified tissues. Microradiography[221] or backscattered electron SEM images show a hypercalcified junction, which correlates with the basophilic line seen in routine decalcified sections. The repairing cementum may be cellular or, less frequently, acellular and may not always initially incorporate Sharpey's fibers. When dentin resorption is repaired from the pulpal aspect, a bony tissue forms.

ACKNOWLEDGMENTS

This work was supported by grants from the Medical Research Council and the Science Research Council. We would also like to thank Elaine Maconnachie for technical assistance and Penny Hand for typing the manuscript.

REFERENCES

1. **Ruch, J. V., Karcher-Djurick, V., and Gerber, R.,** Problèmes et hypothèses concernant la différentiation dentaire, *C. R. Soc. Biol.,* 165, 2425, 1971.
2. **Takuma, S.,** Ultrastructure of dentinogenesis, in *Structural and Chemical Organization of Teeth,* Vol. 1, Miles, A. E. W., Ed., Academic Press, New York, 1967, 325.
3. **Slavkin, H. C., Bringas, P., Cameron, J., LeBaron, R., and Bavetta, L. A.,** Epithelial and mesenchymal cell interactions with extracellular matrix material in vitro, *J. Embryol. Exp. Morphol.,* 22, 395, 1969.
4. **Slavkin, H. C., Croissant, R. D., and Guenther, H.,** The role of extracellular matrix macromolecules upon cell differentiation, in *Protides of the Biological Fluids,* 22nd Colloquium, Peeters, H., Ed., Pergamon Press, New York, 1975, 23.
5. **Slavkin, H. C., Bringas, P., LeBaron, R., Cameron, J., and Bavetta, L. A.,** The fine structure of the extracellular matrix during epithelio-mesenchymal interactions in the rabbit embryonic incisor, *Anat. Rec.,* 165, 237, 1969.

6. **Kollar, E. J.,** The role of collagen during tooth morphogenesis: some genetic implications, in *Development, Function and Evolution of Teeth,* Butler, P. M. and Joysey, K. A., Eds., Academic Press, New York, 1978, 1.
7. **Gerber, R., Karcher-Djurick, V., and Ruch, J. V.,** Collagénase et différentiation des adamantoblastes, *C. R. Soc. Biol.,* 165, 2173, 1971.
8. **Thesleff, I.,** Role of the basement membrane in odontoblast differentiation, *J. Biol. Buccale,* 6, 241, 1978.
9. **Orams, H. J. and Snibson, K. J.,** Ultrastructural localization and gradient of activity of alkaline phosphatase activity during rodent odontogenesis, *Calcif. Tissue Int.,* 34, 273, 1982.
10. **Meyer, J. M., Fabre, M., Staubli, A., and Ruch, J. V.,** Relations cellulaires au cour de l'odontogenèse, *J. Biol. Buccale,* 5, 107, 1977.
11. **Slavkin, H. C.,** Intercellular communication during odontogenesis, in *Developmental Aspects of Oral Biology,* Slavkin, H. C. and Bavetta, L. A., Eds., Academic Press, New York, 1972, 165.
12. **Slavkin, H. C.,** The isolation and characterization of calcifying and non-calcifying matrix vesicles from dentine, in *International Colloquium on Physical Chemistry and Crystallography of Apatites of Biological Interest,* No. 230, Montel. G., Ed., C. N. R. S., Paris, 1973, 161.
13. **Slavkin, H. C. and Croissant, R.,** Intercellular communication during odontogenic epithelial-mesenchymal interactions: isolation of extracellular matrix vesicles containing RNA, in *The Role of RNA in Reproduction and Development,* Niu, C. and Segal, S. J., Eds., North-Holland, Amsterdam, 1973, 247.
14. **Silva, D. G. and Kailis, D. G.,** Ultrastructural studies on the cervical loop and the development of the amelodentinal junction in the cat, *Arch. Oral Biol.,* 17, 279, 1972.
15. **Katchburian, E. and Burgess, A. M. C.,** Fine structure of contacts between ameloblasts and odontoblasts in the rat tooth germ, *Arch. Oral Biol.,* 22, 551, 1977.
16. **Slavkin, H. C., Zeichner-David, M., and Siddiqui, M. A. Q.,** Molecular aspects of tooth morphogenesis and differentiation, *Molec. Aspects Med.,* 4, 125, 1981.
17. **Takuma, S. and Nagai, N.,** Ultrastructure of rat odontoblasts in various stages of their development and maturation, *Arch. Oral Biol.,* 16, 993, 1971.
18. **Slavkin, H. C. and Bringas, P.,** Epithelial-mesenchymal interactions during odontogenesis. IV. Morphological evidence for direct heterotypic cell-cell contacts, *Dev. Biol.,* 50, 428, 1976.
19. **Larsson, A. and Bloom, G. D.,** Studies on dentinogenesis in the rat: fine structure of developing odontoblasts and predentine in relation to the mineralization process, *Z. Anat. Entwickl-Gesch.,* 139, 227, 1973.
20. **Kiely, M. L. and Wilde, J. L.,** Circadian mitotic rhythms in the cervical tissues of the rat maxillary incisor, *J. Dent. Res.,* 53, 1432, 1974.
21. **Leblond, C. P. and Weinstock, M.,** Comparative study of dentin and bone formation, in *The Biochemistry and Physiology of Bone,* Vol. 4, Calcification and Physiology, 2nd ed., Bourne, G. H., Ed., Academic Press, New York, 1976, chap. 12.
22. **Frank, R. M.,** Electron microscopy autoradiography of calcified tissues, *Int. Rev. Cytol.,* 56, 183, 1979.
23. **Nagai, N.,** Electron microscopy of the cytoplasmic bodies in the odontoblasts of young rat incisors, *Bull. Tokyo Dent. Coll.,* 11, 47, 1970.
24. **Goldberg, M., Escaig, F., and Septier, D.,** Etude par cryofracture et sur coupes fines des jonctions intercellulaires entre les odontoblastes de l'incisive de rat. Modifications induites par la vinblastine, *J. Biol. Buccale,* 9, 141, 1981.
25. **Weinstock, M. and Leblond, C. P.,** Synthesis, migration and release of precursor collagen by odontoblasts as visualized by radioautography after [^{3}H] proline administration, *J. Cell Biol.,* 60, 92, 1974.
26. **Weinstock, A., Weinstock, M., and Leblond, C. P.,** Autoradiographic detection of ^{3}H-fucose incorporation into glycoprotein by odontoblasts and its deposition at the site of the calcification front in dentin, *Calcif. Tissue Res.,* 8, 181, 1972.
27. **Weinstock, M. and Leblond, C. P.,** Radioautographic visualization of the deposition of a phosphoprotein at the mineralization front in the dentine of the rat incisor, *J. Cell Biol.,* 56, 838, 1973.
28. **Nikiforuk, G. and Fraser, D.,** Etiology of enamel hypoplasia and interglobular dentin: the roles of hypocalcemia and hypophosphatemia, *Metab. Bone Dis. Rel. Res.,* 2, 17, 1979.
29. **Fitzgerald, M.,** Cellular mechanics of dentinal bridge repair using ^{3}H-thymidine, *J. Dent. Res.,* 58(D), 2198, 1979.
30. **Jones, S. J. and Boyde, A.,** Experimental study of changes in osteoblastic shape induced by calcitonin and parathyroid extract in an organ culture system, *Cell Tissue Res.,* 169, 449, 1976.
31. **Garant, P. R., Szabo, G., and Nalbandian, J.,** The fine structure of the mouse odontoblast, *Arch. Oral Biol.,* 13, 857, 1968.
32. **Frank, R. M.,** Ultrastructural relationship between the odontoblast, its processes and the nerve fiber, in *Dentin and Pulp: Their Structure and Reactions,* Symons, N. B. B., Ed., University of Dundee Press, Dundee, Scotland, 1968, 115.
33. **Holland, G. R.,** Membrane junctions on cat odontoblasts, *Arch. Oral Biol.,* 20, 551, 1975.
34. **Boyde, A., Reith, E. J., and Jones, S. J.,** Intercellular attachments between calcified collagenous tissue forming cells in the rat, *Cell Tissue Res.,* 191, 507, 1978.

35. **Boyde, A. and Reith, E. J.,** Cyclical uptake pattern of tetracycline in post-secretory maturation phase enamel demonstrated in rooted teeth, *Calcif. Tissue Int.,* submitted.
36. **Jessen, H.,** The ultrastructure of odontoblasts in perfusion-fixed, demineralized, incisors of adult rats, *Acta Odont. Scand.,* 25, 491, 1967.
37. **Fromme, H. G., Höhling, H. J., and Riedel, H.,** Elektronenmikroskopische studien über die Dentinbildung II, *Dtsch. Zahnarztliche Z.,* 27, 6, 1972.
38. **Reith, E. J.,** Ultrastructural aspects of dentinogenesis, in *Dentine and Pulp,* Symons, N. B. B., Ed., University of Dundee Press, Dundee, Scotland, 1968, 19.
39. **Hall, D. M. and Schroff, F. R.,** The study of dental ultrastructure by freeze-etching, *Arch. Oral Biol.,* 13, 703, 1968.
40. **Katchburian, E. and Holt, S. J.,** Ultrastructural studies on lysosomes and acid phosphatase in odontoblasts, in *Dentine and Pulp,* Symons, N. B. B., Ed., University of Dundee Press, Dundee, Scotland, 1968, 43.
41. **Costacurta, L., Ferraz de Carvalho, C. A., and Konig, B.,** Electron microscope study of dentin matrix fibrogenesis, *Acta Anat.,* 90, 310, 1974.
42. **Nygren, H., Hansson, A., and Linde, A.,** Ultrastructural localization of proteoglycans in the odontoblast-predentin region of rat incisor, *Cell Tissue Res.,* 168, 277, 1976.
43. **Holland, G. R.,** An ultrastructural survey of cat dentinal tubules, *J. Anat.,* 122, 1, 1976.
44. **Baume, L. J.,** *The Biology of Pulp and Dentine: Monographs in Oral Science,* Vol. 8, S. Karger, Basel, 1980.
45. **Goldberg, M., Escaig, F., and Septier, D.,** Rôle de flux sécréteur dans la dynamique de maturation de la prédentine. Étude morphologique, autoradiographique et par cryofracture chez le rat; modifications induites par la vinblastine, *C.R. Acad. Sci. (Paris),* 291, 287, 1980.
46. **Linde, A. and Persliden, B.,** Cathepsin D activity in isolated odontoblasts, *Calcif. Tissue Res.,* 23, 33, 1977.
47. **Feichtinger, C. and Rossiwall, B.,** Taurodontism in human sex chromosome aneuploidy, *Arch. Oral Biol.,* 22, 327, 1977.
48. **Fox, A. G. and Heeley, J. D.,** Histological study of pulps of human primary teeth, *Arch. Oral Biol.,* 25, 103, 1980.
49. **Johansen, E. and Parks, H. F.,** Electron microscopic observations on sound human dentine, *Arch. Oral Biol.,* 7, 185, 1962.
50. **Frank, R. M.,** Etude au microscope électronique de l'odontoblaste et du canalicule dentinaire humain, *Arch. Oral Biol.,* 11, 179, 1966.
51. **Frank, R. M., Sauvage, C., and Frank, P.,** Morphological basis of dental sensitivity, *Int. Dent. J.,* 22, 1, 1972.
52. **Tsatsas, B. G. and Frank, R. M.,** Ultrastructure of the dentinal tubular substances near the dentino-enamel junction, *Calcif. Tissue Res.,* 9, 238, 1972.
53. **Garant, P. R.,** The organization of microtubules within rat odontoblast processes revealed by perfusion fixation with glutaraldehyde, *Arch. Oral Biol.,* 17, 1047, 1972.
54. **Holland, G. R.,** The dentinal tubules and odontoblast process in the cat, *J. Anat.,* 120, 169, 1975.
55. **Holland, G. R.,** The extent of the odontoblast process in the cat, *J. Anat.,* 121, 133, 1976.
56. **Toda, Y., Shimauchi, K., Takagi, M., Suzuki, M., Toda, M., Kasahara, Y., and Yokoyama, K.,** Scanning electron microscopic studies of the peritubular dentin in dogs, *J. Nihon Univ. Sch. Dent.,* 17, 122, 1975.
57. **Brännström, M. and Garberoglio, R.,** The dentinal tubule and the odontoblast process. A scanning electron microscopic study, *Acta Odont. Scand.,* 30, 291, 1972.
58. **Kubota, K., Sekikawa, M., Shimamura, M., and Nakajima, T.,** A scanning electron microscope consideration of the structure of peritubular dentin, *J. Nihon Univ. Sch. Dent.,* 20, 1, 1978.
59. **Thomas, H. F.,** The extent of the odontoblast process in human dentin, *J. Dent. Res.,* 58, 2207, 1979.
60. **Kelley, K. W., Bergenholtz, G., and Cox, C. F.,** The extent of the odontoblast process in rhesus monkeys *(Macaca mulatta)* as observed by scanning electron microscopy, *Arch. Oral Biol.,* 26, 893, 1981.
61. **Maniatopoulos, C. and Smith, D. C.,** A SEM study of the extent of the odontoblast process in human coronal dentine, *J. Dent. Res.,* 61, 313, 1982.
62. **Kuwajima, K., Ajisaka, M., Oyanagi, T., Aoki, K., and Asano, T.,** Scanning electron microscope study of Tomes' fibres, *J. Nihon Univ. Sch. Dent.,* 12, 112, 1970.
63. **Isokana, S., Yoshida, M., Komuro, A., and Iwatake, Y.,** A preliminary study on the peritubular structure of human dentinal tubules by scanning electron microscopy, *J. Nihon Univ. Sch. Dent.,* 14, 122, 1972.
64. **Lester, K. S. and Boyde, A.,** Electron microscopy of predentinal surfaces, *Calcif. Tissue Res.,* 1, 44, 1967.
65. **Brännström, M., Johnson, G., and Garberoglio, R.,** Ulteriori osservazioni sulle strutture fibro membranose dei tubuli dentinali e della parete pulpare, *Estratto da Mondo Odontostom.,* Jan./Feb., 3, 1974.
66. **Mendis, B. R. R. N. and Darling, A. I.,** A scanning electron microscope and microradiographic study of closure of human coronal dentinal tubules related to occlusal attrition and caries, *Arch. Oral Biol.,* 24, 725, 1979.

67. **Tronstad, L.,** Scanning electron microscopy of attrited dentinal surfaces and subjacent dentine in human teeth, *Scand. J. Dent. Res.*, 81, 112, 1973.
68. **Hansson, H. A., Linde, A., and Nygren, H.,** Scanning electron microscopic studies of the rat incisor odontoblastema, *Cell Tissue Res.*, 159, 233, 1975.
69. **Garberoglio, R. and Brännström, M.,** Scanning electron microscopic investigation of human dentinal tubules, *Arch. Oral Biol.*, 21, 355, 1976.
70. **Arwill, T., Edwall, L., Lilja, J., Olgart, L., and Svensson, S-E.,** Ultrastructure of nerves in the dentinal-pulp border zone after sensory and autonomic nerve transection in the cat, *Acta Odont. Scand.*, 31, 273, 1973.
71. **Corpon, R. E. and Avery, J. K.,** The ultrastructure of intradental nerves in developing mouse molars, *Anat. Rec.*, 175, 585, 1973.
72. **Fearnhead, R. W.,** Innervation of dental tissues, in *Structural and Chemical Organization of Teeth,* Vol. 1, Miles, A. E. W., Ed., Academic Press, New York, 1967, 247.
73. **Frank, R. M.,** Attachment sites between the odontoblast process and the intradental nerve fiber, *Arch. Oral Biol.*, 13, 833, 1968.
74. **Dahl, E. and Mjör, I. A.,** The structure and distribution of nerves in the pulp-dentin organ, *Acta Odont. Scand.*, 31, 349, 1973.
75. **Byers, M. R. and Kish, S. J.,** Delineation of somatic nerve endings in rat teeth by radioautography of axon-transported protein, *J. Dent. Res.*, 55, 419, 1976.
76. **Takuma, S., Yanagisawa, T., and Lin, W. L.,** Ultrastructural and microanalytical aspects of developing osteodentin in rat incisors, *Calcif. Tissue Res.*, 24, 215, 1977.
77. **Munhoz, C. O. G. and Leblond, C. P.,** Deposition of calcium phosphate into dentine and enamel as shown by radioautography of sections of incisor teeth following injection of Ca^{45} into rats, *Calcif. Tissue Res.*, 15, 221, 1974.
78. **Nagai, N. and Frank, R. M.,** Electron microscopic autoradiography of Ca^{45} during dentinogenesis, *Cell Tissue Res.*, 155, 513, 1974.
79. **Boyde, A. and Shapiro, I. M.,** Energy dispersive X-ray elemental analysis of isolated epiphyseal growth plate chondrocyte fragments, *Histochemistry,* 69, 85, 1980.
80. **Reith, E. J.,** The binding of calcium within the Golgi saccules of the rat odontoblast, *Am. J. Anat.*, 147, 267, 1976.
81. **Reith, E. J.,** Collagen formation in developing molar teeth of rats, *J. Ultrastruct. Res.*, 21, 383, 1968.
82. **Boyde, A. and Reith, E. J.,** Quantitative electron probe analysis of secretory ameloblasts and odontoblasts in the rat incisor, *Histochemistry,* 50, 347, 1977.
83. **Schenk, R. K., Hunziker, E., and Hermann, W.,** Structural properties of cells related to tissue mineralization, in *Biological Mineralization and Demineralization,* Life Sciences Res. Rep. No. 23, Nancollas, G. H., Ed., Springer-Verlag, Berlin, 1982, 143.
84. **Sisca, R. F. and Provenza, D. Y.,** Initial dentine formation in human deciduous teeth, *Calcif. Tissue Res.*, 9, 1, 1972.
85. **Katchburian, E.,** Role of extracellular bodies in calcification of dentine, *J. Anat.*, 115, 151, 1973.
86. **Katchburian, E.,** Membrane-bound bodies as initiators of mineralization of dentine, *J. Anat.*, 116, 285, 1973.
87. **Katchburian, E.,** Initiation of mineral deposition in dentine, *Calcif. Tissue Res.*, 22(Suppl.), 179, 1977.
88. **Bernard, G. W.,** Ultrastructural observations of initial calcification in dentine and enamel, *J. Ultrastruct. Res.*, 41, 1, 1972.
89. **Larsson, A. L.,** Studies on dentinogenesis in the rat. Ultrastructural observations on early dentine formation with special reference to dentinal globules and alkaline phosphotase activity, *Z. Anat. Entwicklungsgesch.*, 142, 103, 1973.
90. **Eisenmann, D. R. and Glick, P. L.,** Ultrastructure of initial crystal formation in dentine, *J. Ultrastruct. Res.*, 41, 18, 1972.
91. **Garside, J.,** Nucleation, in *Biological Mineralization and Demineralization,* Life Sciences Res. Rep. No. 23, Nancollas, G. H., Ed., Springer-Verlag, Berlin, 1982, 143.
92. **Linde, A. and Granström, G.,** Odontoblast alkaline phosphatases and Ca^{2+} transport, *J. Biol. Buccale,* 6, 293, 1978.
93. **Simmons, D. J.,** Experimental design and the implication of circadian skeletal rhythmicity, in *Skeletal Research,* Simmons, D. Y. and Kunin, A. S., Eds., Academic Press, New York, 1979, 567.
94. **Yilmaz, S., Newmann, H. N., and Poole, D. F. G.,** Diurnal periodicity of von Ebner growth lines in pig dentine, *Arch. Oral Biol.*, 22, 511, 1977.
95. **Rosenberg, G. D. and Simmons, D. J.,** Rhythmic dentinogenesis in the rabbit incisor: circadian, ultradian, and infradian periods, *Calcif. Tissue Int.*, 32, 29, 1980.
96. **Rosenberg, G. D. and Simmons, D. J.,** Rhythmic dentinogenesis in the rabbit incisor: allometric aspects, *Calcif. Tissue Int.*, 32, 45, 1980.

97. **Gotjamanos, T.,** Cellular organization in the subodontoblastic zone of the dental pulp. I. A study of cell-free and cell-rich layers in pulps of adult rat and deciduous monkey teeth, *Arch. Oral Biol.,* 14, 1007, 1969.
98. **Gotjamanos, T.,** Cellular organization in the subodontoblastic zone of the dental pulp. II. Period and mode of development of the cell-rich layer in rat molar pulps, *Arch. Oral Biol.,* 14, 1011, 1969.
99. **Cahen, P. and Frank, R. M.,** Microscopie electronique de la pulpe dentaire humaine normale, *Bull. Group. Int. Rech. Sci. Stomatol.,* 13, 421, 1970.
100. **Orams, H. J., Zybert, J. J., Phakey, P. P., and Rachinger, W. A.,** Ultrastructural study of human dental enamel using selected-area argon-ion-beam thinning, *Arch. Oral Biol.,* 21, 663, 1976.
101. **Miyauti, T.,** Zur Morphologie der Schmelz-Dentingreze bei menschlichen und tierischen Zähnen, *Jpn. J. Med. Sci. Part IX, Surg. Orthoped. Odontol.,* 6, 20, 1942.
102. **Staley, R. N.,** Dentin crown surface of human adult incisor teeth, *J. Dent. Res.,* 47, 824, 1968.
103. **Whittaker, D. K.,** The enamel-dentine junction of human and *Macaca irus* teeth: a light and electron microscopic study, *J. Anat.,* 125, 323, 1978.
104. **Wright, T. and Gantt, D.,** Ultrastructure of teeth affected by dentinogenesis imperfecta, *J. Dent. Res.,* 61, 312, 1982.
105. **Sela, J., Sela, M., Lustmann, J., and Ulmansky, M.,** Dentinoenamel junction area of a resorbing permanent incisor studied by means of scanning electron microscopy, *J. Dent. Res.,* 54, 110, 1975.
106. **Svejda, J. and Bures, H.,** Rasterelektronmikroskopische Untersuchungen der Schmelzdentingrenze der menschlichen Zähne, *Dtsch. Zahnaerztl. Mund. Kieferhk.,* 60, 158, 1973.
107. **Hurmerinta, K. and Thesleff, I.,** Ultrastructure of the epithelial-mesenchymal interface in the mouse tooth germ, *J. Craniofacial Genet. Dev. Biol.,* 1, 191, 1981.
108. **Lester, K. S. and Boyde, A.,** The question of von Korff fibers in mammalian dentine, *Calcif. Tissue Res.,* 1, 273, 1968.
109. **Risnes, S. and Fosse, G.,** The origin of marsupial enamel tubules, *Acta Anat. (Basel),* 87, 275, 1974.
110. **Palamara, J., Phakey, P., Rachinger, W. A., and Orams, H. J.,** Electron-microscope study of the dentine-enamel junction of kangaroo *(Macropus giganteus)* teeth using selected-area-argon-ion-beam thinning, *Cell Tissue Res.,* 221, 405, 1981.
111. **Johansen, E.,** Ultrastructure of dentine, in *Structural and Chemical Organization of Teeth,* Vol. 2, Miles, A. E. W., Ed., Academic Press, New York, 1967, chap. 13.
112. **Ten Cate, A. R.,** An analysis of Tomes' granular layer, *Anat. Rec.,* 172, 137, 1972.
113. **Hopewell-Smith, A.,** *The Histology and Patho-histology of the Teeth and Associated Parts,* The Dental Manufacturing Co., London, 1903.
114. **Bradford, E. W.,** Microanatomy and histochemistry of dentine, in *Structural and Chemical Organization of Teeth,* Vol. 2, Miles, A. E. W., Ed., Academic Press, New York, 1967, 3.
115. **Owens, P. D. A.,** Light microscopic observations on the formation of the layer of Hopewell-Smith in human teeth, *Arch. Oral Biol.,* 17, 1785, 1972.
116. **Owens, P. D. A.,** A light microscope study of the development of the roots of premolar teeth in dogs, *Arch. Oral Biol.,* 19, 525, 1974.
117. **Owens, P. D. A.,** The fine structure of the coronal root region of premolar teeth in dogs, *Arch. Oral Biol.,* 20, 705, 1975.
118. **Lindskog, S. and Hammarstrom, L.,** The possible origin and nature of Tomes' granular layer, *J. Dent. Res.,* 61, 589, 1982.
119. **Hughes, K., Mead, R., and Adams, D.,** A scanning electron microscope study of root development in human unerupted wisdom teeth, *J. Dent. Res.,* 61, 557, 1982.
120. **Shellis, P.,** Dentine, in *A Companion to Dental Studies,* Vol. 1, Book 2, Osborn, J. W., Ed., Blackwell Scientific, Oxford, 1981, 166.
121. **Dreyfuss, F. and Frank, R.,** Microradiographie et microscopie électronique du cément humain, *Bull. Group Int. Rech. Sci. Stomatol.,* 7, 167, 1964.
122. **Furseth, R. and Johansen, E.,** A microradiographic comparison of sound and carious human dental cementum, *Arch. Oral Biol.,* 13, 1197, 1968.
123. **Neiders, M. E., Eick, J. D., Miller, W. A., and Leitner, J. W.,** Electron probe microanalysis of cementum and underlying dentin in young permanent teeth, *J. Dent. Res.,* 51, 122, 1972.
124. **Mjör, I. A., and Fejerskov, O.,** *Histology of the Human Tooth,* 2nd Ed., Munksgaard, Copenhagen, 1979.
125. **Ten Cate, A. R.,** A fine structural study of coronal and root dentinogenesis in the mouse: observations on the so-called "von Korff fibres" and their contribution to mantle dentine, *J. Anat.,* 125, 183, 1978.
126. **Selvig, K. A.,** An ultrastructural study of cement formation, *Acta Odont. Scand.,* 22, 105, 1964.
127. **Moss, M. L.,** Studies on dentin. I. Mantle dentin, *Acta Anat.,* 87, 481, 1974.
128. **Lester, K. S. and Boyde, A.,** Scanning electron microscopy of developing roots of molar teeth of the laboratory rat, *J. Ultrastruct. Res.,* 33, 80, 1970.

129. **Schmidt, W. J. and Keil, A.,** *Polarizing Microscopy of Dental Tissues,* Pergamon Press, New York, 1971.
130. **Ten Cate, A. R., Melcher, A. H., Pudy, G., and Wagner, D.,** The non-fibrous nature of the von Korff fibers in developing dentine. A light and electron microscope study, *Anat. Rec.,* 168, 491, 1970.
131. **Isokawa, S., Uchino, S., Morimoto, K., Kobayashi, Y., and Hasegawa, S.,** On the so-called von Korff fibres as seen on the human predentinal surface, *J. Nihon Univ. Sch. Dent.,* 14, 12, 1972.
132. **Whittaker, D. K. and Adams, D.,** Electron microscopic studies on von Korff fibres in the human developing tooth, *Anat. Rec.,* 174, 175, 1972.
133. **Nalbandian, J.,** The ultrastructure of odontoblasts and dentinogenesis, in *Biology of the Dental Pulp Organ. A Symposium,* Finn, S. B., Ed., University of Alabama Press, Tuscaloosa, 1968, 195.
134. **Hans, S. S.,** Discussion in *Biology of the Dental Pulp Organ. A Symposium,* Finn, S. B., Ed., University of Alabama Press, Tuscaloosa, 1968, 211.
135. **Herold, R. C.,** Fine structure of tooth dentine in human dentinogenesis imperfecta, *Arch. Oral Biol.,* 17, 1009, 1972.
136. **Portilla, J.,** Comparative light and electron microscopic studies of von Korff fibres, *J. Dent. Res.,* 61, 205, 1982.
137. **Boyde, A.,** Histological studies of dental tissues of odontocetes, *Rep. Int. Whaling Comm.,* Spec. Issue 3, 65, 1980.
138. **Wigglesworth, D. J. and Hayward, A. F.,** The ultrastructure of dentinogenesis and amelogenesis in rat molar tooth germs grown as organ cultures, *in vitro, Z. Zellforsch.,* 138, 171, 1973.
139. **Shackleford, J. M.,** The structure of Tomes' granular layer in dog premolar teeth, *Anat Rec.,* 170, 357, 1971.
140. **Lavelle, C. L. B., Shellis, R. P., and Poole, D. F. G.,** *Evolutionary Changes to the Primate Skull and Dentition,* Charles C Thomas, Springfield, Ill., 1977.
141. **Munksgaard, E. C. and Moe, D.,** Types of collagen in an extract of odontoblasts and dentine from developing bovine teeth, *Arch. Oral Biol.,* 25, 485, 1980.
142. **Kawasaki, K., Tanaka, S., and Ishikawa, T.,** On the incremental lines in human dentine as revealed by tetracycline labelling, *J. Anat.,* 123, 427, 1977.
143. **Furseth, R.,** The structure of peripheral root dentine in young human premolars, *Scand. J. Dent. Res.,* 82, 557, 1974.
144. **Scott, J. H. and Symons, N. B. B.,** *Introduction to Dental Anatomy,* 8th ed., E. & S. Livingstone, Edinburgh, 1977.
145. **Bhaskar, S. N., Ed.,** *Orban's Oral Histology and Embryology,* C. V. Mosby, St. Louis, 1976.
146. **Heritier, M. and Fernandez, J. P.,** Etude en microscopie photonique et électronique de la gaine de Hertwig chez la souris, *J. Biol. Buccale,* 9, 319, 1981.
147. **Larsson, A. and Helander, H. F.,** Studies on dentinogenesis in the rat. Light, electron microscopic and histochemical studies on the interaction between lead pyrophosphate solutions and the dentine producing tissues, *Calcif. Tissue Res.,* 14, 87, 1974.
148. **Lenz, H.,** Elektronenmikroskopische Untersuchungen der Dentinentwicklung, *Dtsch. Zahnaerztl. Mund. Kieferhk,* 9, 367, 1959.
149. **Höhling, H. J., Steffens, H., Ashton, B. A., and Nicholson, W. A. P.,** Molekularbiologie der Hartgewebsbildung, *Verh. Dtsch. Ges. Pathol.,* 58, 54, 1974.
150. **Almuddaris, M. F., and Dougherty, W. J.,** The association of amorphous mineral deposits with the plasma membrane of pre and young odontoblasts and their relationship to the origin of dentinal matrix vesicles in rat incisor teeth, *Am. J. Anat.,* 155, 223, 1979.
151. **Boyde, A.,** Scanning electron microscopy of collagen-free calcified connective tissues, *Beitr. Elektronenmikroskop. Direktabb. Oberl. (Münster),* 1, 213, 1968.
152. **Boyde, A.,** Studies on the mineralizing fronts in calcified connective tissues using the scanning electron microscope, in *Electron Microscopy 1968,* Vol. 2, Borianelli, D. S., Ed., Tipografia Poliglotta Vaticana, Rome, 1968, 427.
153. **Boyde, A. and Reith, E.,** The pattern of mineralization of rat molar dentine, *Z. Zellforsch,* 94, 479, 1969.
154. **Boyde, A. and Jones, S. J.,** Scanning electron microscopic studies of the formation of mineralized tissues, in *Developmental Aspects of Oral Biology,* Slavkin, H. C. and Bavetta, L. A., Eds., Academic Press, New York, 1972, chap. 11.
155. **Tronstad, L.,** Optical and microradiographic appearance of intact and worn human coronal dentine, *Arch. Oral Biol.,* 17, 847, 1972.
156. **Kawasaki, K. and Fearnhead, R. W.,** On the relationship between tetracycline and the incremental lines in dentine, *J. Anat.,* 119, 49, 1975.
157. **Owens, P. D. A.,** Patterns of mineralization in the roots of premolar teeth in dogs, *Arch. Oral Biol.,* 20, 709, 1975.
158. **Owens, P. D. A.,** Ultrastructure of Hertwigs epithelial root sheath during early root development in premolar teeth in dogs, *Arch. Oral Biol.,* 23, 91, 1978.

159. **Owens, P. D. A.,** A light and electron microscopic study on the early stages of root surface formation in the molar teeth in the rat, *Arch. Oral Biol.*, 24, 901, 1979.
160. **Slavkin, H. C. and Boyde, A.,** Cementum: an epithelial secretory product?, *J. Dent. Res.*, 53 (Special issue), 157, 1974.
161. **Katz, E. P. and Li, S.,** The molecular packing of collagen in mineralized and non-mineralized tissues, *Biochem. Biophys. Res. Commun.*, 46, 1368, 1972.
162. **Warshawsky, H.,** The presence of atypical collagen fibrils in EDTA decalcified predentine and dentine of rat incisors, *Arch. Oral Biol.*, 17, 1745, 1972.
163. **Weinstock, M.,** Centrosymmetrical cross banded structures in the matrix of rat incisor predentine and dentine, *J. Ultrastruct. Res.*, 61, 218, 1977.
164. **Johnson, N. W. and Poole, D. F. G.,** Orientation of collagen fibers in dentine, *Nature (London)*, 213, 695, 1967.
165. **Boyde, A.,** The contribution of the scanning electron microscope to dental histology, *Apex*, 4(3), 15, 1970; (4), 9, 1970.
166. **Goldberg, M. and Escaig, F.,** Odontoblastes: collagène dans la prédentine et la dentine de l'incisive de rat: étude par cryofracture, *Biol. Cell*, 40, 203, 1981.
167. **Miles, A. E. W. and Boyde, A.,** Observations on the structure of elephant ivory, *J. Anat.*, 95, 450, 1961.
168. **Kaye, H. and Herold, R. C.,** Structure of human dentine. I, *Arch. Oral Biol.*, 11, 355, 1966.
169. **Nagai, S., Takuma, S., Goto, Y., and Ogiwara, H.,** Electron microscopy of dentine and predentine of developing rat molars stained with ruthenium red, *J. Biol. Buccale*, 2, 73, 1974.
170. **Schweighardt, J. and Boyde, A.,** personal communication.
171. **Boyde, A. and Sela, J.,** A scanning electron microscope study of separated calcospherites from the matrices of different mineralizing systems, *Calcif. Tissue Res.*, 26, 47, 1978.
172. **Schmidt, W. J.,** Die Kristalline Struktur der Globuli im Zahnbein des Menschen, *Z. Zellforsch.*, 97, 313, 1969.
173. **Whittaker, D. K. and Kneale, M. J.,** The dentine-predentine interface in human teeth: a scanning electron microscope study, *Br. Dent. J.*, 146, 43, 1979.
174. **Simpson, M. S.,** Effects of demineralizing tetracycline-stained human dentine, *Calcif. Tissue Int.*, 33, 101, 1981.
175. **Eda, S. and Takuma, S.,** Microstructure of the peritubular matrix in horse dentine, *Bull. Tokyo Dent. Coll.*, 6, 1, 1965.
176. **Weber, D. F.,** Human dentine sclerosis: a microradiographic survey, *Arch. Oral Biol.*, 19, 163, 1974.
177. **Steve-Bocciarelli, D.,** Apatite microcrystals in bone and dentine, *J. Microscopie*, 16, 21, 1973.
178. **Posner, A. S. and Tannenbaum, P. J.,** The mineral phase of dentin, in *Dentin and Dentinogenesis*, Linde, A., Ed., CRC Press, Boca Raton, Fla., 1984.
179. **Daculsi, G., Kerebel, B., and Verbaere, A.,** Methode de mesure des cristaux d'apatite de la dentine humaine en microscopie electronique a transmission de haute resolution, *C. R. Acad. Sci. (Paris)*, 286, 1439, 1978.
180. **Johansen, F. J.,** Microstructure of enamel and dentin, *J. Dent. Res.*, 43, 1007, 1964.
181. **Höhling, H. J., Scholz, F., Boyde, A., Heine, H. G., and Reimer, L.,** Electron microscopical and laser diffraction studies of the nucleation and growth of crystals in the organic matrix of dentine, *Z. Zellsforsch.*, 117, 381, 1971.
182. **Boyde, A.,** Transmission electron microscopy of ion-beam thinned dentine, *Cell Tissue Res.*, 152, 543, 1974.
183. **Boyde, A. and Pawley, J. B.,** Transmission electron microscopy of ion erosion thinned hard tissues, in *Calcified Tissues 1975*, (Suppl. to *Calcified Tissue Research 1975 and Alternative Availability*), Pors Nielsen, S. and Hjørting-Hansen, E., Eds., Fadl's Forlag, Copenhagen, 1975, 117.
184. **Höhling, H. J., Ashton, B. A. and Köster, H. D.,** Quantitative electron microscopic investigations of mineral nucleation in collagen, *Cell Tissue Res.*, 148, 11, 1974.
185. **Höhling, H. J., Kreilos, R., Neubauer, G., and Boyde, A.,** Electron microscopy and electron microscopical measurements of collagen mineralization in hard tissues, *Z. Zellforsch.*, 122, 36, 1971.
186. **Höhling, H. J., Steffens, H., and Heuck, F.,** Untersuchungen zur Mineralisierungsdichte im Hartgewebe mit Protein-Polysaccharid bzw. mit Kollagen als Hauptbestandteil der Matrix, *Z. Zellforsch.*, 134, 283, 1972.
187. **Kato, S. and Ohkura, Y.,** Study on the crystal structure of dentine in man and other animals, *J. Nihon Univ. Sch. Dent.*, 3, 141, 1961.
188. **Kerebel, B., Kerebel, L. M., and Billet, J.,** Etude ultrastructurale de l'email de la dentine dans l'odontodysplasie regimale, *J. Biol. Buccale*, 9, 243, 1981.
189. **Shimoyama, T.,** Peritubular hypercalcified zone of mammalian dentin, *Arch. Histol. Jpn.*, 28, 113, 1967.
190. **Remy, J. A.,** Evolution d'une structure histologique chez les périssodactyles: le développement de la dentine pericanaliculaire, *C. R. Acad. Sci. (Paris)*, 274, 2026, 1972.

191. **Takuma, S. and Eda, S.,** Peritubular matrix in mammalian dentin, *Bull. Tokyo Dent. Col.,* 1, 20, 1960.
192. **Lester, K. S. and Boyde, A.,** The surface morphology of some crystalline components of dentine, in *Dentine and Pulp,* Symons, N. B. B., Ed., University of Dundee Press, Dundee, Scotland, 1968, 197.
193. **Takuma, S. and Eda, S.,** Structure and development of the peritubular matrix in dentine, *J. Dent. Res.,* 45, 683, 1966.
194. **Boyde, A.,** Comparative histology of mammalian teeth, in *Dental Morphology and Evolution,* Dahlberg, A. A., Ed., University of Chicago Press, Chicago, 1971, 81.
195. **Brännström, M. and Garberoglio, R.,** Occlusion of dentinal tubules under superficial attrited dentine, *Swed. Dent. J.,* 4, 87, 1980.
196. **Goldberg, M., Genotellè-Septier, D. and Weill, R.,** Glycoprotéines et protéoglycanes dans la matrice prédentinaire et dentinaire chez le rat: une étude ultrastructurale, *J. Biol. Buccale,* 6, 75, 1978.
197. **Frank, R. M.,** Electron microscopy of undecalcified sections of human adult dentine, *Arch. Oral Biol.,* 1, 29, 1959.
198. **Johanessen, J. V. and Bang, G.,** Transmission electron microscopy on sound demineralized guinea pig dentin, *Scand. J. Dent. Res.,* 80, 213, 1972.
199. **Weber, D. F.,** Peritubular matrix: a correlated radiographic and staining study, *Calcif. Tissue Res.,* 8., 17, 1971.
200. **Allred, H.,** The differential staining of peritubular and intertubular matrices in human dentine, *Arch. Oral Biol.,* 13, 1, 1968.
201. **Johnson, N. W., Taylor, B. R., and Berman, D. S.,** The response of deciduous dentine to caries studied by correlated light and electron microscopy, *Caries Res.,* 3, 348, 1969.
202. **Plackova, A., Pribyl, J., and Stepanek, J.,** Eine elektronenmikroskopische Studie der Dentinstruktur, *Dtsch. Zahnartzl. Z.,* 15, 1010, 1959.
203. **Forssell-Ahlberg, K., Brännström, M., and Edwall, L.,** The diameter and number of dentinal tubules in rat, cat, dog, and monkey. A comparative scanning electron microscopic study, *Acta Odont. Scand.,* 33, 243, 1975.
204. **Mendis, B. R. R. N. and Darling, A. I.,** Distribution with age and attrition of peritubular dentine in the crowns of human teeth, *Arch. Oral Biol.,* 24, 131, 1979.
205. **Blake, G. C.,** The peritubular translucent zones in human dentine, *Br. Dent. J.,* 104, 57, 1958.
206. **Tronstad, L.,** Quantitative microradiography of intact and worn human coronal dentine, *Arch. Oral Biol.,* 18, 533, 1973.
207. **Kerebel, B., Daculsi, G., Menanteau, J., and Kerebel, L. M.,** The inorganic phase in dentinogenesis imperfecta, *J. Dent. Res.,* 60, 1655, 1981.
208. **Skinner, H. C. W., Bartz, Z., Ladenbauer-Bellis, I., Pooley, A., and Albright, J. A.,** Scanning electron microscopy of osteogenesis imperfecta and normal deciduous human dentine, *J. Dent. Res.,* 57, 418, 1978.
209. **Boyde, A., Switsur, V. R., and Fearnhead, R. W.,** Application of the scanning electron-probe X-ray microanalyser to dental tissues, *J. Ultrastruct. Res.,* 5, 201, 1961.
210. **Höhling, H. J.,** Elektronenmikroskopische Untersuchungen am Zahnschmelz und Dentin, *Dtsch. Zahnarztl. Z.,* 5, 1, 1961.
211. **Boyde, A. and Lester, K. S.,** An electron microscope study of fractured dentinal surfaces, *Calcif. Tissue Res.,* 1, 122, 1967.
212. **Vahl, J. and Mierau, H. D.,** Feinstrukturelle Untersuchungen an transparenten Wurzeldentin kariesfreier Zähne, *Dtsch. Zahnartzl. Z.,* 26, 365, 1971.
213. **Lefevre, R., Frank, R. M., and Voegel, J. C.,** The study of human dentine with secondary ion microscopy and electron diffraction, *Calcif. Tissue Res.,* 19, 251, 1976.
214. **Frank, R. M., Wolff, E., and Gutmann, E.,** Microscopie électronique de la carie au niveau de la dentine humaine, *Arch. Oral Biol.,* 9, 163, 1964.
215. **Miller, W. A., Eick, J. D., and Neiders, M. E.,** Inorganic components of the peritubular dentin in young human permanent teeth, *Caries Res.,* 5, 264, 1971.
216. **Nalbandian, J., Gonzales, F., and Sognnaes, R. F.,** Sclerotic age changes in root dentin of human teeth as observed by optical, electron and X-ray microscopy, *J. Dent. Res.,* 39, 598, 1960.
217. **Weber, D. F.,** The distribution of peritubular matrix in human coronal dentine, *J. Morphol.,* 126, 435, 1968.
218. **Isokawa, S., Toda, Y., and Kubota, K.,** A scanning electron microscopic observation of etched human peritubular dentine, *Arch. Oral Biol.,* 15, 1303, 1970.
219. **Lester, K. S. and Boyde, A.,** Electron microscopy of resorbing surfaces of dental hard tissues, *Z. Zellforsch.,* 83, 538, 1967.
220. **Lester, K. S. and Boyde, A.,** Some preliminary observations on caries (''remineralization'') crystals in enamel and dentine by surface electron microscopy, *Virchow's Arch. Abt. A. Pathol. Anat.,* 344, 196, 1968.

221. **Furseth, R.,** The resorption processes of human deciduous teeth studied by light microscopy, microradiography and electron microscopy, *Arch. Oral Biol.,* 13, 417, 1968.
222. **McEvoy, S. A.,** The organic matrix of resorbing root dentin in human primary teeth, *J. Int. Assoc. Dent. Child.,* 10, 11, 1979.
223. **Langeland, K.,** Response of the adult tooth to injury, in *Biology of the Dental Pulp Organ: A Symposium,* Finn, S. B., Ed., University of Alabama Press, Tuscaloosa, 1968, 169.
224. **Jones, S. J. and Boyde, A.,** Coronal cementogenesis in the horse, *Arch Oral Biol.,* 19, 605, 1974.
225. **Holtrop, M. E. and King, G. J.,** The ultrastructure of the osteoclast and its functional implication, *Clin. Orthop. Rel. Res.,* 123, 177, 1977.
226. **Raisz, L. G.,** Mechanisms and regulation of normal and pathological demineralization, in *Biological Mineralization and Demineralization,* Nancollas, G. H., Ed., Springer-Verlag, Berlin, 1982, 287.
227. **Jones, S. J., Hogg, N. M., Shapiro, I. M., Slusarenko, M., and Boyde, A.,** Cells with Fc receptors in the cell layer next to osteoblasts and osteoclasts on bone, *Metab. Bone Dis. Rel. Res.,* 2, 357, 1981.
228. **Boyde, A. and Jones, S. J.,** Estimation of the size of resorption lacunae in mammalian calcified tissues using SEM stereophotogrammetry, in *SEM/1979/II,* Johari, O., Ed., SEM Inc., AMF O'Hare, Chicago, 1979, 393.
229. **Jones, S. J. and Boyde, A.,** unpublished findings.

Chapter 5

MATRIX VESICLES: THEIR ROLE IN CALCIFICATION*

Ermanno Bonucci

TABLE OF CONTENTS

* Dedicated to Professor Rodolfo Amprino on his 70th birthday, as an acknowledgment of his fundamental scientific contributions to the knowledge of bone structure, and of his essential role in proposing and stimulating research activity by the Italian Group for Calcified Tissue Research.

I. INTRODUCTION

In biological systems, calcification is a very complicated process where many general and local physicochemical factors interact to induce or prevent the deposition of inorganic substance in organic matrices. Of the local factors involved, those affecting the structure of the calcifying organic matrix, the biochemical composition of its constituents, and the spatial organization of its molecules seem to play a leading role.[1] Besides this, the calcification process may be stimulated or inhibited by cellular activity. The recent discovery of *matrix vesicles* (MVs) has shown the need to take into consideration an additional important local factor — one which may constitute another indirect way in which the calcification process can be controlled by cells. Many investigators have, in fact, provided evidence that MVs are involved in the early stages of the calcification process, and there now seems to be a firm consensus that they are sites of early crystal formation in many normally and pathologically calcifying tissues.

II. DEFINITION OF MATRIX VESICLES

MVs are roundish bodies consisting of an amorphous substance surrounded by a membrane. They are of cellular origin, but have no direct connection with the cells, since they lie in the intercellular matrix between, and in contact with, collagen fibrils and proteoglycans. MVs represent the early locus of calcification in cartilage, bone, mantle dentin, and many calcifying extraskeletal tissues. They must be differentiated from cross sections of cell processes, whose matrix is usually less electron-dense and more granular than that of MVs, and from proteoglycan aggregates which in cartilage and in other tissues may appear as roundish, electron-dense structures resembling MVs but possessing no peripheral membrane. They should probably be differentiated also from Thyberg's Type II vesicles (see Section V) and from Slavkin's RNA-containing vesicles (see Section IV.B.) .

III. HISTORY OF MATRIX VESICLES

The literature on MVs goes back only as far as 1967. In that year, electron microscope investigations of calcifying epiphyseal cartilage led to the discovery of electron-dense, roundish, osmiophilic bodies which sometimes contained inorganic crystals. This led to their being considered the locus of initial calcification.[2] In the same year, membrane-bound cytoplasmic fragments were observed in the matrix of hypertrophic cartilage induced by the injection of cultured, human amniotic cells into the thigh muscles of cortisone-conditioned mice.[3] A year later, "vesicles" (similar to the previously reported "cytoplasmic fragments") were found in the epiphyseal plate of normal mice,[4] where they showed the same close association with inorganic crystals as that previously reported for the electron-dense bodies. The same association was found in epiphyseal cartilage of scorbutic guinea pigs, giving additional support to the concept that the locus of initial calcification in epiphyseal cartilage consists of electron-dense bodies which, when sectioned according to their equatorial plane, are surrounded by a trilaminar membrane.[5] Moreover, serial sectioning showed that these are true spherical bodies which have no connection with chondrocytes,[5] a finding later confirmed in epiphyseal cartilage[6,7] and in dentin.[8] These early results were greatly developed in investigations by Anderson[9] and Bonucci,[6,7] whose results unequivocally showed that "electron-dense bodies",[2] "matrix vesicles",[4,9] and "calcifying globules"[6] do not differ substantially and that they are membrane-bound structures which derive from chondrocytes and are the locus of initial calcification in cartilage.

After the demonstration of MVs in cartilage, they were recognized in bone. Electron microscope investigations had already suggested that in areas of ossification early inorganic crystals can be found in connection with the cytoplasmic processes of osteoblasts[10] and with the "buds" or "extensions" of osteoblasts[11,12] and odontoblasts.[13] It was later shown that early crystal formation in bone occurs within roundish, membrane-bound bodies similar to cartilage MVs.[14-16]

MVs were isolated from cartilage for the first time in 1970 by enzymatic digestion and differential centrifugation.[17] This method led to the direct chemical analysis of MVs and to the conclusion that alkaline phosphatase is an enzymatic marker of these structures,[17] an observation confirmed soon after by electron microscopy histochemical findings.[18]

From 1971 on, the literature on MVs became copious, and extensive reviews on their morphology, composition, and function are now available.[15,16,19-26] Moreover, the interest in MVs is documented by three International Conferences on Matrix Vesicles, held in 1974 (see *Fed. Proc.*, 35, 105, 1976), 1978 (see *Metab. Bone Dis. Rel. Res.*, 1, 83, 1978), and 1981 (see *Matrix Vesicles,* Wichtig, Milan, 1981).

IV. LOCALIZATION OF MATRIX VESICLES

MVs have been repeatedly described in calcifying cartilage, in several types of bone, in mantle dentin, and in many extraskeletal, normally or pathologically calcifying tissues. MVs have not been described in enamel or calcifying turkey tendons.

A. Matrix Vesicles in Cartilage

Most of our knowledge of MVs derives from investigations on epiphyseal cartilage, probably because it is this, of all the calcifiable tissues, which can most easily be studied by morphological and biochemical methods.

Because of their small size (from 250 to 2500 Å), MVs can hardly be seen under the light microscope: they sometimes appear as very fine granules around chondrocyte lacunae,[2] but more often they are not visible at all, and only a slight change in matrix stainability shows the area where they are collected. This area corresponds to a thin portion of the longitudinal intercellular septa lying near the cell columns, but not in direct contact with the cell lacunae. This area, which roughly corresponds to the limit between the territorial and interterritorial matrix, is the place where the first aggregates of inorganic substance can be demonstrated.

MVs are easier to study under the electron microscope. This shows that they are distributed throughout the epiphyseal plate, but most of them are found in longitudinal intercellular septa, a few microns away from the border of the cell lacunae, i.e., between the territorial and interterritorial matrix (Figure 1). Only a very few of them are found in transversal intercellular septa.

In epiphyseal cartilage MVs are roundish, globular structures whose matrix is homogeneous and electron-dense, and is surrounded by a trilaminar membrane (Figures 1, 2). They are sometimes connected to collagen fibrils, either directly or by the interposition of proteoglycan components of the matrix (Figure 2).[27]

Cartilage MVs can be completely uncalcified, can contain very small inorganic granules (Figure 1),[7] or can be more or less completely masked by inorganic crystals (Figure 3). Single crystals, often placed on and deforming the outer outline of MVs, can be present in them (Figure 3).

MVs can be irregularly scattered throughout the cartilage matrix, or can be collected in groups whose shape is sometimes similar to that of chondrocyte lacunae (Figure 4).[6,7] This finding suggests that these groups of MVs can derive from the disruption of degenerate chondrocytes, as discussed further below.

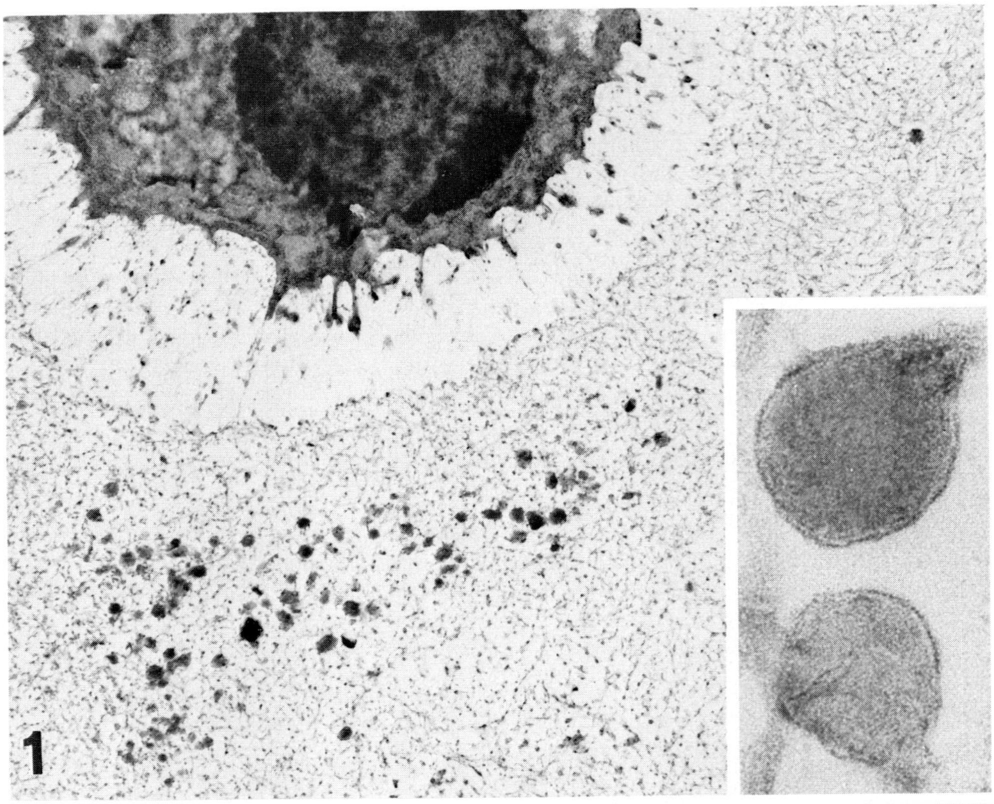

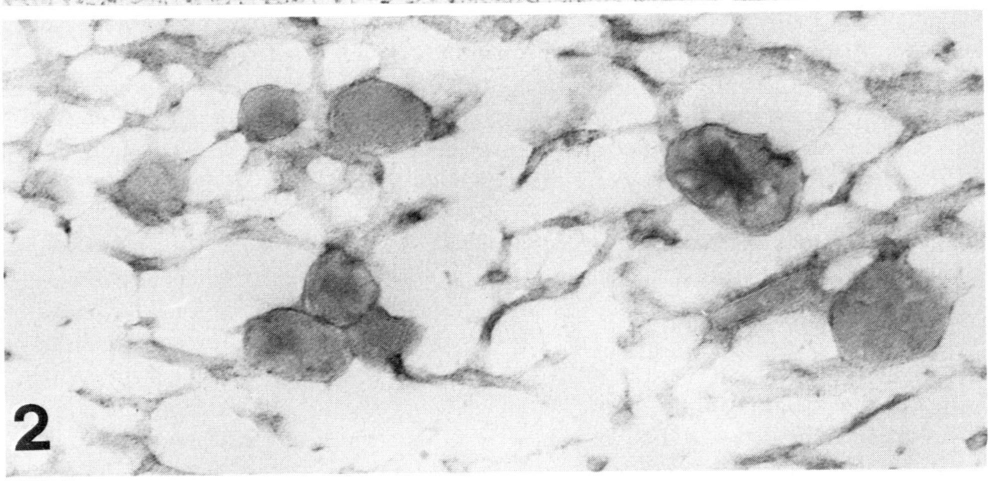

FIGURE 1. Group of MVs around a maturing chondrocyte in epiphyseal cartilage; MVs are located about at the limit between territorial and interterritorial matrix. Inset: detail of two cartilage MVs; their trilaminar membrane is evident. (Uranyl acetate and lead citrate, magnification × 15,000; inset, magnification × 130,000.) FIGURE 2. MVs of epiphyseal cartilage; note their links with collagen fibrils. (Uranyl acetate and lead citrate, magnification × 90,000.)

B. Matrix Vesicles in Bone

Structures similar to cartilage MVs were first found in the calvaria and tibiae of newborn rats, the long bones of chick embryos, and the medullary bone of pigeons,[14-16] and in repairing drill holes of rat femurs.[28] Since then, MVs have been described in areas of osteogenesis in embryonic chick femurs,[22,29-31] the tibial diaphysis and metaphysis of mature thyro-

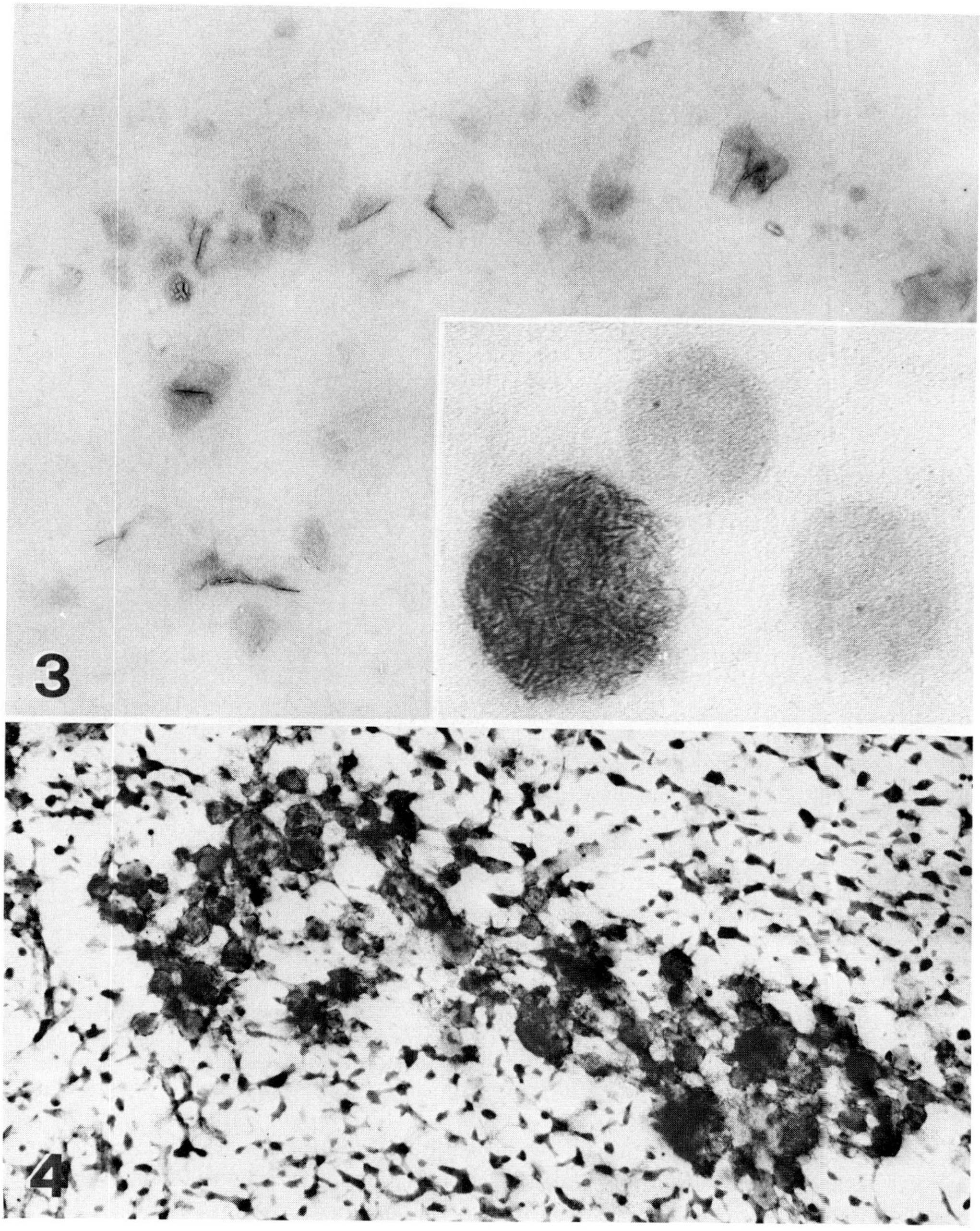

FIGURE 3. Group of cartilage MVs at an initial stage of calcification; single crystals are contained within MVs and on their outer border. Inset: three MVs, one completely filled with crystals, and two containing very small, electron-dense granules. (Unstained, magnification × 92,000; inset, magnification × 150,000.) FIGURE 4. Group of cartilage MVs probably derived by fragmentation of a degenerate chondrocyte. (Uranyl acetate and lead citrate, magnification × 44,000.)

parathyroidectomized rats,[32] the medullary bone of pigeons,[33] rat alveolar bone,[34] explants of fetal mice calvaria grown in vitro,[35] and in the tibiae of young rats[36] and puppies (Figure 5). It must be added that the osteoblast extrusions, extensions, or buds described by Bernard[11] and Bernard and Pease[12] in membrane and endochondral bone are very probably the same structures as MVs. This shows that MVs have been found in areas of osteogenesis in a wide variety of bone types.

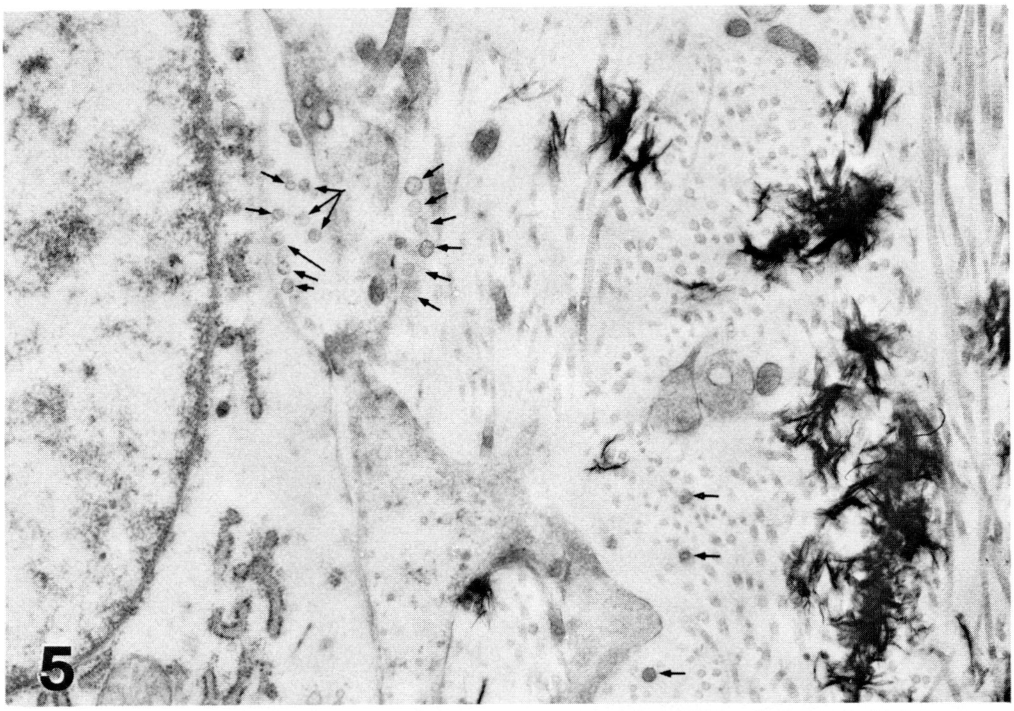

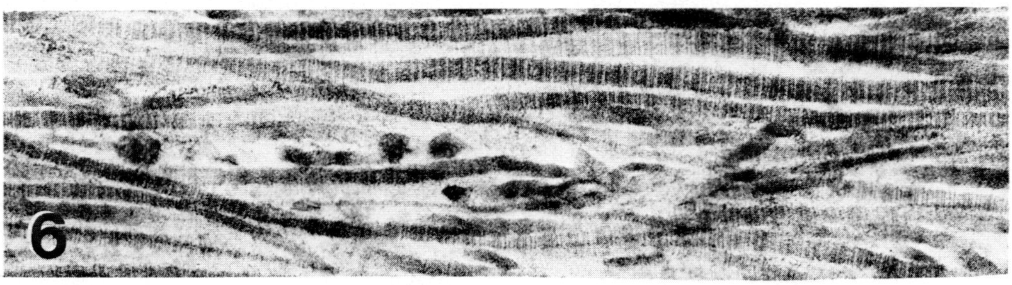

FIGURE 5. Front of calcification in puppy femoral metaphysis. Groups of MVs (arrows) are present in intercellular interstice and between uncalcified collagen fibrils. (Uranyl acetate and lead citrate, magnification × 27,000.)
FIGURE 6. MVs between uncalcified collagen fibrils of compact bone. (Uranyl acetate and lead citrate, magnification × 30,000).

It must be noted, however, that on the basis of results obtained both with conventional electron microscope techniques and after tissue processing in anhydrous organic solvents, it has been suggested that MVs may have a role in the calcification of embryonic bones, but not in that of mature compact bone.[37] MVs, in reality, are found in all types of bone at any age,[38,39] and are present also in compact bone (Figure 6), but they become less frequent as the compactness of the collagen fibrils of the matrix increases[20] so that, unless a careful search is made, they may be overlooked in bone with a compact matrix.

MVs have been found in bone in several pathological conditions. They have been described in osteoid tissue in rickets (Figure 7),[40-43] nutritional osteomalacia[44] and renal osteodystrophy,[45] exostosis developing in osteolathyrism,[46] heterotopic cartilage and bone induced by transplantation of transitional epithelium,[47] membranous bone in the cloverskull syndrome,[48] metaphyseal bone in osteopetrosis fetalis,[49] and in bone in several types of skeletal tumors such as osteosarcoma,[50-52] "cementoma" of long bones,[53] enchondroma,[54] and osteoblastoma.[55]

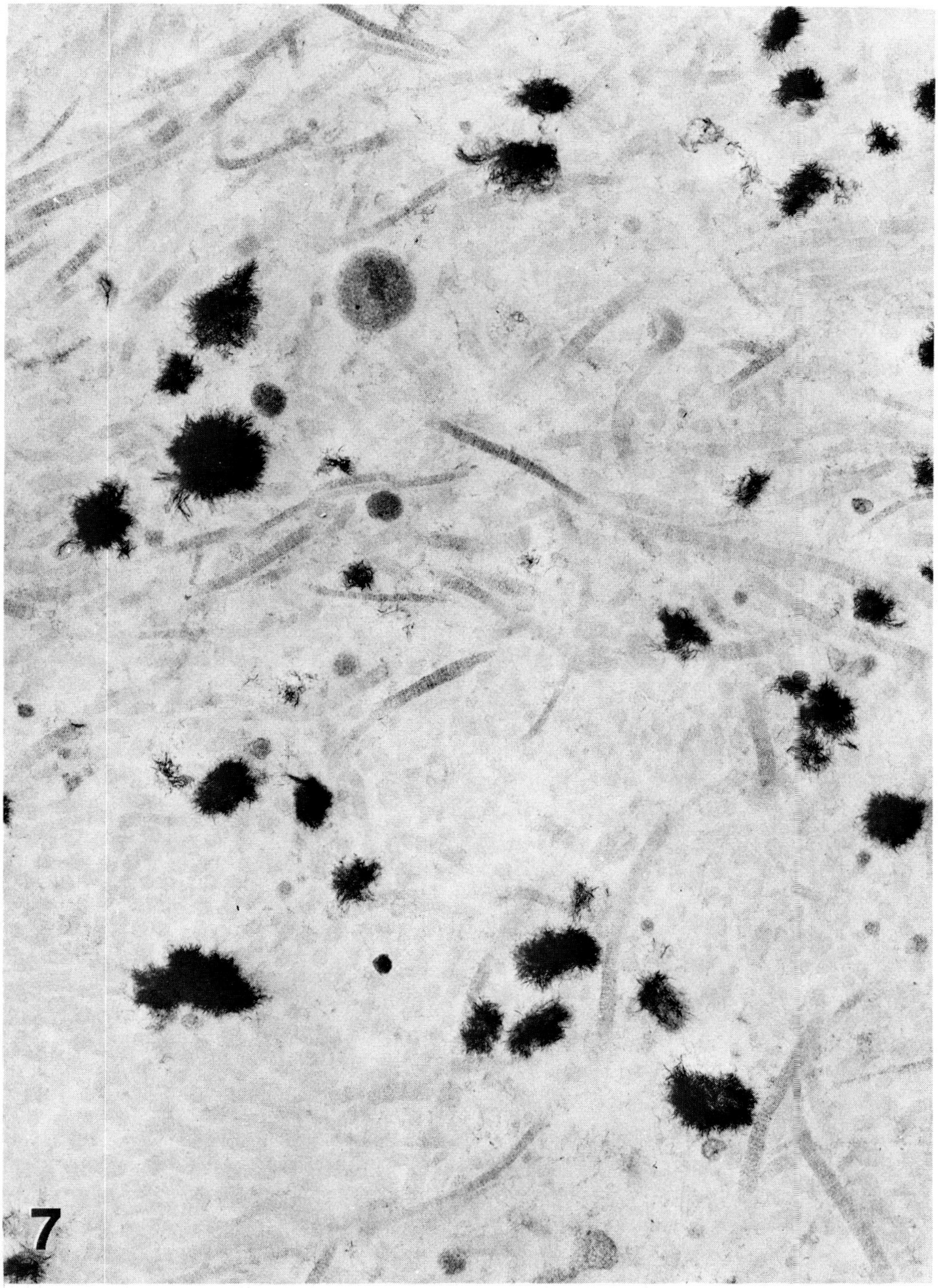

FIGURE 7. Uncalcified and calcified MVs in the osteoid tissue of rachitic rats. (Uranyl acetate and lead citrate, magnification × 30,000.)

C. Matrix Vesicles in Dentin

The earliest mentions of vesicle-like structures in dentin are probably those of Bernard[13] and Croissant,[56] who described membrane-bound bodies or odontoblast "buds" in primary, mantle dentin. The first descriptions of true MVs in dentin were made independently in

1972 by a number of authors.[57-61] Vesicles similar to those found in calcifying cartilage and bone were reported in so-called *mantle dentin,* that is, the dentin that is formed first in the zone located between odontoblasts and the developing ameloblasts.[58] These vesicles have almost the same ultrastructural morphology as those in cartilage and bone (Figures 8-12). They are roundish bodies surrounded by a membrane, and are placed between the collagen fibrils of the dentin matrix (Figures 8-10). They already contain variable amounts of inorganic crystals (Figures 11 and 12) when the adjacent collagen fibrils are still uncalcified.

Slavkin et al.[62] have reported that a number of the vesicles which are located in the extracellular matrix interposed between primary enamel epithelium and mesenchymal cells contain RNA. They have suggested that these vesicles have morphogenetic functions and can mediate developmental information from mesenchyme to epithelia during early tooth development. It is not known whether these RNA-containing vesicles are the same structures as calcifying MVs.

Dentin MVs are initially found in mantle dentin. As a layer of dentin is formed, the number of dentin MVs decreases and they are no longer visible in the so-called *circumpulpal dentin,* where calcification seems to be closely related to collagen fibrils. These early results have been confirmed by a number of later investigations.[8,62-66] The presence of MVs has also been reported in the repairing dentin of healing pulps in rats and dogs.[67,68] MVs have also been found in dentin in the tooth germ of the killifish *Oryzias latipes.*[69]

D. Matrix Vesicles in Calcifying Extraskeletal Tissues

Several studies have been devoted to an investigation of the presence and structure of MVs in calcifying extraskeletal tissues. In most of these tissues the early deposition of inorganic substance occurs directly within the cells, usually beginning in mitochondria, but a number of electron microscope investigations have reported that this process occurs in MVs in many normal and pathological conditions. In the former, MVs have been observed in calcifying deer antlers,[70,71] fish scales,[72,73] fibrocartilage of tendon-bone joints,[74] aging articular,[75] and tracheal and costal cartilage;[76-78] in the latter, MVs have been found in cutaneous calcinosis,[79-81] areas of lung calcification,[82] human aortic valve and aortic media,[83] experimentally calcified rat aorta,[84] cartilage in osteoarthritis,[85] and articular cartilage grafts.[86]

Structures resembling MVs have also been reported in the regenerating shell of *Helix pomatia*[87] and on the surface of calcifying *Bacterionema matruchotii.*[88]

V. THE MORPHOLOGY OF MATRIX VESICLES

As reported above, MVs are roundish bodies whose amorphous, osmiophilic matrix is surrounded by a trilaminar membrane (Figure 1). MVs in bone and mantle dentin are similar to, but sometimes smaller than those in calcifying cartilage. In bone and dentin, especially, but in cartilage, too, MVs resemble cross-sectioned cell processes and may be confused with them. Serial sections carried out on epiphyseal cartilage[5-7,89] and dentin[8] undoubtedly show that MVs are roundish bodies without any direct contact with chondrocytes or odontoblasts, or with their processes. So far, no serial sections have been made of MVs in bone. Even so, the fact that, as reported below, bone MVs can be isolated by homogenization and differential centrifugation provides independent confirmation that they are roundish bodies not directly connected with cells.

FIGURES 8—10. Groups of MVs in mantle dentin (newborn rats); note that some of them are calcified, whereas collagen fibrils are completely free of mineral substance. (Uranyl acetate and lead citrate, magnification × 70,000.) FIGURE 11. Detail of Figure 8, showing crystals within MVs. (Uranyl acetate and lead citrate, magnification × 140,000.) FIGURE 12. Almost completely calcified MVs in mantle dentin (newborn rat). (Uranyl acetate and lead citrate, magnification × 180,000.)

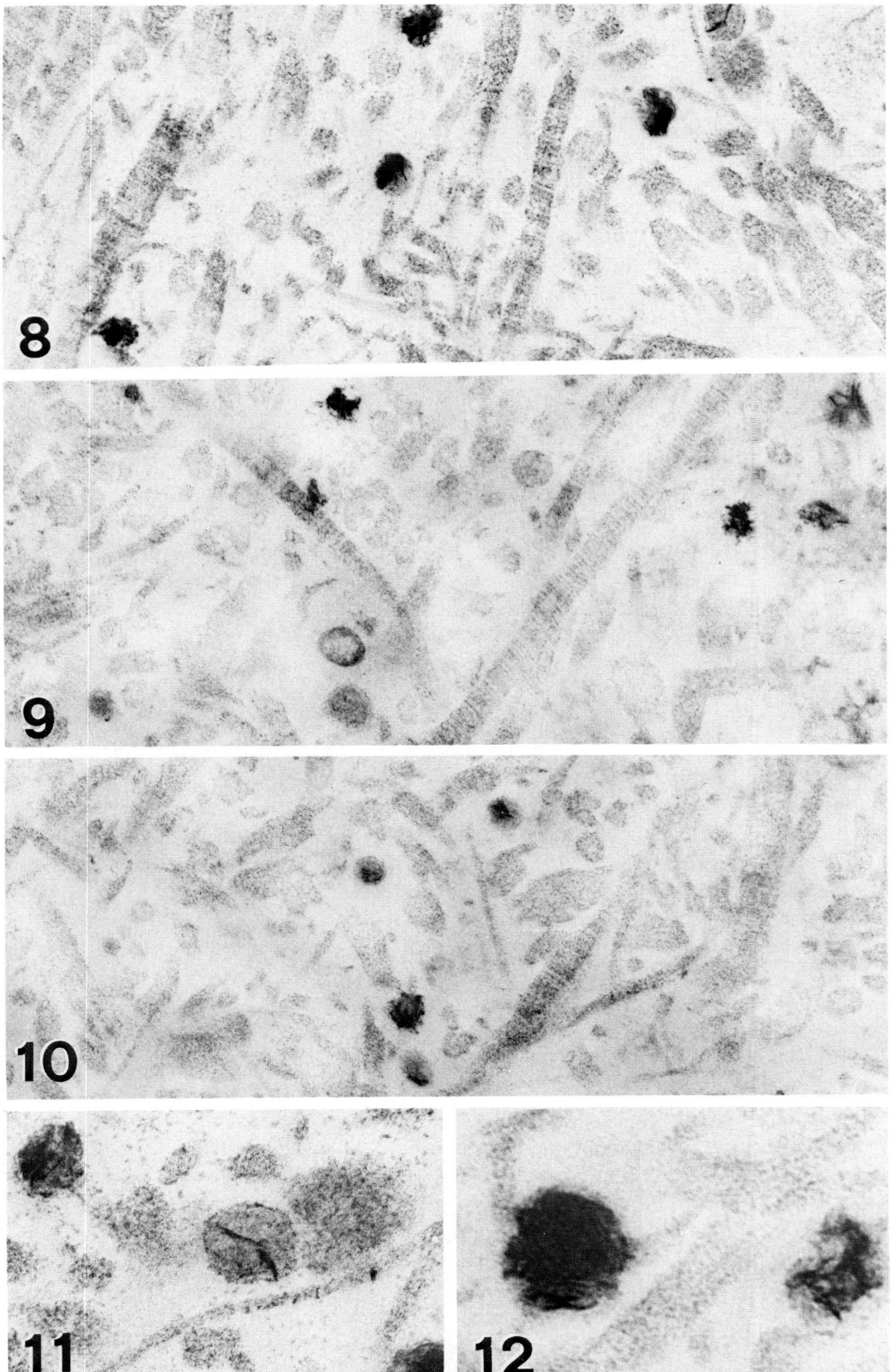

FIGURES 8—12.

No great differences in the morphology of MVs are observed in different calcifying tissues, but some heterogeneity has been reported. In particular, two different types of MVs (Type I and II) have been described in the epiphyseal cartilage of guinea pigs.[90-92] *Type I MVs* resemble the MVs described by others in cartilage, bone, and mantle dentin. *Type II MVs* are irregularly shaped and have a matrix that is less electron-dense than that of Type I MVs and similar to chondrocyte cytoplasm. Type II MVs appear to consist of fragments of budding cytoplasmic processes of degenerating cells,[25] probably of the same type as that described in the cartilage of scorbutic guinea pigs.[89] Since serial sections have not been made, it is difficult to say whether Type II MVs are true MVs as defined above, or whether they are simply cross-sectioned cell processes.

Recently, the possiblity that three types of vesicle-like structures are present in the hypertrophic cartilage has been suggested by Takagi et al.[93] on the basis of the density and distribution of particles on the P-face of the vesicle membrane.

VI. ISOLATION OF MATRIX VESICLES

MVs have been isolated from cartilage,[17,94] dentin,[61] and bone[95,96] by digestion with collagenase and separation by differential centrifugation (up to 300,000 g for 60 min). MVs are found chiefly in the fifth (150,000 g for 30 min) of the seven fractions usually obtained. This fraction is characterized by high alkaline phosphatase activity. To avoid the possible artifactual extraction arising from enzymatic digestion, a nonenzymatic isolation method has been developed.[97] Cartilage slices are homogenized twice; after differential centrifugation, the microsomal pellet is resuspended in a 10% sucrose solution and centrifuged again to separate the various density fractions. The collected fractions are pooled and diluted 1:4 with buffer and then sedimented again by centrifugation at 100,000 g for 2 hr.

Vesiculation of MVs from chondrocytes has recently been reported.[98,99] Freshly isolated chondrocytes are exposed to several vesiculating agents at 37° for 90 min. They are then sedimented by centrifugation and the supernatant collected. First MVs, and then vesicles, are separated by centrifugation after they have been loaded with calcium phosphate in the presence of ATP. The richest vesicle fraction is obtained after treatment with a salt solution whose composition is similar to that of the growth plate extracellular fluid. Isolated vesicles have high alkaline phosphatase activity and bind calcium ions.

It may be noted that the fluid aspirated by micropuncture from the cartilage of vitamin D- and phosphate-deficient rats contains a particulate fraction which, after sedimentation at 140,000 g for 4 hr, reveals electron microscope images consistent with MVs, and has mineral-forming properties.[100]

VII. HISTOCHEMICAL PROPERTIES OF MATRIX VESICLES

MVs contain glycoproteins, as shown by the PAS method under the light microscope[2] and by the periodic acid-silver nitrate method under the electron microscope.[6,101] Moreover, the outer layer of the MV membrane is coated with acidic proteoglycans, as shown by the colloidal iron[6,101] and colloidal thorium methods.[102] This proteoglycan coat can form spikes projecting radially into the surrounding matrix[102] and linking MVs to collagen fibrils.[27]

Electron microscope histochemical methods have demonstrated the presence of alkaline phosphatase and ATPase activities within and in close juxtaposition to the investing membrane of MVs in cartilage, bone, and dentin.[18,62,69,103-105] Interestingly, MVs in the elastic cartilage of the epiglottis, which does not calcify, show no phosphatase activity.[106]

Thyberg and Friberg[91] have reported acid phosphatase activity in their Type I MVs, which also appear to display aryl sulfatase activity.[92] Similar results have been obtained by Meikle[105,107] by electron microscope histochemical studies on the mandibular condyle cartilage of 1-week-old rats: acid phosphatase and aryl sulfatase activities were present in intracellular lysosome-like bodies, whereas only acid phosphatase activity was present in the same bodies in the extracellular matrix.

The results just reported are not in agreement with those of other investigators who state that MVs display no acid phosphatase activity.[18] The question is discussed further below.

VIII. BIOCHEMICAL PROPERTIES OF MATRIX VESICLES

The fact that MVs can be isolated means that biochemical analysis can be performed on them directly. Of the results so obtained, those concerning the composition of MVs are particularly interesting.

It has been repeatedly documented that MVs contain a variety of lipids, such as free fatty acids, cholesterol, sphingomyelin, glycolipids, lysophospholipids, and phosphatidylserine, whose composition is similar to that of the plasma membrane.[108-112]

As far as their enzymatic properties are concerned, biochemical analyses have clearly shown that alkaline phosphatase is the most typical marker of MVs.[17,94,113-117] Isolated MVs also display pyrophosphatase, ATPase, and 5′AMP-ase activity.[17,34,113,118-120] Biochemical data show that alkaline phosphatase, ATPase, and pyrophosphatase activities share a number of properties; such data are consistent with the view that ATPase and pyrophosphatase activities stem from one enzyme, that is, alkaline phosphatase.[113,121] These biochemical investigations do not support Thyberg's hypothesis that some MVs are lysosome-like bodies, because they do not contain biochemically demonstrable acid phosphatase activity.

In this connection, it should be recalled that, in a study on isolated MVs, lysosomal enzymatic activity was reported in the vesicle fraction.[122] This was later shown to be due to contamination, since the use of a different density gradient medium let to the complete separation of lysosomal and alkaline phosphatase activity, the latter being the only one associated with the vesicle fraction.[121]

Mitochondrial respiratory enzymes are not present in MVs.[123]

IX. THE ORIGIN OF MATRIX VESICLES

The presence of a peripheral membrane, and its morphological and biochemical similarity with the membrane of chondrocytes, suggest that MVs are of cellular origin. However, the way MVs are generated is still uncertain.

In a review on the biogenesis of cartilage MVs, Rabinovitch and Anderson[124] hypothesized that there are four different ways in which MVs may be formed:

1. Budding from cells and cellular processes
2. Extrusion of preformed structures
3. Disintegration of degenerate cells
4. Extracellular assembly of secreted subunits

Hypothesis 4 still appears to be dubious,[125] and hypothesis 2 is probably valid for bone only.[20] Many morphological findings support hypotheses 1 and 3. Budding from cells and cellular processes has been documented several times by conventional electron microscopy[6,7,65,89,125] and freeze-fracture studies[126] in epiphyseal cartilage and dentin, and by scanning electron microscopy in epiphyseal cartilage[127,128] and bone.[36] Similarly, the origin of MVs from degenerate, disrupted chondrocytes (so-called "Verdammerung der Zellen") has been amply documented (Figure 4).[6,7,78,89,93,129] It is interesting to note that the formation of MVs is enhanced by treatment with glucocorticoids both in vivo[130,131] and in vitro.[132]

X. MATRIX VESICLES AND CALCIFICATION

There is conclusive evidence that MVs are the loci of initial calcification in epiphyseal cartilage, bone, mantle dentin, and several other calcifying tissues.

Electron microscope investigations have repeatedly shown that early crystals can be found within MVs (Figures 3,11,12).[2,6-9,15,16,19,20,22,29,30,58,63,65,78,89,101,129] It has also been shown that the first crystals are often closely related to the membrane of MVs (Figure 3)[17,19,20,23,27,133] and that the appearance of the crystals may be preceded by the formation of very small, electron-dense granules (Figure 3, inset).[6,7,20] In addition, it has been shown by frozen thin sectioning and conventional embedding methods that MVs may contain both amorphous and crystalline mineral substance.[31,134] It has, however, recently been reported that in ultrathin sections prepared by ultracryomicrotomy and other nonaqueous techniques there is no relationship between MVs and solid phase particles of calcium phosphate.[37,135,136] These results have led to the conclusion that the presence of mineral particles found in the MVs of tissues exposed to aqueous solvents is artifactual and that the proposed role of MVs as loci of early calcification is questionable.[136]

Such a line of reasoning is, however, difficult to accept. First, it leads to the paradoxical conclusion that with the classic techniques, which are based on the use of aqueous solvents and should therefore induce a drastic removal of calcium and phosphate, a better demonstration of amorphous and crystalline mineral substance can be obtained than with more sophisticated, apparently less wasteful techniques, such as cryofixation. In theory, the view that anhydrous techniques should give better results than the classic methods is correct, but theory and practice often diverge. Judging by the fact that ultrastructural components, especially the cells and cellular organelles, may be seriously damaged by ultracryomicrotomy, often so severely that they become completely unrecognizable, and accepting the evidence that during cryofixation ion diffusion may not only occur, but may actually induce artifactual accumulation of mineral clusters in mitochondria,[137] it should be concluded that at present there are no grounds for the claim that ultracryomicrotomy offers better results than conventional techniques as far as calcium and phosphate ions are concerned.

Secondly, it must be considered that the negative results mentioned above[37,135,136] are in evident contrast with those obtained by other investigators using the same technique[31,66,134] and using high pressure freezing (which is a purely physical method of tissue stabilization) with subsequent freeze substitution.[27] Furthermore, the results obtained by ultracryomicrotomy and ultramicroincineration, showing that MVs contain a crystalline and amorphous mineral material,[30] seem to conflict with the above reported contrasting findings.

On the other hand, the role of MVs as the earliest loci of calcification is supported not only by the presence of crystals within them, when the adjacent matrix is still uncalcified, but also by a number of other findings. Biochemical investigations have shown that the concentration of Ca^{2+} in MVs is between 25 and 50 times higher than in adjacent chondrocytes, and that the intravesicular concentration of Ca^{2+} increases as the hypertrophic cartilage is approached.[138] This is in agreement with the observation that MVs can concentrate $^{45}Ca^{2+}$ in vitro.[139-142] Electron-probe analysis, even when carried out on cryosections,[143] shows that MVs accumulate calcium in passing from the proliferative to the hypertrophic zone of the epiphyseal cartilage.[144-146] Moreover, the potassium pyroantimonate-osmium method shows not only that MVs contain calcium ions,[147] but also that as the calcification zone is approached, the Ca^{2+} concentration increases in MVs and simultaneously decreases in mitochondria.[148,149]

These results suggest that calcium ions are initially accumulated in mitochondria and are later released into the extracellular space, where they are accumulated in MVs. The possibility that MVs themselves function as carriers of calcium ions from the cells into the matrix calls for further investigation.

XI. MECHANISM(S) OF MATRIX VESICLE CALCIFICATION

Most of the theories proposed to explain MV calcification are based on their high phosphatase activities. In this connection, Ali et al.[17,94] have suggested that MV calcification could occur by three possible mechanisms:

1. Hydrolysis of phosphate esters, which induces an increase in the local Pi concentration.
2. Increase in calcium or phosphate concentration by active transport, with energy supplied by the hydrolysis of ATP.
3. Removal of calcification inhibitors by hydrolysis of pyrophosphates.

It seems, however, that MVs can induce calcium phosphate precipitation, whether hydrolyzable phosphates are available or not,[118] and that MVs do not concentrate calcium ions via an energy-dependent ion transport system.[118,150]

One interesting hypothesis is that MV calcification may be mediated not by energy from ATP, but by the exhaustion of this substance.[151] In fact, since an MV membrane has the same structure and orientation as a chondrocyte membrane,[126] it may be presumed to possess a Ca^{2+}-extrusion pump. Within the confined space of an MV, however, such a pump would quickly become unworkable through the exhaustion of oxidizable substances, so leading to an equalization of calcium concentration inside and outside MVs, that is to an increment of calcium within MVs which facilitates the formation of mineral precipitates.[151]

MV calcification might also be achieved in a series of steps, including Ca^{2+}-loading and unloading of mitochondria, the transport of nascent calcium phosphate precipitates in the cytosol, the blebbing of calcium phosphate-primed MVs from the cellular membrane, the accumulation of inorganic ions by intravesicle diffusion, the accumulation of noncrystalline mineral, the degradation of the membrane of the MVs with release of soluble Mg^{2+}, and the conversion of nascent calcium phosphate precipitates into apatite.[152]

Clearly, the mechanism(s) of MV calcification are not yet fully understood. In this connection, it cannot be overlooked that Ca^{2+} accumulation might simply depend on the chemical properties of the MV constituents. A leading role could, for instance, be played by the formation of calcium-acidic phospholipid phosphate complexes.[108,153-157] Incidentally, this would explain the frequent finding that inorganic crystals are closely related to the membrane of MVs.[7,17,19,20,23,27,133] The findings that MVs contain glycoproteins,[2,7,101] that MV alkaline phosphatase is a glycoprotein with strong Ca^{2+} affinity,[151] and that the same enzyme may represent a carrier of inorganic phosphate into MVs[158] cannot be a simple coincidence and suggests that the enzyme plays a basic role in MV calcification. Furthermore, the presence of proteoglycans on the outer surface of the membrane of MVs[6,101] and their arrangement into spikes radiating from MVs into the surrounding matrix[102] might represent, simply throught their aggregation or hydrolysis, a further element of regulation of Ca^{2+} concentration in and around MVs.

The mechanism(s) of MV calcification, and of the spread of the calcification process from MVs into the surrounding matrix,[159] certainly require further investigation.

XII. CONCLUSIONS

In spite of remaining uncertainties and of isolated contrasting reports, the concept that MVs are the loci of initial calcification in cartilage, bone, mantle dentin and several extraskeletal soft tissues may by now be considered to have been definitively proven. Their role in the early phases of the calcification process, however, seems to differ in different calcifying tissues. There is no doubt that MVs are active in epiphyseal cartilage, in mantle dentin, and in embryonic and other types of bone. On the other hand, they are not found in circumpulpal dentin and in enamel, and few or very few of them are observed in compact bone. The fact that MVs are not present at the same concentration in all calcifying tissues does not mean, as is sometimes claimed, that they must be denied any role in calcification. The question arises why some calcifying tissues contain plenty of MVs and others very few or none. One possible explanation is that MVs are needed for the calcification of rapidly mineralizing tissues, whereas their role is less important when calcification occurs slowly, such as in compact bone, in which case cells may have enough time to regulate matrix calcification by themselves through their cytoplasmic processes.

Conversely, it cannot be concluded that MVs are the only structures involved in early mineralization, since other matrix components certainly play a role as important as theirs in inducing and regulating the calcification process. Further studies, and above all open, unprejudiced minds are needed to assign MVs their right place in the complicated puzzle called biological calcification.

REFERENCES

1. **Bonucci, E.,** The structural basis of calcification, in *Connective Tissue Matrix,* Ruggeri, A., Ed., Martinus Nijhoff, The Hague, in press.
2. **Bonucci, E.,** Fine structure of early cartilage calcification, *J. Ultrastruct. Res.,* 20, 33, 1967.
3. **Anderson, H. C.,** Electron microscopy studies of induced cartilage development and calcification, *J. Cell Biol.,* 35, 81, 1967.
4. **Anderson, H. C.,** Vesicles in the matrix of epiphyseal cartilage: fine structure, distribution and association with calcification, in *Electron Microscopy 1968,* Vol. 2, Steve Bocciarelli, D., Ed., Tipografia Poliglotta Vaticana, Rome, 1968, 437.
5. **Bonucci, E. and De Matteis, A.,** Ultrastruttura della cartilagine epifisaria nello scorbuto sperimentale. II. La matrice organica ed il processo di calcificazione, *Ortop. Traumat. Appar. Motore,* 36, 293, 1968.
6. **Bonucci, E.,** Fine structure and histochemistry of "calcifying globules" in epiphyseal cartilage, *Z. Zellforsch.,* 103, 192, 1970.
7. **Bonucci, E.,** Fine structure of epiphyseal cartilage in experimental scurvy, *J. Pathol.,* 102, 219, 1970.
8. **Katchburian, E.,** Membrane-bound bodies as initiators of mineralization of dentine, *J. Anat.,* 116, 285, 1973.
9. **Anderson, H. C.,** Vesicles associated with calcification in the matrix of epiphyseal cartilage, *J. Cell Biol.,* 41, 59, 1969.
10. **Hancox, N. M. and Boothroyd, B.,** Electron microscopy of the early stages of osteogenesis, *Clin. Orthop.,* 40, 153, 1965.
11. **Bernard, G. W.,** The ultrastructural interface of bone crystals and organic matrix in woven and lamellar endochondral bone, *J. Dent. Res.,* 48(Suppl.), 781, 1969.
12. **Bernard, G. W. and Pease, D. C.,** An electron microscopic study of initial intramembraneous osteogenesis, *Am. J. Anat.,* 125, 271, 1969.
13. **Bernard, G. W.,** Initial calcification of dentin and enamel: an electron microscopic view, *Int. Assoc. Dent. Res.,* 47th General Meet., Abstr. 305, Houston, 1969.
14. **Ascenzi, A. and Bonucci, E.,** Etude compareé au microscope électronique des phases initiales de la calcification de l'os et du cartilage, in *Phosphate et Metabolisme Phosphocalcique,* Hioco, D. J., Ed., Sandoz Editions, Paris, 1971, 65.
15. **Bonucci, E.,** The locus of initial calcification in cartilage and bone, *Clin. Orthop.,* 78, 108, 1971.
16. **Bonucci, E.,** Problemi attuali attinenti all'istochimica di talune matrici calcificanti normali e patologiche, *Riv. Istochim. Norm. Pat.,* 17, 153, 1971.
17. **Ali, S. Y., Sajdera, S. W., and Anderson, H. C.,** Isolation and characterization of calcifying matrix vesicles from epiphyseal cartilage, *Proc. Nat. Acad. Sci. U.S.A.,* 67, 1513, 1970.
18. **Matsuzawa, T. and Anderson, H. C.,** Phosphatase of epiphyseal cartilage studied by electron microscopic cytochemical methods, *J. Histochem. Cytochem.,* 19, 801, 1971.

19. **Bonucci, E.,** The organic-inorganic relationships in calcified organic matrices, in *Physico-chimie et Cristallographie des Apatites d'Intérêt Biologique,* Colloque Int. du C.N.R.S. n. 230, Centre Nat. Rech. Sci., Paris, 1975, 231.
20. **Bonucci, E.,** The origin of matrix vesicles and their role in the calcification of cartilage and bone, in *International Cell Biology 1980-81,* Schweiger, H. G., Ed., Springer-Verlag, Berlin, 1981, 993.
21. **Alcoock, N. W.,** Calcification of cartilage, *Clin. Orthop.,* 86, 287, 1972.
22. **Anderson, H. C.,** Calcium-accumulating vesicles in the intercellular matrix of bone, in *Hard Tissue Growth, Repair and Remineralization,* Ciba Found. Symp. 11, Elsevier, Excerpta Medica, North-Holland, 1973, 213.
23. **Anderson, H. C.,** Matrix vesicles of cartilage and bone, in *The Biochemistry and Physiology of Bone,* Vol. 4, 2nd ed., Bourne, G. H., Ed. Academic Press, New York, 1976, 135.
24. **Irving, J. T.,** Theories of mineralization of bone, *Clin. Orthop.,* 97, 225, 1973.
25. **Thyberg, J. and Friberg, U.,** The lysosomal system in endochondral growth, *Prog. Histochem. Cytochem.,* 10, 1, 1978.
26. **Boskey, A. L.,** Models of matrix vesicle calcification, *Inorg. Perspect. Biol. Med.,* 2, 51, 1979.
27. **Hunziker, E. B., Herrmann, W., Schenk, R. K., Marti, M., and Moor, H.,** Structural integration of matrix vesicles in calcifying cartilage after cryofixation and freeze substitution, in *Matrix Vesicles,* Ascenzi, A., Bonucci, E., and De Bernard, B., Eds., Wichtig, Milan, 1981, 25.
28. **Schenk, R. K., Müller, J., Zinkernagel, R., and Willenegger, H.,** Ultrastructure of normal and abnormal bone repair, *Calcif. Tissue Res.,* 4(Suppl.), 110, 1970.
29. **Anderson, H. C. and Reynolds, J. J.,** Pyrophosphate stimulation of calcium uptake into cultured embryonic bones. Fine structure of matrix vesicles and their role in calcification, *Dev. Biol.,* 34, 211, 1973.
30. **Schraer, H. and Gay, C. V.,** Matrix vesicles in newly synthesizing bone observed after ultracryotomy and ultramicroincineration, *Calcif. Tissue Res.,* 23, 185, 1977.
31. **Gay, C. V., Schraer, H., and Hargest, T. E., Jr.,** Ultrastructure of matrix vesicles and mineral in unfixed embryonic bone, *Metab. Bone Dis. Rel. Res.,* 1, 105, 1978.
32. **Weisbrode, S. E., Capen, C. C., and Nagoda, L. A.,** Fine structural and enzymatic evaluation of bone in thyroparathyroidectomized rats receiving various levels of vitamin D, *Lab. Invest.,* 28, 29, 1973.
33. **Bonucci, E. and Gherardi, G.,** Histochemical and electron microscope investigations on medullary bone, *Cell Tissue Res.,* 163, 81, 1975.
34. **Bab, I. A., Muhlrad, A., and Sela, J.,** Ultratructural and biochemical study of extracellular matrix vesicles in normal alveolar bone of rats, *Cell Tissue Res.,* 202, 1, 1979.
35. **Marvaso, V. and Bernard, G. W.,** Initial intramembranous osteogenesis in vitro, *Am. J Anat.,* 149, 453, 1977.
36. **Ornoy, A., Atkin, I., and Levy, J.,** Ultrastructural studies on the origin and structure of matrix vesicles in bone of young rats, *Acta Anat.,* 106, 450, 1980.
37. **Landis, W. J., Paine, M. C., and Glimcher, M. J.,** Electron microscopic observations of bone tissue prepared anhydrously in organic solvents, *J. Ultrastruct. Res.,* 59, 1, 1977.
38. **Bonucci, E.,** Are there matrix vesicles in bone? Studies in normal and pathological conditions, *Abstr. 4th Int. Workshop on Calcified Tissues,* Kiriat Anavim, Israel, 1980, 10.
39. **Sela, J., Bab, I. A., and Muhlrad, A.,** A comparative study on the occurrence and activity of extracellular matrix vesicles in young and adult rat maxillary bone, *Calcif. Tissue Int.* 33, 129, 1981.
40. **Simon, D. R., Berman, I., and Howell, D. S.,** Relationship of extracellular matrix vesicles to calcification in normal and healing rachitic epiphyseal cartilage, *Anat. Rec.,* 176, 167, 1973.
41. **Anderson, H. C., Cecil, R., and Sajdera, S. W.,** Calcification of rachitic rat cartilage *in vitro* by extracellular matrix vesicles, *Am. J. Pathol.,* 79, 237, 1975.
42. **Anderson, H. C., Hsu, H. H. T., Johnson, T. F., Murphee, S. S., and Stein, R.,** Matrix vesicles in rickets, in *Matrix Vesicles,* Ascenzi, A., Bonucci, E., and De Bernard, B., Eds., Wichtig, Milan, 1981, 233.
43. **Krempien, B.,** In vitro effects of $1,25(OH)_2D_3$ and of $24,25(OH)_2D_3$ on matrix vesicles of cartilage and on the endosteal cell envelope of bone, in *Matrix Vesicles,* Ascenzi, A., Bonucci, E., and De Bernard, B., Eds., Wichtig, Milan, 1981, 123.
44. **Dopping-Hepenstal, P. J. C., Ali, S. Y., and Stamp, T. C. B.,** Matrix vesicles in the osteoid of human bone, in *Matrix Vesicles,* Ascenzi, A., Bonucci, E., and De Bernard, B., Eds., Wichtig, Milan, 1981, 229.
45. **Bonucci, E., Gherardi, G., Faraggiana, T., Mioni, G., Cannella, G., Castellani, A., and Maiorca, R.,** Bone changes in hemodialyzed uremic subjects, *Virchows Arch.,* 371A, 183, 1976
46. **Martino, L. J., Yeager, V. L., and Taylor, J. J.,** An ultrastructural study of the role of calcification nodules in the mineralization of woven bone, *Calcif. Tissue Int.,* 27, 57, 1979.
47. **Dziedzic-Goclawska, A., Bonucci, E., Lamprecht, J., Wojtowicz, A., Wlodarski, K., and Ostrowski, K.,** Matrix vesicles in heterotopic enchondral and mesenchymal osteogenesis induced by the transplants of transitional epithelium, in *Matrix Vesicles,* Ascenzi, A., Bonucci, E., and De Bernard, B., Eds., Wichtig, Milan, 1981, 209.

48. **Bonucci, E. and Nardi, F.,** The cloverleaf skull syndrome, *Virchows Arch.*, 357A, 199, 1972.
49. **Bonucci, E., Sartori, E., and Spina, M.,** Osteopetrosis fetalis. Report on a case, with special reference to ultrastructure, *Virchows Arch.*, 368A, 109, 1975.
50. **Sela, J. and Boyde, A.,** Further observations on the relationship between the matrix and the calcifying fronts in osteosarcoma, *Virchows Arch.*, 376A, 175, 1977.
51. **Muhlrad, A., Stein, H., Bab, I. A., and Sela, J.,** Fine structure and enzymes of matrix vesicles in osteosarcoma: possible occurrence of contractile proteins, *Metab. Bone Dis. Rel. Res.*, 1, 277, 1978.
52. **Sela, J., Bab, I. A., Muhlrad, A., and Stein, H.,** Extracellular matrix vesicles in human osteogenic neoplasms: an ultrastructural and enzymatic study, *Cancer*, 48, 1602, 1981.
53. **Mirra, J. M., Bernard, G. W., Bullough, P. G., Johnston, W., and Mink, G.,** Cementum-like production in solitary bone cysts (so called "cementoma" of long bones), *Clin. Orthop.*, 135, 295, 1978.
54. **Steiner, G. C.,** Ultrastructure of benign cartilaginous tumors of intraosseous origin, *Human Pathol.*, 10, 71, 1979.
55. **Bonucci, E. and De Santis, E.,** Ultratructure of osteoblastoma, with particular reference to calcification and matrix vesicles, in *Bone and Tumors*, Donath, A. and Courvoisier, B., Eds., Médecine et Hygiène, Geneva, 1980, 232.
56. **Croissant, R. D.,** Isolation of an intercellular matrix "RNA-protein complex" during odontogenesis, *J. Dent. Res.*, 50, 1065, 1971.
57. **Bernard, G. W.,** Ultrastructural observations of initial calcification in dentine and enamel, *J. Ultrastruct. Res.*, 41, 1, 1972.
58. **Eisenmann, D. R. and Glick, P. L.,** Ultrastructure of initial crystal formation in dentin, *J. Ultrastruct. Res.*, 41, 18, 1972.
59. **Ozawa, H. and Yajima, T.,** Ultrastructure and cytochemistry of matrix vesicles in the developing cartilage and tooth germ, *4th Int. Congr. Histochemistry and Cytochemistry*, Kyoto, Japan, 1972, 311.
60. **Sisca, R. F. and Provenza, D. V.,** Initial dentin formation in human deciduous teeth. An electron microscope study, *Calcif. Tissue Res.*, 9, 1, 1972.
61. **Slavkin, H. C., Croissant, R., and Bringas, P., Jr.,** Epithelial-mesenchymal interactions during odontogenesis. III. A simple method for the isolation of matrix vesicles, *J. Cell Biol.*, 53, 841, 1972.
62. **Slavkin, H. C., Croissant, R. C., Bringas, P., Matosian, P., Wilson, P., Mino, W., and Guenther, H.,** Matrix vesicles heterogeneity: possible morphogenetic functions for matrix vesicles, *Fed. Proc. Fed. Am. Soc. Exp. Biol.*, 35, 127, 1976.
63. **Larsson, Å.,** Studies on dentinogenesis in the rat. Ultrastructural observations on early dentin formation with special reference to "dentinal globules" and alkaline phosphatase activity, *Z. Anat. Entwickl. Gesch.*, 142, 103, 1973.
64. **Larsson, Å.,** Studies on dentinogenesis in the rat. The interaction between lead-pyrophosphate solutions and dentinal globules, *Calcif. Tissue Res.*, 16, 93, 1974.
65. **Almuddaris, M. F. and Dougherty, W. J.,** The association of amorphous mineral deposits with the plasma membrane of pre- and young odontoblasts and their relationship to the origin of dentinal matrix vesicles in rat incisor teeth, *Am. J. Anat.*, 155, 223, 1979.
66. **Ozawa, H., Yamada, M., and Yamamoto, T.,** Ultrastructural observations on the location of lead and calcium in the mineralizing dentine of rat incisors, in *Matrix Vesicles*, Ascenzi, A., Bonucci, E., and De Bernard, B., Eds., Wichtig, Milan, 1981, 179.
67. **Sela, J., Tamari, I., Hirschfeld, Z., and Bab, I.,** Transmission electron microscopy of reparative dentin in rat molar pulps. Primary mineralization via extracellular matrix vesicles, *Acta Anat.*, 109, 247, 1981.
68. **Hayashi, Y.,** Ultrastructure of initial calcification in wound healing following pulpotomy, *J. Oral Pathol.*, 11, 174, 1982.
69. **Yamada, M. and Ozawa, H.,** Ultrastructual and cytochemical studies on the matrix vesicle calcification in the teeth of the killifish,*Oryzias latipes*, *Arch. Histol. Jpn.*, 41, 309, 1978.
70. **Sayegh, F. S., Solomon, G. C., and Davis, R. W.,** Ultrastructure of intracellular mineralization in the deer's antler, *Clin. Orthop.*, 99, 267, 1974.
71. **Newbrey, J. W. and Banks, W. J.,** Characterization of developing antler cartilage matrix. II. An ultrastructural study, *Calcif. Tissue Res.*, 17, 289, 1975.
72. **Maekawa, K. and Yamada, J.,** Some histochemical and fine structural aspects of growing scales of the rainbow trout, *Bull. Fac. Fish. Hokkaido Univ.*, 21, 70, 1970.
73. **Schönbörner, A. A., Boivin, G., and Baud, C. A.,** The mineralization process in teleost fish scales, *Cell Tissue Res.*, 202, 203, 1979.
74. **Yamada, M.,** Ultrastructural and cytochemical studies on the calcification on the tendon-bone joint, *Arch. Histol. Jpn.*, 39, 347, 1976.
75. **Shitama, K.,** Calcification of aging articular cartilage in man, *Acta Orthop. Scand.*, 50, 613, 1979.
76. **Bonucci, E., Cuicchio, M., and Dearden, L. C.,** Investigations of ageing in costal and tracheal cartilage of rats, *Z. Zellforsch.*, 147, 505, 1974.

77. **Dearden, L. C., Bonucci, E., and Cuicchio, M.,** An investigation of ageing in human costal cartilage, *Cell Tissue Res.,* 152, 305, 1974.
78. **Bonucci, E. and Dearden, L. C.,** Matrix vesicles in aging cartilage, *Fed. Proc. Fed. Am. Soc. Exp. Biol.,* 35, 163, 1976.
79. **Plackovà, A. and Vahl, J.,** The ultrastructure of topical cutaneous calcinosis, *Cell Tissue Res.,* 159, 523, 1975.
80. **Boivin, G.,** Etude chez le rat d'une calcinose cutanée induite par calciphylaxie locale. I. Aspects ultrastructuraux, *Arch. Anat. Microsc. Morphol. Exp.* 64, 183, 1975.
81. **Boivin, G., Baud, C. A., and Walzer, C.,** Matrix vesicles in ectopic calcification, in *Matrix Vesicles,* Ascenzi, A., Bonucci, E., and De Bernard, B., Eds., Wichtig, Milan, 1981, 235.
82. **Le Bouffant, L., Bruyère, S., Martin, J. C., Normand, C., and Tichoux, G.,** Aspects, composition et croissance des calcifications pulmonaires pathologiques, in *Physico-chimie et Cristallographie des Apatites d'Intérêt Biologiques,* Colloque Int. du C.N.R.S. n. 230 Paris, 1975, 323.
83. **Kim, K. M.,** Calcification of matrix vesicles in human aortic valve and aortic media, *Fed. Proc. Fed. Am. Sec. Exp. Biol.,* 35, 156, 1976.
84. **Bonucci, E. and Sadun, R.,** Dihydrotachysterol-induced aortic calcification, *Clin. Orthop.,* 107, 283, 1975.
85. **Ali, S. Y. and Griffiths, S.,** Matrix vesicles and apatile deposition in osteoarthritis, in *Matrix Vesicles,* Ascenzi, A., Bonucci, E., and De Bernard, B., Eds., Wichtig, Milan, 1981, 241.
86. **Sela, J. and Bab, I.,** Extracellar matrix vesicles in articular cartilage grafts and reparative dentin, in *Matrix Vesicles,* Ascenzi, A., Bonucci, E., and De Bernard, B., Eds., Wichtig, Milan, 1981, 257.
87. **Saleuddin, A. S. M. and Chan W.,** Shell regeneration in *Helix* shell matrix composition and crystal formation, *Can. J. Zool.,* 47, 1107, 1976.
88. **Lie, T. and Selvig, K. A.,** Effect of salivary proteins on calcification of oral bacteria, *Scand. J. Dent. Res.,* 82, 135, 1974.
89. **Bonucci, E.,** Matrix vesicle formation in cartilage of scorbutic guinea pigs: electron microscope study of serial sections, *Metab. Bone Dis. Rel. Res.,* 1, 205, 1978.
90. **Thyberg, J. and Friberg, U.,** Ultrastructure and acid phosphatase activity of matrix vesicles and cytoplasmic dense bodies in the epiphyseal plate, *J. Ultrastruct. Res.,* 33, 554, 1970.
91. **Thyberg, J. and Friberg, U.,** Electron microscopic enzyme histochemical studies on the cellular genesis of matrix vesicles in the epiphyseal plate, *J. Ultrastruct. Res.,* 41, 43, 1972.
92. **Thyberg, J.,** Ultrastructural localization of aryl sulfatase activity in the epiphyseal plate, *J. Ultrastruct. Res.,* 38, 332, 1972.
93. **Takagi, M., Kasahara, Y., Takagi, H., and Toda, Y.,** Freeze-fracture images of matrix vesicles of epiphyseal cartilage and non-calcified tracheal cartilage. *J. Electron Micros.,* 28, 165, 1979.
94. **Ali, S. Y., Anderson, H. C., and Sajdera, S. W.,** Enzymic and electron-microscopic analysis of extracellular matrix vesicles associated with calcification in cartilage, *Biochem. J.,* 122, 56P, 1971.
95. **Bab, I., Deutsch, D., Muhlrad, A., and Sela, J.,** Quantitative morphology of isolated bone matrix vesicles, in *Matrix Vesicles,* Ascenzi, A.,Bonucci, E., and De Bernard, B., Eds., Wichtig, Milan, 1981, 59.
96. **Deutsch, D., Sela, J., Bab, I., Setton, A. J., and Muhlrad, A.,** A comparative biochemical study of extracellular matrix vesicles isolated from bone and cartilage, in *Matrix Vesicles,* Ascenzi, A., Bonucci, E., and De Bernard, B., Eds., Wichtig, Milan, 1981, 53.
97. **Wuthier, R. E., Linder, R. E., Warner, G. P., Gore, S. T., and Borg, T. K.,** Non-enzymatic isolation of matrix vesicles: characterization and initial studies on ^{45}Ca and ^{32}P-orthophosphate metabolism, *Metab. Bone Dis. Rel. Res.,* 1, 125, 1978.
98. **Golub, E. E., Schattschneider, S., McArthur, W. P., Burke, A., and Shapiro, I. M.,** Induction of vesiculation by cultured chondrocytes, in *Matrix Vesicles,* Ascenzi, A., Bonucci, E., and De Bernard, B., Eds., Wichtig, Milan, 1981, 41.
99. **Shapiro, I. M., Burke, A., Schattschneider, S., and Golub, E. E.,** Vesiculation of chondrocytes in vitro: a new technique for isolating vesicles from chondrocytes, in *Matrix Vesicles,* Ascenzi, A., Bonucci, E., and De Bernard, B., Eds., Wichtig, Milan, 1981, 33.
100. **Howell, D. S., Pita, J. C., and Alvarez, J.,** Possible role of extracellular matrix vesicles in initial calcification of healing rachitic cartilage, *Fed. Proc. Fed. Am. Soc. Exp. Biol.,* 35, 122, 1976.
101. **Dearden, L. C. and Espinosa, T.,** Comparison of mineralization of the tibial epiphyseal plate in immature rats following treatment with cortisone, propylthiouracil or after fasting, *Calcif. Tissue Res.,* 15, 93, 1974.
102. **Scherft, J. P. and Groot, C. G.,** The development of matrix vesicles into bone nodules, studied with colloidal thorium dioxide, in *Matrix Vesicles,* Ascenzi, A., Bonucci, E., and De Bernard, B., Eds., Wichtig, Milan, 1981, 173.
103. **Göthlin, G. and Ericsson, J. L. E.,** Fine structural localization of alkaline phosphomonoesterase in the fracture callus of the rat, *Israel J. Med. Sci.,* 7, 488, 1971.

104. **Bernard, G. W.,** Ultrastructural localization of alkaline phosphatase in initial intramembranous osteogenesis, *Clin. Orthop.*, 135, 218, 1978.
105. **Meikle, M. C.,** The mineralization of condylar cartilage in the rat mandible: an electron microscopic enzyme histochemical study, *Arch. Oral Biol.*, 21, 33, 1976.
106. **Nielsen, E. H.,** Ultrahistochemistry of matrix vesicles in elastic cartilage, *Acta Anat.*, 100, 268, 1978.
107. **Meikle, M. C.,** The distribution and function of lysosomes in condylar cartilage, *J. Anat.*, 119, 85, 1975.
108. **Majeska, R. J., Holwerda, D. L., and Wuthier, R. E.,** Localization of phosphatidylserine in isolated chick epiphyseal cartilage matrix vesicles with trinitrobenzenesulfonate, *Calcif. Tissue Int.*, 27, 41, 1979.
109. **Peress, N. S., Anderson, H. C., and Sajdera, S. W.,** The lipids of matrix vesicles from bovine fetal epiphyseal cartilage, *Calcif. Tissue Res.*, 14, 275, 1974.
110. **Wuthier, R. E.,** Lipid composition of isolated epiphyseal cartilage cells, membranes and matrix vesicles, *Biochim. Biophys. Acta,* 409, 128, 1975.
111. **Wuthier, R. E.,** Lipids of matrix vesicles, *Fed. Proc. Fed. Am. Soc. Exp. Biol.*, 35, 117, 1976.
112. **Glaser, J. H. and Conrad, H. E.,** Formation of matrix vesicles by cultured chick embryo chondrocytes, *J. Biol. Chem.*, 256, 12607, 1981.
113. **Majeska, R. J. and Wuthier, R. E.,** Studies on matrix vesicles isolated from chick epiphyseal cartilage. Association of pyrophosphatase and ATPase activities with alkaline phosphatase, *Biochim. Biophys. Acta,* 391, 51, 1975.
114. **Fortuna, R., Anderson, H. C., Carty, R. P., and Sajdera, S. W.,** The purification and molecular characterization of alkaline phosphatases from chondrocytes and matrix vesicles of bovine fetal epiphyseal cartilage, *Metab. Bone Dis. Rel. Res.*, 1, 161, 1978.
115. **Kahn, S. E., Jafri, A. M., Lewis, N. J., and Arsenis, C.,** Purification of alkaline phosphatase from extracellular vesicles of fracture callus cartilage, *Calcif. Tissue Res.*, 25, 85, 1978.
116. **Väänänen, H. K. and Korhonen, L. K.,** Purification of matrix-vesicle alkaline phosphatase from chicken epiphyseal cartilage and experiments on its ATP-hydrolyzing properties, *Clin. Orthop.*, 148, 291, 1980.
117. **Watkins, E. L., Stillo, J. V., and Wuthier, R. E.,** Subcellular fractionation of epiphyseal cartilage. Isolation of matrix vesicles and profiles of enzymes, phospholipids, calcium and phosphate, *Biochim. Biophys. Acta,* 631, 289, 1980.
118. **Felix, R. and Fleisch, H.,** Pyrophosphatase and ATPase of isolated cartilage matrix vesicles, *Calcif. Tissue Res.*, 22, 1, 1976.
119. **Sela, J., Bab, I. A., and Muhlrad, A.,** Ultrastructural and biochemical characterization of extracellular matrix vesicles in healing alveolar bone sockets: preliminary indications for the presence of contractile proteins, *Metab. Bone Dis. Rel. Res.*, 1, 185, 1978.
120. **Fortuna, R., Anderson, H. C., Carty, R. P., and Sajdera, S. W.,** Enzymatic characterization of the matrix vesicles alkaline phosphatase isolated from bovine fetal epiphyseal cartilage, *Calcif. Tissue Int.*, 30, 217, 1980.
121. **Väänänen, H. K. and Korhonen, L. K.,** Phosphatases of matrix vesicles, in *Matrix Vesicles,* Ascenzi, A., Bonucci, E., and De Bernard, B., Eds., Wichtig, Milan, 1981, 111.
122. **Väänänen, H. K. and Korhonen, L. K.,** Matrix vesicles in chicken epiphyseal cartilage. Separation from lysosomes and the distribution of inorganic pyrophosphatase activity, *Calcif. Tissue Int.*, 28, 65, 1979.
123. **Person, P., Papierman, S., Zipper, H., and Libbin, R. M.,** Absence of mitochondrial terminal respiratory enzymes in cartilage matrix vesicles, *Calcif. Tissue Res.*, 24, 37, 1977.
124. **Rabinovitch, A. L. and Anderson, H. C.,** Biogenesis of matrix vesicles in cartilage growth plates, *Fed. Proc. Fed. Am. Soc. Exp. Biol.*, 35, 112, 1976.
125. **Dickson, G. R.,** The role of matrix vesicles in the calcification of amphibian growth cartilage, in *Matrix Vesicles,* Ascenzi, A., Bonucci, E., and De Bernard, B., Eds., Wichtig, Milan, 1981, 191.
126. **Cecil, R. N. A. and Anderson, H. C.,** Freeze-fracture studies of matrix vesicle calcification in epiphyseal growth plate, *Metab. Bone Dis. Rel. Res.*, 1, 89, 1978.
127. **Ornoy, A. and Langer, Y.,** Scanning electron microscopy studies on the origin and structure of matrix vesicles in epiphyseal cartilage from young rats, *Israel J. Med. Sci.*, 14, 745, 1978.
128. **Ornoy, A., Levy, J., Atkin, I., and Salamon, J.,** Scanning and transmission electron microscopic observations on the origin and structure of matrix vesicles in normal and papain-digested epiphyseal cartilage of young rats, *Israel J. Med. Sci.*, 15, 928, 1979.
129. **Dearden, L. C.,** Enhanced mineralization of the tibial epiphyseal plate in the rat following propylthiouracil treatment: a histochemical light, and electron microscopic study, *Anat. Rec.*, 178, 671, 1974.
130. **Silbermann, M., Lewinson, D., and Toister, Z.,** Early cartilage response to systemic glucocorticoid administration: an ultrastructural study, *Metab. Bone Dis. Rel. Res.*, 2, 267, 1980.
131. **Dearden, L. C., Mosier, H. D., Jr., and Jaffe, N. R.,** The effect of glucocorticoids on calcification of the fetal rat skeleton, in *Matrix Vesicles,* Ascenzi, A., Bonucci, E., and De Bernard, B., Eds., Wichtig, Milan, 1981, 135.

132. **Silbermann, M., Lewinson, D., Toister, Z., Gonen, H., and Gitai, H.,** An in vitro study on the effects of various steroid hormones upon the ultrastructure of young cartilage with special reference to the induction of matrix vesicles, in *Matrix Vesicles,* Ascenzi, A., Bonucci, E., and De Bernard, B , Eds., Wichtig, Milan, 1981, 129.
133. **Morris, D. C., and Appleton, J.,** Ultrastructural localization of calcium in the mandibular condylar growth cartilage of the rat, *Calcif. Tissue Int.,* 30, 27, 1980.
134. **Gay, C. V.,** The ultrastructure of the extracellular phase of bone as observed in frozen thin sections, *Calcif. Tissue Res.,* 23, 215, 1977.
135. **Landis, W. J., Paine M. C., and Glimcher, M. J.,** Use of acrolein vapors for the anhydrous preparation of bone tissue for electron microscopy, *J. Ultrastruct. Res.,* 70, 171, 1980.
136. **Landis, W. J. and Glimcher, M. J.,** Electron optical and analytical observations of rat growth plate cartilage prepared by ultracryomicrotomy: the failure to detect a mineral phase in matrix vesicles and the identification of heterodispersed particles as the initial solid phase of calcium phosphate deposited in the extracellular matrix, *J. Ultrastruct. Res.,* 78, 227, 1982.
137. **Barnard, T. and Sevéns, L.,** Do dense particle clusters in mitochondrial profiles of frozen-dried thin cryosections of unfixed tissue represent *in vivo* mitochondrial electrolyte pools? *J. Ultrastruct. Res.,* 66, 81, 1979.
138. **Wuthier, R. E.,** Electrolytes of isolated epiphyseal chondrocytes, matrix vesicles, and extracellular fluid, *Calcif. Tissue Res.,* 23, 125, 1977.
139. **Ali, S. Y. and Evans, L.,** The uptake of [^{45}Ca] calcium ions by matrix vesicles isolated from calcifying cartilage, *Biochem. J.,* 134, 647, 1973.
140. **Ali, S. Y.,** Analysis of matrix vesicles and their role in the calcification of epiphyseal cartilage, *Fed. Proc. Fed. Am. Soc. Exp. Biol.,* 35, 135, 1976.
141. **Hsu, H. H. T. and Anderson, H. C.,** A simple and defined method to study calcification by isolated matrix vesicles. Effect of ATP and vesicle phosphatase, *Biochim. Biophys. Acta,* 500, 162, 1977.
142. **Väänänen, H. K.,** Calcium incorporation in matrix vesicles isolated from chicken epiphyseal cartilage, *Calcif. Tissue Int.,* 30, 227, 1980.
143. **Ali, S. Y., Wisbi, A., and Gray, J. C.,** Electron probe analysis of cryosections of epiphyseal cartilage, *Metab. Bone Dis. Rel. Res.,* 1, 97, 1978.
144. **Hall, T. A., Höhling, H. J., and Bonucci, E.,** Electron probe X-ray analysis of osmiophilic globules as possible sites of early mineralization in cartilage, *Nature (London),* 231, 535, 1971.
145. **Althoff, J., Quint, P., Barckhaus, R. H., Krefting, E. R., Lissner, G., and Höhling, H. J.,** Combined microprobe and topochemical analyses on the epiphyseal growth plate, in *Matrix Vesicles,* Ascenzi, A., Bonucci, E., and De Bernard, B., Eds., Wichtig, Milan, 1981, 79.
146. **Barckhaus, R. H., Krefting, E. -R., Althoff, J., Quint, P., and Höhling, H. J.,** Electron-microscopic microprobe analysis on the initial stages of mineral formation in the epiphyseal growth plate, *Cell Tissue Res.,* 217, 661, 1981.
147. **Burger, E. H. and Matthews, J. L.,** Cellular calcium distribution in fetal bones studied with K-pyroantimonate, *Calcif. Tissue Res.,* 26, 181, 1978.
148. **Brighton, C. T. and Hunt, R. M.,** The role of mitochondria in growth plate calcification as demonstrated in a rachitic model, *J. Bone Joint Surg.,* 60A, 630, 1978.
149. **Lewinson, D. and Silbermann, M.,** Chondrocyte involvement in condylar cartilage calcification utilizing potassium pyroantimonate-osmium tetroxide, *Metab. Bone Dis. Rel. Res.,* 1, 243, 1978.
150. **Sajdera, S. W., Franklin, S., and Fortuna, R.,** Matrix vesicles of bovine fetal cartilage: metabolic potential and solubilization with detergents, *Fed. Proc. Fed. Am. Soc. Exp. Biol.,* 35, 154, 1976.
151. **Stagni, N., Tavagnacco, C., Vittur, F., and De Bernard, B.,** Glycoproteins and phosphatases of epiphyseal cartilage, in *Matrix Vesicles,* Ascenzi, A., Bonucci, E., and De Bernard, B., Eds., Wichtig, Milan, 1981, 149.
152. **Wuthier, R. E.,** Proposed mechanism of matrix vesicle formation and vesicle-mediated mineralization, in *Matrix Vesicles,* Ascenzi, A., Bonucci, E., and De Bernard, B., Eds., Wichtig, Milan, 1981, 103.
153. **Wuthier, R. E. and Gore, S. T.,** Partition of inorganic ions and phospholipids in isolated cell, membrane and matrix vesicle fractions evidence for Ca-Pi-acidic phospholipid complexes, *Calcif. Tissue Res.,* 24, 163, 1977.
154. **Boskey, A. L.,** The role of calcium-phospholipid-phosphate complexes in tissue mineralization, *Metab. Bone Dis. Rel. Res.,* 1, 137, 1978.
155. **Boskey, A. L.,** The role of Ca-phospholipid-phosphate complexes, membrane lipids, and matrix vesicles in calcification, in *Matrix Vesicles,* Ascenzi, A., Bonucci, E., and De Bernard, B., Eds., Wichtig, Milan, 1981, 161.
156. **Boyan-Salyers, B. D., Vogel, J. J., Riggan, L. J., Summers, F., and Howell, R. E.,** Application of a microbial model to biologic calcification, *Metab. Bone Dis. Rel. Res.,* 1, 143, 1978.

157. **Vogel, J. J., Boyan-Salyers, B., and Campbell, M. M.,** Protein-phospholipid interactions in biological calcification, *Metab. Bone Dis. Rel. Res.*, 1, 149, 1978.
158. **Warner, G. P. and Wuthier, R. E.,** Metabolism of ^{32}Pi and ^{45}Ca by matrix vesicles isolated from epiphyseal cartilage by nondigestive methods, in *Matrix Vesicles,* Ascenzi, A., Bonucci, E., and De Bernard, B., Eds., Wichtig, Milan, 1981, 47.
159. **Bonucci, E.,** Intra- vs. extra-vesicle calcification in epiphyseal cartilage, in *Matrix Vesicles,* Ascenzi, A., Bonucci, E., and De Bernard, B., Eds., Wichtig, Milan, 1981, 167.

INDEX

A

B

C

H

I

J

L

M

N

O

P

Q

R

S

T

U

V

W

Z